Educating the Young Child

Advances in Theory and Research, Implications for Practice

Volume 14

This academic and scholarly book series will focus on the education and development of young children from infancy through eight years of age. The series will provide a synthesis of current theory and research on trends, issues, controversies, and challenges in the early childhood field and examine implications for practice. One hallmark of the series will be comprehensive reviews of research on a variety of topics with particular relevance for early childhood educators worldwide. The mission of the series is to enrich and enlarge early childhood educators' knowledge, enhance their professional development, and reassert the importance of early childhood education to the international community. The audience for the series includes college students, teachers of young children, college and university faculty, and professionals from fields other than education who are unified by their commitment to the care and education of young children. In many ways, the proposed series is an outgrowth of the success of *Early Childhood Education Journal* which has grown from a quarterly magazine to a respected and international professional journal that is published six times a year.

More information about this series at http://www.springer.com/series/7205

Hannah Brewer • Mary Renck Jalongo
Editors

Physical Activity and Health Promotion in the Early Years

Effective Strategies for Early Childhood Educators

Springer

Editors
Hannah Brewer
Department of Physical and Health Education
Slippery Rock University of Pennsylvania
Slippery Rock, PA, USA

Mary Renck Jalongo
Journal and Book Series Editor Springer
Emerita, Indiana University of Pennsylvania
Indiana, PA, USA

Educating the Young Child
ISBN 978-3-030-09377-8 ISBN 978-3-319-76006-3 (eBook)
https://doi.org/10.1007/978-3-319-76006-3

Printed on acid-free paper

This Springer imprint is published by the registered company Springer International Publishing AG part of Springer Nature.
The registered company address is: Gewerbestrasse 11, 6330 Cham, Switzerland

Foreword

In recent years, I served as a content advisor for the longest-running children's television program, *Sesame Street.* Although I was well-acquainted with the Muppets and the program that airs weekly in my community, delving further into the group's work made me aware not only of the international footprint of *Sesame Street* but also their work in health and wellness. It was interesting to discover that they had produced a series of programs on "heart healthy" habits that aired in the USA, Canada, and Columbia. Underlying this initiative were at least two assumptions. First, that the early years are an opportunity to teach wellness concepts and establish healthy habits, and second, that encouraging regular physical activity and minimizing sedentary behavior are ways to counteract obesity and disease. This volume in the *Educating the Young Child Series* adopts a similar stance. The distinguished and diverse group of authors assembled here is unified by the conviction that the habit of physical activity, launched during in the early years, can exert a powerful and positive impact on young children's health and fitness.

Why Be Concerned About Young Children's Physical Activity?

Where physical activity is concerned, there exists a persistent misconception that young children are "naturally" active and require no systematic opportunities, encouragement, or instruction to have a healthy lifestyle. Clearly, this is not the case. Internationally, there is concern that children are leading more sedentary lives, have much higher rates of obesity, and are setting in motion habits that will lead to compromised health (Carson et al., 2010; World Health Organization, 2012). It has been argued that contemporary young children are less fit and less active than ever before (American Academy of Pediatrics, 2016). How has this happened? Outside of school, vigorous activity for children often is restricted for a variety of reasons. Concerns about safety often keep children indoors rather than outdoors playing with neighborhood children. Once inside, children tend to devote many hours to "screen time" with television, computers, smartphones, and electronic games, making them sedentary for much of the day. Moreover, many parents/guardians work long hours or multiple jobs, continue to be "wired in" and work after they arrive home, have household duties to perform, or are just too exhausted to be physically active after work. As a result, adults in the home may not provide models of moderate-to-vigorous physical activity on a regular basis. Studies also have suggested that many parents feel that they lack knowledge about how to encourage physical activity in their children, other than enrolling them in some sort of class or organized sports. Many of these programs are not well-suited for very young children

Opportunities to be physically active in educational settings are restricted as well. Few programs are meeting the "minimum daily requirement" of exercise for children. The Institute of Medicine (2011) recommends at least 15 minutes of physical activity for every hour spent in child care in order to prevent obesity. Yet, at the very time when research clearly documents the positive effects of both planned and informal physical activity on children's overall health, many schools are reducing the amount of time allocated to vigorous physical activity (Ramstetter, Murray & Garner, 2010). In addition, both the pressure to attain higher academic standards and pressing budgetary considerations have reduced or eliminated many physical education classes. Few early childhood programs have the services of teachers with specialized expertise in physical education so this responsibility frequently is relegated to teachers who lack the preparation, skills, confidence, materials, and environments to lead children in physical activity.

Another damaging attitude toward children's physical activity is a "talent scout" mentality in which only those children who appear to be gifted and talented athletically are given extensive support to develop their skills. Too often, children whose physical skills are regarded by adults as ordinary or deficient in some way are excluded if, for example, play areas are inaccessible to young children with special needs or if teachers fail to make the necessary accommodations that give everyone a chance to participate. Even adults who are physically active themselves may be misguided and focus on competition with others rather than performing at one's personal best. This type of bias should be no more tolerated in the realm of opportunities for physical skill development than it is in opportunities for intellectual skill development. Collectively, these influences can undermine the goal of promoting active lifestyles for everyone.

What Is the Contribution of This Volume?

An appreciation for the healthy mind and body connection has existed for centuries. In ancient Rome *Mens sana in corpore sano* ("a sound mind in a sound body") was a goal for all citizens. This volume takes that ancient wisdom, applies it to the youngest children, and supports it with current empirical and international evidence—all with an eye toward improving wellness across the lifespan. The benefits of physical activity for young children have attracted national attention as countries take action to promote health in their youngest citizens (Alberta Accreditation of Early Learning and Care Services, 2013; Centers for Disease Control, 2010). For example, when it was determined that one in five young children in New South Wales, Australia is obese, the country launched the Healthy Kids Eat Well, Be Active (New South Wales Ministry of Health, 2013) initiative. Their team concluded that more active, healthy habits benefit children by:

- Promoting healthy growth and development
- Helping to achieve and maintain a healthy weight
- Building strong bones and muscles
- Improving cardiovascular fitness
- Improving balance, coordination, and strength
- Maintaining and developing flexibility
- Improving posture
- Assisting with the development of gross motor and fine motor skills
- Providing the opportunity to develop fundamental movement skills
- Helping to establish connections between different parts of the brain
- Improving concentration and thinking skills
- Improving confidence and self-esteem
- Relieving stress and promoting relaxation
- Providing opportunities to develop social skills and make friends
- Improving sleep

Empirical evidence from various fields to support such assertions is mounting (Bowers, Green, Hemme & Chalip, 2014; Jensen, 2005; Mayo Clinic Staff, 2011). Collectively, these sources document that participation not only in structured but also in informal physical activity can set in motion habits and attitudes that affect all areas of development commencing in early childhood and continuing throughout life (Lu and Montague, 2016; Spark!, 2016).

Audience for the Book

In reviewing the literature on physical activity and wellness, we identified two major shortcomings. First of all, there were very few books on the topic that focused on the age group of this volume, birth to eight years. This made most of the publications less applicable to the youngest children who are acquiring fundamental movement abilities. These include locomotor (e.g., walking, running, jumping, skipping), nonlocomotor (e.g., turning, twisting, nodding), and manipulative (e.g., throwing, catching, dribbling) (Robinson, 2011) (e.g., walk, hop, skip) rather than orchestrating sophisticated physical behavior repertoires, such as those required for participation in organized sports. Secondly, of the few books published, many of them were written for an audience of educators specializing in physical education rather than a more general population of teachers. Given that it is the "regular" early childhood educator who most often is expected to plan and provide physical activity for young children, we saw a need to gather together experts in the field who could make the theory, research, and practice accessible to those without specialized preparation in physical education. Ideally, physical activity and healthful eating initiatives at home and at school during the early years would:

- Support development of "fundamental movement abilities" that affect coordination, balance, and attainment of physical education goals
- Contribute to every child's self-concept and self-expression
- Enhance the development of academic skills as children learn to self-monitor and solve problems
- Build social skills as children learn to interpret gestures and the physical movements of others
- Address the "obesity epidemic" in a proactive way
- Shape the young child's attitudes, values, beliefs, and habits about physical activity in ways that affect lifelong habits (Isenberg & Jalongo, 2016)

Organization of the Volume

The book is organized into three sections: (1) Foundations of Physical Activity and Health Promotion in Early Childhood, (2) Research-Based Teaching Strategies to Promote Physical Activity and Health During Early Childhood, and (3) Physical Activity Programs and Preservice/Inservice Teacher Education. The chapters are replete with evidence-based strategies that support the efforts of early childhood educators in various roles, including child care providers, classroom teachers, pre-service educators, parent/family educators, and higher education faculty members.

Conclusion

Increasingly, it is being argued that there is yet another type of literacy: physical literacy (McNulty & Prosser, 2011). It includes a repertoire of behaviors, habits, and wisdom about what bodies need to be healthy and well and, as with other types of literacy (e.g., print, information, technology), physical literacy requires major investments of time and support. Young children need much more than admonitions from adults in order to achieve this goal. To illustrate, I observed two preschool girls playing together in the block center. They had built a school and a home, and now a small wooden figure, used to represent a child, was returning home for an after-school snack. The child playing the mother's role said, "Annah, let's get a good snack for you" to which the preschooler playing the role of the child said, "OK, I want candy." The first child protested, saying, "No, Annah. You have to say something that's *good for* you" and her playmate answered, "But I like candy. It's good."

As the second child's candid comment suggests, it is not enough to tell children to be active and make more healthful choices. We need to practice it ourselves because it is one of those dispositions that is acquired, over time, primarily by emulating positive role models. This means that early childhood educators will need to reach out to families and communities. Early childhood educators worldwide will need to work together to advocate for the young child's wellness of body just as assiduously as they have advocated for developing the young child's intelligence and socioemotional skills. To that end, we bring to you this informative, expert, and interesting volume of the *Educating the Young Child*. We chose the edited book format so that we could bring together a chorus of expert opinion from different areas of specialization, all united by a focus on promoting the young child's physical literacy. In keeping with the goal of the series, our distinguished group of authors discusses advances in theory and research and demonstrates how they are using that evidence to improve professional practice and collaborate with families.

Journal and Book Series Editor Springer
Emerita, Indiana University of Pennsylvania
Indiana, PA, USA

Mary Renck Jalongo

References

Alberta Acreditation of Early Learning and Care Services. (2013). *The importance of physical literacy*. Retrieved November 1, 2016, from http://www.aelcs.ca/Announcements/Reflective_Bulletins/Documents/The Importance of Physical Literacy.pdf

American Academy of Pediatrics. (2016). *Early Childhood: 1–4 years*. Retrieved November 1, 2016 from http://www.brightfutures.org/physicalactivity/pdf/EarlyChild.pdf

Bowers, M. T., Green, B. C., Hemme, F., & Chalip, L. (2014). Assessing the relationship between youth sport participation settings and creativity in adulthood. *Creativity Research Journal, 26*(3), 314–327.

Carson, V., Clark, D., Ogden, N., Harber, V., & Kuzik, N. (2010). Short-term influence of revised provincial accreditation standards on physical activity, sedentary behavior, and weight status in Alberta, Canada child care centers. *Early Childhood Education Journal, 43*(6), 459–465. https://doi.org/10.1007/s10643-015-0688-3

Centers for Disease Control. (2010). *The association between school-based physical activity, including physical education and academic performance*. Atlanta, GA: U.S. Department of Health and Human Services.

Institute of Medicine (IOM). (2011). *Early childhood obesity prevention policies*. Washington, DC: The National Academies Press.

Isenberg, J. P., & Jalongo, M. R. (2016). *Creative thinking and arts-based learning, K-2nd grade* (7th ed.).

Jensen, E. (2005). *Teaching with the brain in mind* (2nd ed.). Alexandria, VA: Association for Supervision and Curriculum Development.

Lu, C., & Montague, B. (2016). Move to learn, learn to move: Prioritizing physical activity in early childhood education programming. *Early Childhood Education Journal, 44*(5), 409–417.

Mayo Clinic Staff. (2011). *7 benefits of regular physical activity*. Retrieved November 1, 2016, from http://www.mayoclinic.com/health/exercise/HQ01676

McNulty, C., & Prosser, T. (2011). Being active together: How to raise a physically educated child. *Childhood Education, 87*(3), 202–203.

New South Wales Ministry of Health. (2013). *Benefits of being active.* Retrieved November 1, 2016, from http://www.healthykids.nsw.gov.au/teachers-childcare/physical-activity.aspx

Ramstetter, C. L., Murray, R., & Garner, A. S. (2010). The crucial role of recess in schools. *Journal of School Health, 80*(11), 517–526.

Robinson, L. E. (2011). The relationship between perceived physical competence and funda-mental motor skills in preschool children. *Child: Care, Health and Development, 37*(4), 589–596.

Spark! (2016). *Early childhood.* Retrieved November 1, 2016, from http://www.sparkpe.org/early-childhood/

World Health Organization. (2012). *Obesity and overweight fact sheet.* Retrieved from http://www.who.int/mediacentre/factsheets/fs311/en/

Contents

Part I
Foundations of Physical Activity and Health Promotion in Early Childhood

Chapter 1
Foundations of Physical Activity and Health Promotion in Early Childhood

Hannah J. Brewer

Cultural Shifts in Daily Physical Activity

In August, the week before Ms. Cook was to begin implementing a structured physical activity program at an early childhood education center, she walked into the center to meet the staff and get acquainted with the facilities. It was early in the morning, and as she entered the facility, she saw all of the children sitting quietly on mats on the floor. With their eyes wide, all of the children were attentive and contently watching morning television. The early childhood educators were getting materials ready for the day, greeting children and their caregivers as they came through the door, and helping each child store their personal belongings in the nearby cubbies.

As Ms. Cook gazed around the room, she couldn't help but think that all of the children looked healthy – healthy and happy. This scene is all too common in today's society. Children who are calm, quiet, and engrossed with technology appear to be safe and comfortable, making it sometimes difficult for parents and early childhood educators to see the negative ramifications of too much screen time – or other sedentary behaviors.

It became very clear to Ms. Cook that movement, in today's society, may not happen naturally among children and needs to be purposefully incorporated into daily routines.

Physical activity and quality of life have gone hand-in-hand for centuries. Physical activity during early childhood is imperative for optimal growth and development, and the relationship between physical activity and quality of life dates back to the 1800s (Dauer & Pangrazi, 1975). Despite substantial evidence linking the importance of physical activity to optimal child development, according to Le Masurier and Corbin (2006), physical activity has been replaced by modern day conveniences and "engineered out of most aspects of daily life" (p. 44). This poses real and lasting

H. J. Brewer (✉)
Department of Physical and Health Education, Slippery Rock University of Pennsylvania, Slippery Rock, PA, USA
e-mail: Hannah.brewer@sru.edu

H. Brewer, M. R. Jalongo (eds.), *Physical Activity and Health Promotion in the Early Years*, Educating the Young Child 14,
https://doi.org/10.1007/978-3-319-76006-3_1

challenges for children growing up in the twenty-first century. To combat these challenges, children must be provided with opportunities to be physically active throughout the day that help them develop motor skills, reduce their risk for chronic disease, understand the relationship between movement and wellness, and develop an appreciation for physical activity.

Childhood sedentary behavior is a complex system problem that emerged during the economic growth and globalization of the marketplace. Before 1990, movement was more or less engrained into everyday life – walking to school, riding bicycles through the neighborhood, and playing outside until dusk were common childhood activities. In today's society, meeting physical activity guidelines no longer happens without concentrated efforts. Movement must be planned and purposefully incorporated into one's daily routine. This does not mean that movement must be structured, but that children must be given proper time, space, equipment and skills to facilitate physical activity.

Today, meeting physical activity guidelines is often a learned and intentional behavior. Therefore, caregivers and early childhood educators must value health as a key part of learning and promote physical activity in early childhood settings. Helping children shape positive attitudes about physical activity is as important as incorporating adequate opportunities for physical activity into the daily routine. Shaping positive attitudes and embedding physical activity into a child's day can be accomplished in a variety of ways, but the evidence is clear that physical activity needs to be considered a priority in early childhood education (Javanainen-Levonen, Poskiparta, Rintala, & Satomaa, 2009; Vidoni & Ignico, 2011).

A number of early childhood researchers suggest that both structured and unstructured physical activity are essential for proper physical, social, and cognitive development (Hinkley et al., 2014). This chapter investigates the importance of physical activity for (1) improved cognitive health and development, (2) better physical health, and (3) improved emotional well-being. The following section defines physical activity and sedentary behavior and provides an overview of the differences between structured and unstructured physical activity.

Physical Activity Defined

Physical activity is defined as "any bodily movement produced by skeletal muscles that results in energy expenditure" (Meeks, Heit, & Page, 2013, p. 240). While a significant proportion of children do not meet daily physical activity recommendations (Colley et al., 2011; Townsend, Wickramasinghe, Williams, Bhatnagar, & Rayner, 2015), physical activity in itself is enjoyable for most children. Young children are naturally inclined to move freely and explore spaces around them by jumping, spinning, and clapping. These are just a few of the unstructured movements young children typically enjoy.

Although children naturally enjoy physical activity, there is a misconception that because they enjoy it, they are "naturally" active and do not require any encouragement or support to be physically active. This is far from the truth. In England, in 2012, only one in ten children aged 2–4 years met the recommended levels of physical activity (Townsend et al., 2015). In the United States, approximately one in four children met the age-specific Physical Activity Guidelines for Americans in 2008, and in Canada, less than 7% of children met the Canadian Physical Activity Guidelines on at least six days per week in 2009 (Colley et al., 2011). Although physical activity guidelines vary slightly from country to country, one common theme prevails: Most children today are not getting enough physical activity.

Unstructured Physical Activity

Unstructured physical activity is self-directed and allows children to explore their environment without restraint. Giving children time to engage in unstructured physical activity enhances creativity, self-expression, and cooperation (SPARK, 2016). Although unstructured physical activity is just that – unstructured, young children need to be presented with situations that encourage them to move in their own exploratory ways. This brings some sense of "structure" to unstructured physical activity in today's early childhood environments. For example, 20 children moving freely through an open space with a scarf or ribbon while music plays in the background are engaging in unstructured physical activity, even though a teacher planned this experience into the day.

Structured Physical Activity

Structured physical activity is planned, directed, and has an instructional purpose. The purpose may be to develop gross motor skills, develop health-related physical fitness, or improve object control skills (Stodden & Goodway, 2007). Structured physical activity is specifically designed with the child's developmental level in mind and can ensure that children are learning fundamental skills essential for Activities of Daily Living (ADL) such as coordination, stability, and spatial awareness. Specifically, structured physical activity would assist young children in developing the skills needed to alternate their feet as they walk up and down stairs and swing their arms as they walk or run to improve efficiency. Physical activity that is planned and purposeful assists children with object control and manipulation by helping them develop the proper form, stance, and follow-through for throwing or catching. Structured physical activity is also beneficial to ensure that young children are engaged in moderate-to-vigorous physical activity for the recommended amount of time (60 min for children ages 3–5 and children ages 6–17). During unstructured physical activity, children can generally choose the intensity level at which they would like to move at, oftentimes resulting in light or moderate physical activity.

Structured physical activity may more readily encourage children to move at a faster or more vigorous pace.

Physical activity recommendations for both children and adults often make reference to light, moderate, and vigorous physical activity. Casual walking or light dancing are considered light intensity physical activity, brisk walking, walking uphill, or using most playground equipment is considered moderate physical activity, and running or jumping rope are considered vigorous physical activity (Lee & Paffenbarger, 2000). The phrase moderate-to-vigorous physical activity (MVPA) describes bodily movement fast enough to burn three to six times as many calories per minute than would be burnt at rest (sitting quietly). Specifically, MVPA refers to activities that burn three to six METs (metabolic equivalent) while vigorous-intensity activities burn more than six METs. One MET stands for the amount of oxygen consumed and the number of calories burnt at rest (Harvard School of Public Health, 2016).

Physical Activity Guidelines

Physical activity guidelines vary slightly between states and countries, but recommendations internationally require that children (up to 8 years of age) obtain a minimum of 60 min of physical activity each day (Centers for Disease Control and Prevention, 2016). The National Association for Sport and Physical Education (NASPE) recommends that children receive 60 min of unstructured physical activity per day in addition to 60 min of structured physical activity per day. The only difference in physical activity guidelines for children ages 3–5 and children ages 6–17 is that 3–5 year olds need 60 min of unstructured physical activity in addition to 60 min of structured physical activity each day. Further, children should not be sitting or lying for more than 60 min at a time unless they are sleeping. This recommendation confirms that young children (ages 3–5 specifically) should engage in at least 2 h of physical activity per day. Hinkley et al. (2014) summarized physical activity and sedentary behavior guidelines from Canada, Australia, the United Kingdom, and the United States and concluded that for optimal health, children need even more than 2 h of physical activity per day. Specifically, "children younger than school age and capable of walking should accumulate 3 hours of physical activity (PA) each day" (Hinkley et al., 2014, p. 183).

Although past research suggests that most of the health-enhancing benefits of physical activity are gained through moderate-to-vigorous physical activity, new research suggests that activities that feel even mildly uncomfortable for children may discourage future participation in physical activity (Seger, 2015). In support of this finding, identifying physical activities that are pleasurable for children– whether light, moderate, vigorous, or a combination of intensity levels, may be more important in early childhood than ensuring children engage in moderate-to-vigorous physical activity for a certain period of time.

Sedentary Behavior

Sedentary behaviors are associated with adverse health outcomes in children. Sedentary behavior requires little energy expenditure and refers to any activity completed in a seated posture or lying posture while the body is awake. Sleeping is not considered sedentary behavior unless the individual is sleeping repeatedly during the day or oversleeping. More specifically, sedentary behavior is defined as an energy expenditure of less than or equal to 1.5 metabolic equivalents during a waking activity (Australian Department of Health, 2014a, b). Common sedentary behaviors among children include watching television, computer, video game, and internet use, and riding in a car. The term sedentary is sometimes used interchangeably with the term inactive.

Sedentary behavior is difficult to quantify, but research suggests there is a dose-response relationships between sedentary behavior and risks for overweight and obesity, metabolic syndrome, type 2 diabetes, and cardiovascular disease (Colberg, 2012; Matthews et al., 2008). This means, the more time a child spends is sedentary behaviors, the higher his or her risk becomes for these chronic conditions. Because of this dose-response relationship, many countries have created sedentary behavior guidelines to supplement physical activity guidelines. A child who engages in 60 min of structured physical activity per day but spends the rest of the day sitting will be more at-risk for chronic health conditions than a child who takes activity breaks throughout the day in addition to his or her 60 min of physical activity. Brain breaks, movement breaks, walking, or simply standing instead of sitting provide clear health benefits, even if just completed for a short amount of time. All movement counts. All movement is beneficial, even if it is just 30 s of walking between learning stations or 3 min of using the whole body to spell words between sedentary classroom activities.

A recent report by Pate, Mitchell, Byun, and Dowda (2011) found that higher levels of sedentary behavior were reported in non-white children, children from lower socioeconomic backgrounds, and children from households with more access to televisions, computers, or the internet. When parents or caregivers set rules or limitations on screen time, lower levels of sedentary behavior were reported. These health disparities should be considered when working with children who are more at-risk for sedentary behavior.

Acknowledging the importance of not only increasing physical activity but also decreasing sedentary behavior has led to new health campaigns such as "Sitting is the New Smoking" and "Limit Sit Time to Increase Fit Time" (Yoder-Wise, 2014). These two campaigns portray the importance of all movement throughout the day and the risks associated with a sedentary lifestyle. To truly meet early childhood activity guidelines, movement must become engrained into children's everyday experiences instead of being taught exclusively during exercise time/physical education class. Australia's Physical Activity and Sedentary Behavior Guidelines for Children recommend breaking up long periods of sitting as much as possible, and provide the following specific suggestions for decreasing sedentary behavior among children: (1) Reward positive behavior with active family time instead of with electronic media use, (2) Allocate specific time periods for electronic media use, preferably not during daylight hours, (3) Turn the television and other electronic media devices off during meal times, (4.) Make bedrooms electronic media-free zones, (5) Store portable electronic devices out of sight, and (6) Set a good example by reducing media use for entertainment.

Reducing screen time and sedentary behavior among children is a simple, yet tangible way to improve health and well-being. In addition to reducing screen time, Castelli and Ward (2012) presented several ways to reduce sedentary behavior in early childhood settings and elementary schools outside of structured physical education classes. It is important to recognize that physical education classes taught by certified Physical Education Teachers are a key component to quality education. Yet, time spent in physical education classes, especially in early childhood, rarely provides adequate physical activity time to meet physical activity guidelines. To complement physical education classes, Castelli and Ward (2012) recommend: (1) Morning physical activity, (2) Physical activity breaks in the classroom, (3) Physical activity rewards and incentives, and (4) Content-rich physical activity. In addition, all early childhood educators must value and promote physical activity since health and learning are intimately linked. The next section will discuss why attitudes associated with physical activity and the methods used to introduce and encourage physical activity in early childhood are as important as meeting the time requirements or "minutes of physical activity required per day."

Early Enjoyment of Physical Activity and Lifelong Health

Despite countless interventions designed to increase physical activity and combat obesity in children, Michelle Segar, behavior expert and author of No Sweat, reports that enjoyment of physical activity, not short-term weight loss or knowledge of how physical activity benefits health, is the strongest predictor for maintaining a health-enhancing level of physical activity throughout the lifespan. Physical activity must be enjoyable in order for it to be sustainable. Experiences during early childhood have the power to shape individuals' views about physical activity for a lifetime. These views can be positive or negative, depending on each child's unique experience. Take, for example, the child who remembers finishing last in a relay race and feeling as though she is the reason her team does not win the race. This experience may cause the child to avoid running, skipping, galloping, or whatever movement she associates with that particular event. The negative image accrued through this specific life experience has the potential to impact other types of physical activity as well, causing the individual to avoid all types of physical activity in the future – even ones completely unassociated with the relay event (Seger, 2015). Most adults who have a negative perception of physical activity can identify one or more events in their past that shaped these negative views. Physical activity experiences during childhood have a powerful influence on future behaviors.

In contrast to this example, imagine a child who loves music and is given permission to listen to headphones while walking around the perimeter of the playground. This child who associates positive feelings with physical activity is more likely to choose walking or other forms of physical activity in the future to reduce stress, or just for fun. He enjoys music and feels good about being able to walk while listening to something important to him. Although he may never reach his target heart rate training zone during the walk, he is much more likely to pick up his headphones and head out for a walk in the future than the child who associates negative feelings with physical activity. The Surgeon General created a call to action to increase walking as a form of physical activity for all age groups (US Department of Health and Human Services, 2016). Walking does not require special skills, facilities, or expensive equipment and is accessible to most children. Walking also assists children in beginning and maintaining a physically active lifestyle. Although some fitness enthusiasts may still believe that vigorous physical activity is essential, Seger (2015) stated that "the 20 minute walk you are doing every day is more beneficial than the five mile run you are not doing" (p. 117). Because humans are hard wired to repeat behaviors that feel good to them and avoid behaviors that are unpleasant, fostering enjoyment of physical activity in early childhood provides both immediate and long-term benefits.

A child's decision to continue to be active on his own is often based on how he perceives physical activity. If it feels as though physical activity is a chore, he will avoid it until a teacher, parent, coach, or doctor prescribes it. If he feels like physical activity is a gift or a treat, he will find ways to incorporate physical activity into his day without hesitation. This approach uses emotion and personal fulfillment as a means for encouraging physical activity instead of desired health outcomes or weight loss as the end goal. Research consistently shows that engaging in physical activity specifically to address health outcomes (body composition, blood pressure, cholesterol, blood sugar, triglyceride levels, etc.,) can be effective in the short term but generally does not lead to lifelong behavioral change (Jakicic et al., 2015). On the contrary, engaging in physical activity because it feels good, clears one's mind, provides enjoyment, or reduces stress is much more likely to lead to sustainable physical activity habits. Although this text will include the importance of physical activity in early childhood for improving children's physical health, the primary focus will be on creating a culture of wellness in early childhood education where physical activity (both structured and unstructured) is not seen as an add-on or "break" from learning, but instead, as an integral part of the learning and living process.

Children's Cognitive Health and Development

Early childhood is a time when experiences in physical activity can be broadened, pleasure can be found in movement, and realistic ways physical activity can be incorporated into everyday lives can be discovered. This section will focus on how physical activity is associated with improved cognitive health among children.

A number of researchers and psychologists conclude that strong connections exist between movement and learning. In fact, healthy brain development is incumbent upon physical activity (Davis et al., 2011; Gartrell & Sonsteng, 2008). Critical parts of the body develop at different rates, and certain childhood physical activities facilitate the development of sensory organs.

Specifically, the vestibular, also known as the inner-ear, is the first sensory organ to mature. The inner-ear and the cerebellar system serve to help gather information about movement and send messages to other parts of the body. The vestibular and cerebellar system helps children maintain focus and attention. They are highly important for assisting with proper delivery of impulses traveling through the nervous system. Stimulation of the inner-ear during early childhood (through physical activity) improves the development of these sensory functions (Jensen, 2005). Movements such as swinging, rolling, jumping, tumbling, and rocking strengthen the ability of the sensory system to respond quickly to stimuli.

The reticular activating system (RAS) consists of a set of connected nuclei in the brain, and also benefits from these types of physical movement. A well-developed RAS helps children with balance, responding to impulses, and initiating movements. The RAS, which is found in the brainstem, serves as an essential neural component of the sleep/wake cycle (Jensen, 2005). Playground equipment is often constructed intentionally to encourage children to participant in activities that stimulate the inner ear and the RAS. Providing opportunities for children to spin, rock, tumble, flip upside down, and use playground facilities that encourage these movements is supportive of improving their cognitive health.

Palmer (2003) conducted several studies examining the effect of early motor stimulation on listening skills, reading comprehension, and writing ability. Almost universally, children in her Smart Start program which focused on improving children's sensory motor system at an early age demonstrated better attention and listening skills than children in the control group (Palmer, 2003). This is one example of how physical movements improve cognition. Hung, Chang, Tang, & Shih (2008) conducted a study with a population of 5 year olds to examine the effect of physical activity on brain development in young children. An equally matched experimental and control group were used to ensure that the results could be attributed to the addition of physical activity and not other confounding factors. After a 6 month structured physical activity program, children in the physical activity group had higher electroencephalography (EEG) power in the delta bands for the frontal, temporal, and central areas of the brain than children in the control group. The physical activity group also had higher EEG power at the theta band for the frontal area. EEG is a relatively noninvasive method used to track and record electrical activity of the brain that places electrodes along the scalp. This example demonstrates that physical activity is linked not only to brain development, but also to brain activity and responsiveness.

Further research suggests that the cerebellum, the part of the brain known for regulating motor control, is also responsible for processing learning (or academic content). Thinking, anticipating movements, and making predictions before carrying out actions are primary functions of the cerebellum. This thought-action process suggests that movement and cognition are intricately linked because engaging in physical activity often requires young children to make quick decisions about how they will move. This includes body awareness, movement, and reaction time—all of which improve the reactivity of the cerebellum. Jensen (2005) reported that "the cerebellum can make predictive and corrective actions regardless of whether it's dealing with a gross-motor task sequence or a mentally rehearsed task sequence" (p. 62). This concept implies that engaging in activities that encourage mental processes of the cerebellum such as prediction, sequencing, ordering, and rehearsing (often achievable through sports, motor skills, and other forms of physical activity) not only enhances coordination of physical movements, but also improves receptiveness to cognitive functions.

More evidence supporting physical activity as part of human development was offered by Anderson, Eckburg, and Relucio (2002). Their research discovered that people who were physically active had more cortical mass than those who were sedentary. Cortical mass refers to the weight and thickness of the brain's cortex. Physical activity increases oxygen flow to the brain, and as blood flow increases, more nutrients are transported to the brain. Neurotropins, also referred to as "brain food" are carried in the blood, and sitting still for extended periods of time weakens the flow of blood, oxygen, and neurotropins to the brain. This is another example of how physical activity plays a key role in healthy brain development and may explain why, in addition to accumulating 2 h of physical activity per day, the NASPE recommends that "preschoolers should not be sedentary for more than 60 minutes at a time except when sleeping" (NASPE, 2010). Since the benefits of physical activity extend well beyond cognitive development, the following section presents the positive impact physical activity has on physical health and well-being.

Children's Physical Health

Individuals begin to develop physical activity habits at a young age (Eliassen, 2011). Improving physical activity habits during childhood and before profound health complications have the opportunity to surface has become an international priority. Healthy People (2020) Objectives include reducing the proportion of children ages 2–5 who are overweight or obese, reducing the percent of children ages 6–11 who are overweight or obese, and preventing inappropriate weight gain in children ages 2–5 and 6–11 (Healthy People 2020). These national objectives were developed specifically to improve health outcomes based on epidemiological data linking the top causes of death in most developed countries (diseases of the heart, malignant neoplasms, and cerebrovascular disease) to modifiable risk-factors, including physical inactivity during childhood (Cottrell, Girvan, McKenzie, & Seabert, 2015).

A primary cause of childhood obesity is lack of physical activity. Recent initiatives have been implemented on the international, national, and local levels to improve the health of the nation starting with the youngest learners- children. As a result of these efforts, obesity rates among children in developed countries have stabilized (Wabitsch, Moss, & Kromeyer-Hauschild, 2014). This was an unexpected finding because in the United States, it was projected that the prevalence of obesity in children would reach 30% by 2030 (Wang, Beydoun, Liang, Caballero, & Kumanyika, 2008). Making physical activity and proper nutrition a high priority in public health today has resulted in minor improvements in the prevalence of childhood obesity.

Despite these improvements, when the data are more closely examined, evidence shows that the heaviest children have become heavier, and obesity rates among children of low socioeconomic backgrounds have not declined (Claire Wang, Gortmaker, & Taveras, 2011). In fact, the prevalence of childhood overweight and obesity in low income families is still increasing. Because of this health disparity, it is important to continue public health programs that prevent childhood obesity and expand programmatic offering for obesity prevention in communities where children are most at-risk for becoming overweight or obese.

Cardiovascular disease is the leading cause of death in the United States, and obese and even slightly overweight children are inclined to cardiovascular risk factors. High blood pressure, high blood triglycerides, and elevated blood sugar are common among children who do not meet daily physical activity requirements (Freedman, Mei, Srinivasan, Berenson, & Dietz, 2007; Kalavainen, Korppi, & Nuutinen, 2007). Although cardiovascular disease has historically been considered a "disease of aging", health experts know that childhood sedentary behaviors contribute to cardiovascular disease becoming a "disease of lifestyle". Hong (2010) reported that atherosclerosis (deposits of plaque on the inner artery walls) typically manifests itself clinically in middle or late adulthood. Yet, the asymptomatic phase of plaque development begins much earlier in life. It begins during childhood. Furthermore, children with hypertension (continually elevated blood pressure) are more likely to have hypertension as an adult and physical activity is one of the most effective ways for young children to reduce their risk for hypertension.

The development of Type 2 Diabetes is complex and linked to multiple modifiable and nonmodifiable risk factors including genetics, the environment, and lifestyle. Yet, strong evidence links childhood obesity and physical inactivity to the development of insulin resistance and Type 2 Diabetes (Bartz & Freemark, 2012). The Bogalusa Heart Study and Cardiovascular Risk in Young Finns Study conducted a longitudinal study that examined a large cohort of children for over 20 years. They concluded that childhood obesity was the strongest predictor for developing insulin resistance or future diabetes later in life. Specifically, obese children had three times the risk of developing Type 2 Diabetes later in life than their healthy-weight counterparts (Bartz & Freemark, 2012).

There is a correlation between physical activity and physical health both during childhood and throughout the lifespan. Concentrated public health efforts to address childhood obesity may have helped put a halt on the climbing obesity rates, but there is still more work to be done. Together, clear recommendations from the United States Department of Agriculture (USDA) to decrease the consumption of sugar-sweetened soft drinks among children and increase physical activity may have helped curb obesity rates.

Research on the complications associated with childhood obesity is abundant. Physicians, early childhood educators, and most caregivers now acknowledge the importance of reducing children's screen time, decreasing children's sugar consumption, and increasing children's opportunities for physical activity. Now, the focus must be directed towards shaping healthy habits during early childhood that are sustainable for a lifetime, and ensuring that early learning centers adhere to the physical activity guidelines that are known to benefit children.

Children's Well-Being

Physical activity is not only a vehicle for improving cognitive and physical health, but also a gift that can help children feel well a regular basis. This includes social and emotional wellness. Although there is little research on how physical activity affects young children's social and emotional health, research relating to adolescents' physical activity and social and emotional well-being is so strong that new standards have been put into place in some public schools to improve emotional health including suicide prevention (Association for Supervision and Curriculum Development, 2014). Specifically, adolescents who were physically active on four or more days per week had a 23% reduction in both suicidal ideation and attempt among bullied adolescents in the United States (Sibold, Edwards, Murray-Close, & Hudziak, 2015). Physical activity frequency was inversely related to sadness and suicidality. There are clear psychological benefits of physical activity and these benefits may extend beyond bullying victims and beyond this specific age group of adolescents.

Although research on young children's emotional health is less robust, there is evidence suggesting that more children may be suffering from anxiety or depression today than in the past. Unicef, the UN children's agency, reported that family life is in crisis and that children's unhappiness may be linked to rampant consumerism and parents' long working hours. Even though Britain is the fifth wealthiest country in the world, British children reportedly suffer from more emotional health issues than any other country in the world. British children are also the most tested in the world which reportedly leads to anxiety at a young age (Livingstone, 2011). Being physically active may improve children's well-being and reduce feelings of stress and anxiety. Greco and Ison (2014) researched the factors that bring happiness to Argentine children. When asking children "what makes you happy" during structured focus groups, most children referred to interpersonal relationships as their first response (i.e., "I am happy when I play with my siblings," or "I am happy when I go to my grandparents"). Second, children began listing recreational activities such as "riding my bike around the neighborhood" "playing with my classmates at break time" or "playing games outside". This research demonstrates the social and emotional benefits of physical activity on children's overall well-being and happiness.

According to the National Center for Infants, Toddlers, and Families, keeping children healthy through adequate nutrition and physical activity is one of the most important roles of parenting (Zero to Three, 2016). Second, Eric Barker (2014) provided a list of ways to raise happy kids. Among this list were (1) creating positive relationships with parents and caregivers, (2) providing opportunities for the child to feel competent in something, or more specifically, mastery, (3) teaching self-care skills including hygiene, healthy eating, adequate sleep, meditation, and regular physical activity, and (4) cultivating fun or enjoying life. Evidence suggests that regular physical activity is not only enjoyable for children, but is required for health, vitality, and happiness.

Early Childhood Educator's Role

National Association for Sport and Physical Education for NASPE and Association for Supervision, Curriculum, and Development for ASCD declares that getting an "active start" is a promising way to promote lifetime physical activity (2010) and health. Having access to safe indoor and outdoor facilities that encourage movement is necessary for young children to gain the full benefits of physical activity. As such, early childhood educators should be cognizant of the indoor and outdoor environments available for children, and maximize the potential of the environment to give children Opportunities to Move (OTMs). This could mean such things as using a hillside next to the playground to march up and down once before going back inside after outdoor play time, bringing ridable or movable toys outside on nice days to encourage young children to be more physically active, writing a grant to request physical activity equipment that promotes gross motor movements, or simply rearranging chairs, desks, and furniture inside to allow for more open space to move in between seated activities without risking injury.

According to the American Heart Association's Physical Activity and Public Health Guidelines (2007), intermittent bouts of physical activity throughout the day can add up to the recommended 1–3 h of daily physical activity recommended for young children. Although there are multiple health benefits associated with elevating the heart rate for an extended period of time, similar benefits can be achieved through engaging in small increments of physical activity. Even brief aerobic activities strengthen the heart and improve the body's ability to deliver oxygen to its cells. Therefore, early childhood educators can utilize small increments of time throughout the day for OTMs. For example, this could be as simple as telling the children they are going to take the long way to the drinking fountain and take a community walk around the outer perimeter of the classroom instead of walking straight to the drinking fountain. Another example is for teachers to lead children through three simple stretches or yoga exercises before nap time or story time. This encourages physical activity and helps them relax and transition into a quieter activity.

Summary

In the opening scenario, the early childhood educators did not see anything immediately wrong with their current educational model because the children were quiet and happy. Although parents, caregivers, and educators have different values, teaching strategies, and parenting styles, one concept all caregivers of young children can agree upon is that they want their children to be happy and healthy (Syrad et al., 2015). Decreasing screen time and sedentary behaviors while providing opportunities for young children to be physically active allows for (1) improved cognitive health and development, (2) better physical health, and (3) improved emotional well-being. Teachers who value physical activity as an integral component of their early childhood curriculum are helping create a better society, starting with our most important resource – our children.

References

American Heart Association. (2007). *Physical activity and public health guidelines.* Retrieved from: http://www.americanheart.org/presenter.jhtml?identifier=1200013

Anderson, B. J., Eckburg, P. B., & Relucio, K. I. (2002). Alterations in the thickness of motor cortical subregions after motor-skill and exercise. *Learning and Memory, 9*(1), 9–1.

Association for Supervision and Curriculum Development. (2014). *Learning and health: Whole School, Whole Community, Whole Child (WSCC).* Retrieved from: http://www.ascd.org/programs/learning-and-health/wscc-model.aspx

Australian Government Department of Health. (2014a). *Sedentary behavior.* Retrieved from: http://www.health.gov.au/internet/main/publishing.nsf/content/sbehaviour

Australian Government Department of Health. (2014b). *Australia's physical activity and sedentary behavior uidelines.* Retrieved from: http://www.health.gov.au/internet/main/publishing.nsf/content/health-pubhlth-strateg-phys-act-guidelines

Barker, E. (2014, March). How to raise happy kids: 10 steps backed my science. *Time Magazine.* http://time.com/35496/how-to-raise-happy-kids-10-steps-backed-by-science/

Bartz, S., & Freemark, M. (2012). Pathogenesis and prevention of type 2 diabetes: Parental determinants, breastfeeding, and early childhood nutrition. *Current Diabetes Reports, 12*(1), 82–87.

Castelli, D. M., & Ward, K. (2012). Physical activity during the school day: Physical activity breaks can help children learn. *Journal of Physical Education, Recreation & Dance, 83*(6), 20.

Centers for Disease Control and Prevention (CDC). (2016). *Division of nutrition, physical activity, and obesity: How much physical activity do children need?* Retrieved from: http://www.cdc.gov/physicalactivity/basics/children

Claire Wang, Y., Gortmaker, S. L., & Taveras, E. M. (2011). Trends and racial/ethnic disparities in severe obesity among US children and adolescents, 1976–2006. *International Journal of Pediatric Obesity, 6*(1), 12–20.

Colberg, S. R. (2012). Physical activity: The forgotten tool for type 2 diabetes management. *Frontiers in Endocrinology, 3*, 70. https://doi.org/10.3389/fendo.2012.00070

Colley, R. C., Garriguet, D., Janssen, I., Craig, C. L., Clarke, J., & Tremblay, M. S. (2011). Physical activity levels of Canadian children and youth. *Health Reports, 22*(1), 15–25.

Cottrell, R., Girvan, J., McKenzie, J., & Seabert, D. (2015). *Principles and foundations of health promotion and education* (6th ed.). Boston, MA: Pearson.

Dauer, V. P., & Pangrazi, R. P. (1975). *Dynamic education for elementary school children* (5th ed.). Minneapolis, MN: Burgess Publishing Company.

Davis, C. L., Tomporowski, P. D., McDowell, J. E., Austin, B. P., Miller, P. H., Yanasak, N. E., … Naglieri, J. A. (2011). Exercise improves executive function and achievement and alters brain activation in overweight children: A randomized, controlled trial. *Health Psychology, 30*(1), 91–98.

Eliassen, E. K. (2011). The impact of teachers and families on young children's eating behaviors. *Young Children, 66*(2), 84–89.

Freedman, D. S., Mei, Z., Srinivasan, S. R., Berenson, G. S., & Dietz, W. H. (2007). Cardiovascular risk factors and excess adiposity among overweight children and adolescents: The Bogalusa Heart Study. *Juvenile Pediatrics, 50*(1), 12–17.

Gartrell, D., & Sonsteng, K. (2008). Promote physical activity- it's proactive guidance. *Young Children, 63*(2), 51–53.

Greco, C., & Ison, M. S. (2014). What makes you happy? Appreciating the reasons that bring happiness to Argentine children living in vulnerable social contexts. *The Journal of Latino-Latin American Studies, 6*(1), 4–18.

Harvard T.H. Chan School of Public Health. (2016). *Obesity Prevention Source*. Examples of Moderate and Vigorous Physical Activity: Retrieved from: http://www.hsph.harvard.edu/obesity-prevention-source/moderate-and-vigorous-physical-activity

Healthy People. (2020). Office of Health Promotion and Disease Prevention. *Nutrition and weight status*. Retrieved from: http://www.healthypeople.gov/2020/topics-objectives/topic/nutrition-and-weight-status/objectives

Hinkley, T., Teychenne, M., Downing, K. L., Ball, K., Salmon, J., & Hesketh, K. D. (2014). Early childhood physical activity, sedentary behaviors and psychosocial well-being: A systematic review. *Preventive Medicine, 62*(2014), 182–192.

Hong, Y. M. (2010). Atherosclerotic cardiovascular disease beginning in childhood. *Korean Circulation Journal, 40*(1), 1–9.

Hung, T. M., Chang, T. C., Tang, H. C., & Shih, H. H. (2008). Does physical activity affect brain development in young children? *International Journal of Psychophysiology, 69*(3), 276–277.

Jakicic, J. M., King, W. C., Marcus, M. D., Davis, K. K., Helsel, D., Rickman, A. D., … Belle, S. H. (2015). Short-term weight loss with diet and physical activity in young adults: The IDEA Study. *Obesity, 23*(12), 2385–2397.

Javanainen-Levonen, T., Poskiparta, M., Rintala, P., & Satomaa, P. (2009). Public health nurses' approaches to early childhood physical activity in Finland. *Journal of Child Health Care, 13*(1), 30–45.

Jensen, E. (2005). *Teaching with the brain in mind* (2nd ed.). Alexandria, VA: Association for Supervision and Curriculum Development.

Kalavainen, M. P., Korppi, M. O., & Nuutinen, O. M. (2007). Clinical efficacy of group-based treatment for childhood obesity compared with routinely given individual counseling. *International Journal of Obesity, 31*, 1500–1508.

Le Masurier, G., & Corbin, C. B. (2006). Top 10 reasons for quality physical education. *Journal of Physical Education Recreation and Dance, 77*(6), 44–53.

Lee, I. M., & Paffenbarger, R. S., Jr. (2000). Associations of light, moderate, and vigorous intensity physical activity with longevity. The Harvard Alumni Health Study. *American Journal of Epidemiology, 151*(3), 293.

Livingstone, T. (2011). What really makes our children happy. *The Telegraph*. http://www.telegraph.co.uk/news/health/children/8771115/What-really-makes-our-children-happy.html

Matthews, C. E., Chen, K. Y., Freedson, P. S., Buchowski, M. S., Beech, B. M., Pate, R. R., … Troiano, R. P. (2008). Amount of time spent in sedentary behaviors in the United States, 2003–2004. *American Journal of Epidemiology, 167*(7), 875–881. https://doi.org/10.1093/aje/kwm390

Meeks, L., Heit, P., & Page, R. (2013). *Comprehensive school health education: Totally awesome strategies for teaching health*. New York, NY: McGraw Hill.

National Association for Sport and Physical Education (NASPE). (2010). *Active start: A statement of physical activity guidelines for children from birth to five* (2nd ed). Retrieved from: http://www.aahperd.org/naspe/standards/nationalGuidelines/ActiveStart.cfm

Palmer, L. (2003). *Developmental brain stimulation in school and day care settings: SMART overview*. Winona, MN: Office of Accelerated Learning, Winona State University.

Pate, R. R., Mitchell, J. A., Byun, W., & Dowda, M. (2011). Sedentary behaviour in youth. *British Journal of Sport Medicine, 45*(11), 906–913.

Seger, M. (2015). *No sweat: How the simple science of motivation can bring you a lifetime of fitness*. New York, NY: AMACOM.

Sibold, J., Edwards, E., Murray-Close, D., & Hudziak, J. (2015). Physical activity, sadness, and suicidality in bullied US adolescents. *Journal of the American Academy of Child and Adolescent Psychiatry, 54*(10), 808–815.

SPARK. (2016). *Early childhood teaching tips: Structured activity vs unstructured activity*. Retrieved from: http://www.sparkpe.org/blog/structured-activity-unstructured-activity/

Stodden, D. F., & Goodway, J. D. (2007). The dynamic association between motor skill development and physical activity. *Journal of Physical Education, Recreation & Dance, 78*(8), 33.

Syrad, H., Falconer, C., Cooke, L., Saxena, S., Kessel, A. S., Viner, R., … Croker, H. (2015). 'Health and happiness is more important than weight': A qualitative investigation of the views of parents receiving written feedback on their child's weight as part of the national child measurement program. *Journal of Human Nutrition and Dietetics, 28*(1), 47–55.

U.S. Department of Health and Human Services (DHHS). (2016). *Step it up! The surgeon general's call to action to promote walking and walkable communities*. Retrieved from: http://www.surgeongeneral.gov/library/calls/walking-and-walkable-communities/exec-summary.html

Townsend, N., Wickramasinghe, K., Williams, J., Bhatnagar, P., & Rayner, M. (2015). *Physical activity statistics 2015*. British Heart Foundation: London.

Vidoni, C., & Ignico, A. (2011). Promoting physical activity during early childhood. *Early Child Development and Care, 181*(9), 1261–1269.

Wabitsch, M., Moss, A., & Kromeyer-Hauschild, K. (2014). Unexpected plateauing of childhood obesity rates in developed countries. *BMC Medicine, 12*(1), 1.

Wang, Y., Beydoun, M. A., Liang, L., Caballero, B., & Kumanyika, S. K. (2008). Will all Americans become overweight or obese? Estimating the progression and cost of the US obesity epidemic. *Obesity, 16*(10), 2323–2330.

Yoder-Wise, P. S. (2014). Sitting is the new smoking. *The Journal of Continuing Education in Nursing, 45*(12), 523–523.

Zero to Three. (2016). National Center for Infants, Toddlers, and Families. *Early Experiences Matter*. Retrieved from: http://www.zerotothree.org

Hannah J. Brewer has been teaching for over 10 years in both P-12 education and higher education. She began her career in early childhood by teaching health and physical education for children in grades K-2. She conducted research on preschoolers' health, nutrition, and physical activity habits and studied the impact of a structured physical activity program on young learners' health and well-being. She has published in peer reviewed journals on these topics, and has presented several of these topics at national conventions.

Chapter 2
Fine Motor Skills, Executive Function, and Academic Achievement

Audrey C. Rule and Latisha L. Smith

Part I: Motor Skills, Executive Function, and Academic Achievement

Attention is crucial to learning and academic achievement. In this chapter, we explore the connections between fine motor skills, academic achievement, and attention. First, we investigate the relationship between motor and cognitive development. This is followed by consideration of specific links between fine motor skills and achievement. Classroom-tested ways to improve fine motor writing skills in kindergarten are considered. Then, we review connections between executive function skills, which include attention, and achievement. Ways to improve executive function skills, including the use of fine motor skill activities, are discussed next. In the last part of the first half of the chapter, we examine how fine motor skills, executive function skills, and school achievement are fundamentally interrelated.

Relationship Between Motor and Cognitive Development

More than a half-century ago, Piaget (1953) proposed that sensory and movement activities during the sensorimotor stage were important for the development of cognitive abilities. Several recent studies provide evidence for this assertion. One study (Bushnell & Boudreau, 1993) investigated the role that motor development might

A. C. Rule (✉)
Department of Curriculum and Instruction, University of Northern Iowa,
Cedar Falls, IA, USA

L. L. Smith
Teacher Education Department, Upper Iowa University, Fayette, IA, USA
e-mail: smithl@uiu.edu

H. Brewer, M. R. Jalongo (eds.), *Physical Activity and Health Promotion in the Early Years*, Educating the Young Child 14,
https://doi.org/10.1007/978-3-319-76006-3_2

play in determining developmental sequences in other domains. Researchers examined the effects of motor achievements on haptic (touch) and depth perception, concluding that object perception occurred as a result of manual tactile exploration of objects and that the various aspects of depth perception entailed a progression of motor skills such as control of the head, oculomotor control, and stereopsis (depth perception through binocular vision). A single, universal, developmental acquisition, such the onset of locomotion, may produce a family of experiences that elevate partially accomplished skills to a much higher level (Campos et al., 2000). For example, in a review of several studies (Campos et al., 2000), investigators observed that crawling or walker-using infants looked back at their mothers for feedback and were able to follow mother's gaze and pointing of her finger to look in the direction of an object being referenced more often than non-mobile infants of the same age. In this way, locomotion provided a set of experiences that allowed infants to develop their ability to follow referential gestural communication. In several additional areas addressed by these authors, such as family social dynamics, wariness of heights, attention to distant space, changes in posture in response to visual changes to tilt or motion of the walls (altered during experiment), and spatial search performance, locomotor experience dramatically changed the relation of the infant to the infant's environment and facilitated social, emotional, or cognitive development.

Motor skills, besides providing opportunities for children to experience situations that support other areas of development, may serve as predictors of future cognitive achievement. Investigators studied the postural control of healthy, six-month-old preterm infants and found that inadequate postural control (neck hyperextension or elbow extension) was a predictor of lower scores on cognitive tasks and less attention to task at age 12 months and age 24 months (Wijnroks & van Veldhoven, 2003). Lack of posture control may disrupt the development of arm and hand functions, including reaching. Through visual and tactile attention to objects, manipulation of objects' properties, and exploration of the infants' effects upon the objects, infants progress in their cognitive development. Therefore, lack of posture control may directly delay cognitive development. Poor posture control may also impede social interaction, infant-caregiver communication, and parental attachment. Because the social environment mediates learning, infants with less sensitive maternal responses may not develop as quickly socially and cognitively. Another possibility is that poor posture control, poor cognitive functioning, and inattention are all symptoms of lack of integrity of the central nervous system. Other researchers investigated the relationship of motor function of children of low-birthweight from age 1 year to cognitive development at age 4 years, finding that comprehensive testing results of motor development at 12 months was strongly predictive of the same child's general cognitive score 3 years later (Burns, O'Callaghan, McDonell, & Rogers, 2004). These researchers found that cognitive scores were independent of biological and social measures, making poor social interaction or general lack of integrity of the central nervous system unlikely causes of the observed motor skill-correlated cognitive levels. These findings point to the importance of encouraging and supporting children's motor development while infants for later cognitive achievement.

Early motor development has long-ranging effects that reach into middle adulthood. A random sample of 104 subjects from Northern Finland, who were aged 33–35 years and for whom the age of first independent standing had been recorded in infancy, were examined to determine the relationship of developmental data to neuropsychological test scores (Murray et al., 2006). The researchers found that those who had been able to stand earlier than peers during infancy scored higher on adult tests of executive function and working memory. Another study (Piek, Dawson, Smith, & Gasson, 2008) aimed to determine whether measures of motor performance during preschool years could predict motor and cognitive performance of subjects when they reached school age. Results of analysis of information from 33 subjects indicated a significant predictive relationship between early gross motor skills and later working memory and processing speed, but no significant predictability from early fine motor skill performance. These studies indicate that there is a strong relationship between early motor control and cognitive development, making attention to a child's motor development important to reducing risks of poor cognitive performance. Therefore, child caregivers should plan activities for infants that encourage movement to strengthen muscles and neural movement pathways.

Links Between Fine Motor Skills and Academic Achievement

For decades, human development books have included a table that aligns the achievement of physical milestones with cognitive ones. Research in recent years has provided evidence that a connection exists between fine motor skills and a child's academic achievement (Carlson, Rowe, & Curby, 2013). "Although the link between early motor skills and later cognitive attainment may not be causal, the high levels of association suggest that early intervention by schools… …could be of enormous benefit in, at least, the motor domain" (Brown, 2010, p. 269)." Several researchers have concluded that the fine motor skills children exhibit at the beginning of kindergarten could be used to predict academic achievement as well as attention later on (Grissmer, Grimm, Aiyer, Murrah, & Steele, 2010). Motor development in infancy sets the stage for cognitive development because movement allows children to interact with the environment in new ways that lead to cognitive advances (Bushnell & Boudreau, 1993; Carlson et al., 2013).

Several studies address why lack of fine motor skills is problematic in the educational setting. Teachers have long identified fine motor skills as an important component of school readiness (Roebers & Jäger, 2014). Children who exhibit challenges with fine motor skills are most often at risk for low academic achievement (Carlson et al., 2013). One study (Cameron et al., 2012) identified motor development as a factor of kindergarten performance early on as well as throughout the year in the areas of block building, drawing, and copying designs. In addition, the results of this research indicated that children whose fine motor skills are inadequate, especially design copy skills, are at risk to struggle academically. Several studies have indicated that children with developmental motor problems tend to have difficulties with reading, precipitating the idea that all children with reading difficulties be tested for motor problems (Brown, 2010; Iversen, Berg, Ellertsen, & Tønnessen, 2005; McPhillips & Sheehy, 2004; O'Hare, & Khalid, 2002).

Understanding the link between fine motor skills and academic achievement is critical if the goal of helping all children to have academic success is to be achieved. Rather than a simple correlation of skills, current evidence suggests that the fine motor-academic achievement association is a "complex, brain-based phenomenon" (Dinehart & Manfra, 2013, p. 139). Researchers examined whether two types of preschoolers' fine motor skills, object manipulation and writing, predicted academic achievement in second grade (Dinehart & Manfra, 2013). They determined that both fine motor writing and object manipulation skills were significantly connected to success in second grade mathematics and reading, although writing ability was a stronger predictor. These results were confirmed by a study of 812 South African first grade students: "A strong relationship was indicated between visual-motor integration, visual perception and motor proficiency and early school success in critical school performance areas such as math, reading, and writing" (Pienaar, Barhorst, & Twisk, 2013, p. 376). Analysis of six longitudinal data sets allowed researchers (Grissmer et al., 2010) to identify kindergarten readiness factors and to quantify their importance through determining which predict later math, reading, and science achievement. The set of attention, fine motor skills, and general knowledge were strong overall predictors of later mathematics, reading, and science scores (Grissmer et al., 2010).

Two aspects of fine motor skills, visual-spatial integration and visual-motor coordination, can be differentiated (Carlson et al., 2013). A study was conducted to determine how these two aspects impacted academic achievement later in the schooling years. Each of these two aspects were measured by using a tracing task to determine visual-motor coordination proficiency and by asking the student to copy a figure to assess visual-spatial integration. The findings indicated visual-spatial integration skills (measured by copying a figure), rather than visual motor coordination skills, were associated with fine motor ability and achievement. "Thus it may be that motor coordination drives very early cognitive development, while visual-spatial integration drives later cognitive development throughout childhood" (Carlson et al., 2013, p. 528).

Research in the area of fine motor development has the potential to impact the work of early childhood professionals and should be factored in when curriculum and planning decisions are made. Because research has shown fine motor skills can be a predictor of academic achievement in the elementary years, a focus on fine motor writing skills may provide a way to reduce the achievement gap that exists in children in kindergarten (Dinehart & Manfra, 2013). Children with fine motor problems should receive more opportunities to practice the problematic fine motor skills (Brown, 2010). Intervention at the early childhood level should address attention and fine motor skills as opposed to direct instruction in math and reading (Dinehart & Manfra, 2013; Grissmer et al., 2010). Early childhood students need to have experiences with writing to positively impact academic achievement in later grades (Dinehart & Manfra, 2013). Early childhood curricula that include fine motor writing and copying may improve learning during the early school years (Cameron et al., 2012; Dinehart & Manfra, 2013).

Improving Fine Motor Writing Skills

It is clear that fine motor skills, and writing/copying skills in particular, are important to early school success. How can teachers intervene with students to improve their fine motor writing skills? Two kindergarten teachers have conducted separate action research projects to determine the utility of various fine motor skill interventions with children in their classrooms. These investigations provide ideas for different interventions that should be further tested under more controlled conditions. An action research study of three children in a kindergarten (Keifer, 2015) indicated that interventions tailored to the fine motor needs of students are effective in improving their handwriting. These interventions included using a pinch-type clothespin to pick up cotton balls, peeling stickers, stringing beads, weaving yarn, molding clay, tracing dotted lines, using a single hole punch, and cutting with scissors. In a similar manner, Morrow (2015) investigated the utility of fine motor skill interventions on 14 kindergarten students through an action research project, finding that they were helpful in improving students' fine motor skills. The interventions used in this study included: line tracing, dot-to-dot tracing, pencil mazes, stringing pony beads on pipe cleaners, moving small objects with spoons or chopsticks, attaching chain links, marking numbers with a Bingo stamper, and dough molding activities.

Connections Between Executive Function and Academic Achievement

Executive function is a broad construct involving attention shifting, working memory, and inhibitory control. Executive function may have evolved to anticipate and control humans' continuous sensorimotor interaction with the environment (Koziol, Budding, & Chidekel, 2012). Executive function skills assist children in planning, organizing, prioritizing, focusing attention, remembering, and carrying tasks through to completion, including motor tasks. These executive function tasks are essential to success in school (Brooks & Goldstein, 2007). Children who are able to mentally manipulate ideas through working memory, pay attention to required tasks including resisting distraction or shifting tasks when needed (attentional or cognitive flexibility), and control impulses to initiate more adaptive behaviors (inhibitory control) have greater success in school (Morrison, Ponitz, & McClelland, 2010). A child's inhibitory control is a significant predictor of academic achievement; it also predicts physical and mental health in adulthood, making it a vital part of childhood cognitive development (Diamond, 2013). Children with poor attention and lack of impulse control often are diagnosed with attention deficit hyperactivity disorder. This is discussed in more detail in Part II of this chapter.

Six large longitudinal data sets were used to determine connections of school-entry academic skills, attention, and socioemotional skills with later school reading and mathematics achievement (Duncan et al., 2007). The researchers found that across all six data sets, mathematics skills, reading skills, and attention at school entry were the strongest predictors of later achievement, confirming the importance of attention, an aspect of executive function, to student success. A study using a sample of over 2000 students ranging in age from 5 to 17 years (Best, Miller, & Naglieri, 2011) measured student performance on nine academic tasks and three executive function tasks to investigate the connections between executive function and academic achievement throughout K-12 education. These researchers also examined different aspects of performance such as accuracy, completion time, and their ratio on the executive function tasks using the Cognitive Assessment System standardized test (Naglieri & Das, 1997). Growth in executive function was found to be large across the youngest groups, more moderate during late childhood, and diminished more in adolescence (Best et al., 2011; Romine & Reynolds, 2005). Different developmental patterns were identified by comparing student responses on sections of the test: younger children completing tasks more accurately also completed them faster, but, starting at age 12, accuracy increased very little, while completion time continued to improve (Best et al., 2011). This may indicate that younger children who complete the tasks accurately have better strategies and older students tend to improve through efficiency of those same strategies. The correlation between the executive function tasks and academic achievement was also examined. The researchers found that, overall, this correspondence was similar for both mathematics and reading, indicating that common cognitive processes of planning, self-monitoring, updating, and impulse control are important to both academic domains. These findings build on the work of other researchers (Bull, Espy, & Wiebe, 2008), who studied 124 children, following them through second grade with testing at preschool entrance (mean age 4.5 years), end of kindergarten, and at age 7–8. Through correlational and regression analysis of test data, they determined that visual short-term and working memory specifically predicted mathematics achievement from preschool through second grade (age 8), while executive function skills predicted learning in general. Better executive function skills during preschool, such as inhibition and planning, provide children with a foundation for math and reading leading to better early academic skills, an advantage that is maintained throughout early childhood.

Improving Executive Function

Given the research-backed importance of executive function skills, teachers need strategies or programs for improving executive function. A review (Diamond & Lee, 2011) of programs that improve executive functioning for children found that programs incorporating repeated practice along with constant challenge in executive function skills were the most effective. Among these were computerized training, face-to-face games, aerobic exercise, martial arts, yoga, mindfulness, and certain school curricula such as *Tools of the Mind* (Bodrova & Leong, 2007), a preK-K curriculum that is based on Vygotsky's ideas of social pretend play, and Montessori Education (Montessori, 1949) in which children learn to wait their turn, are individually challenged through a developmental sequence of activities, and cross-age tutored. One of the most researched and successful programs was CogMed©, computerized working memory training, that gradually increased the load on working memory through a games format. Working memory skills learned through the CogMed© games transferred to other working memory tasks but did not generalize to other executive function tasks. Only for those children for whom working memory loads were increased was improvement seen (Dunning, Holmes, & Gathercole, 2013).

Working memory is the cognitive system that temporarily stores information to support mental activities such as instructions, mental arithmetic, and problem-solving. Working memory has three components: (1) concurrent storage and processing, (2) relational integration (discerning relationships between stored pieces of information), and (3) supervision (setting goals, preventing distraction, applying response criteria, and shifting tasks) (Oberauer, Süβ, Wilhelm, & Wittman, 2008).

For example, suppose that a first grader, standing with a marker at a whiteboard, is presented with a story problem in math: two ducks were swimming in a pond and were joined by one more. If another family of four ducks landed on the pond, how many ducks were there altogether? The ***supervision*** aspect of working memory may begin the work by ***deciding the goal*** of this interaction. Do I want to expend the effort to solve the problem or should I just say I can't do it and sit down? Is the problem one at which I can be successful? I probably can handle adding or subtracting one-digit numbers. How does the teacher want me to respond (***applying criteria***)? Probably I should draw a picture on the whiteboard, write an equation, and explain my ideas. The child must ***store*** the problem in working memory while beginning to ***process*** the information. There are three numerical sets of information: the two ducks, the one duck, and the four ducks. ***Relational integration*** occurs as the child realizes that these three numbers representing ducks need to be summed to find out how many there are altogether. The child ***plans (supervision)*** that she will draw little circles for the ducks on the pond, while repeating the problem out loud, then write the equation, and explain her thinking. The child draws the first two ducks on the pond and then the next duck. Another student calls out that the ducks don't look like ducks and the child must ***suppress responding (supervision)*** to it as she continues with her plan of attack on the problem. She mentally adds the first two numbers ***(processing information),*** writes that part of the equation (2+1), and announces (***shifting tasks***) that there are currently three ducks resulting from the first two numbers. She then repeats the last part of the problem from ***stored memory*** and completes solving it by adding the four ducks to the first three ***(processing information)***. Interspersed with these operations, the ***supervision aspect*** of working memory does the following: directs the child to ***focus*** on the problem and ***avoid***

distractions by friends in the class or other mental ideas related to ducks, ***maintains a positive attitude*** so that she has confidence to solve the problem, and ***shifts*** from drawing the ducks to writing parts of the equation to verbalizing and explaining the answer. ***Relational integration*** again plays a part in making sure the visual drawings, written equations, and verbal explanations all relate correctly to the remembered numbers in the story problem. This complex of working memory processes operates smoothly to ensure effective problem solution for this child. However, working memory is not as well-developed in some children. For example, children with ***poor mental supervision*** may become distracted from the problem and begin to tell a story of ducks from a TV show, may become discouraged and quit at the first obstacle, may ignore the needs of the audience and write too small or mumble, or may become engrossed in the drawing and neglect to shift to other needed tasks. Children with ***poor storage and processing*** may become confused about where they are in the problem, may not be able to mentally add the one-digit numbers, instead relying upon counting the drawn ducks, or forget information from the problem. Children with ***poor relational integration*** may be puzzled by whether to add or subtract, may not have drawings and equations that match, or may not be logical in their explanation of the problem's solution.

Researchers (Moreno, Shwayder, & Friedman, 2016) observed preschool classrooms for children's examples of executive function and teachers' strategies for promoting it. These researchers suggest prompting metacognitive thought by asking a child why she likes her picture instead of the teacher providing a judgment. Teachers can offer elaborative utterances to describe aspects of a child's construction or behavior, thereby supporting the child's higher order thinking or problem-solving. Attentional focus might be encouraged when the teacher makes observations of what the child is doing rather than suggesting actions. Organization skills may be refined by the teacher pointing attention to the steps the child took during the process. Working memory may be supported when the teacher talks about strategies she or he has found to be helpful in the past such as drawing a picture, making tally marks, or using manipulatives.

Scholars at the Center on the Developing Child (2014) suggest numerous ways in which early childhood teachers can provide practice to enhance the executive function skills of their students. Activities that are appropriate for 3–5 year olds include imaginary play and obstacle courses. Imaginary play encourages cooperation and increases self-regulation skills, while an obstacle course physically challenges children, requiring them to monitor and adjust their actions as they encounter obstacles. Music and dance are effective activities, particularly when used in games such as *Freeze dance* sometimes called *Musical statues*. In this game, students are asked to dance (move in rhythm to music) and then freeze quickly when the music stops, an action that requires inhibitory control. Songs with repetition and added parts, such as *She'll be coming 'round the mountain* and *Five green and speckled frogs,* allow children to practice memory skills. Puzzles of increasing challenge enhance visual working memory while cooking experiences exercise following directions, waiting, and attention to detail. For 5–7 year olds, card games such as *Go fish* and *Old maid* provide ideal practice for working memory. *Perfection* is a game that challenges students to focus their attention on shapes and the placement of those shapes in a race against the clock to practice focusing attention, quick decisions, and self-control. Popular games including *Sorry!*, *Battleship*, and *checkers*, encourage children to strategize their next move. *Red Light, Green Light* and *Mother May I?* both test inhibition and offer practice with attention skills. Puzzle books are also suitable, especially those that offer matching exercises, word finds, and mazes. *I Spy* and books with a search and find concept help children focus attention as they hunt for items on a page.

Interrelationships

Fine motor skills, executive function, and school achievement may be fundamentally interrelated. Functional neuroimaging studies (Diamond, 2000) consistently have found a strong connection between activation of the dorsolateral prefrontal cortex and activation of the contralateral cerebellum. The former location has been commonly associated with complex cognitive activities, while the latter has been thought to control fine motor functions. When a cognitive task produces increased activation in the prefrontal cortex, it has also been found to increase activation in the cerebellum. Similarly, when a task has been practiced and requires less concentration, or when damage occurs to one of the areas, activation in both locations decreases, indicating coupling of these brain areas. The cerebellum and prefrontal cortex work together especially when a task is difficult, new, changing or unpredictable, requires a quick response, and requires concentration. Association of cognitive disorders with impaired motor functions in Attention Deficit Hyperactivity Disorder and dyslexia provide additional evidence.

During the early school years, most instructional activities have motor as well as cognitive components. An observational study of 10 Head Start and 10 kindergarten classrooms (Marr, Cermak, Cohn, & Henderson, 2003) found that children in Head Start spent a mean of 37% of their day in fine motor activities while children in kindergarten spent a mean of 46% of the day in fine motor activities. Of these tasks, 42% were paper-pencil activities for kindergarten students. Tasks requiring complex motor control put greater burdens on cognitive resources than those with simple motor requirements (Cameron et al., 2012). Children who struggle with handwriting and fine motor tasks devote their brain power to fine motor processing and take longer to complete assignments, therefore missing exposure to some learning experiences (Lawrence et al., 2002). Children with greater automaticity in fine motor movements may be able to learn more complex cognitive concepts because of greater available processing capacity (Berger, 2010).

The importance of fine motor skills to school achievement now becomes clearer as it can be seen as an integral part of thinking, learning, and academic achievement. Because of the pairing of motor and higher cognitive functions during brain activities, fine motor skills acquisition may remove processing burden, thereby allowing energy to be expended on cognitive tasks. Activities that have been shown to improve early childhood students' fine motor skills are discussed in the sections to which the studies were related in Part II of this chapter.

Part II: Psychiatric Disorders Involving Motor Skills

In the second part of this chapter, we address psychiatric disorders that typically involve decreased fine motor skill levels to provide the reader with an awareness of populations who may benefit from activities that improve fine motor skills. These disorders include developmental coordination disorder, attention deficit hyperactivity disorder, autism, and schizophrenia. Additionally, in conjunction with these disorders, we explore some classroom-tested fine motor activities for early childhood that support cognitive skill development and impact student attention.

Developmental Coordination Disorder

Preschooler Andre accidentally bumps into a peer, knocking over her block tower and causing her considerable anguish. Moments later, the teacher encourages Andre to join her at the writing center. He refuses because of the difficulty he experiences while attempting to write his name or use scissors. Before going outside, he asks the teacher for help because he cannot get his arm into the sleeve of his jacket. During outdoor play, he falls while climbing the stairs to the slide and later scrapes his knee when he trips on the sidewalk. As a lunch helper, he becomes distraught when several utensils and cups fall to the floor as he attempts to manipulate them.

Developmental coordination disorder is identified in children through performance in fine and gross motor tasks at a level below that expected for chronological age and intelligence (American Psychiatric Association, 2000). Between 6 and 13% of all school-aged children exhibit developmental coordination disorder with a higher incidence occurring among males (Hadders-Algra, 2000). Developmental coordination disorder is frequently comorbid (existing simultaneously) with attention deficit hyperactivity disorder, dyslexia, and autism spectrum disorders (Dewey, 2002).

A public school study in Greece (Asonitou, Koutsouki, Kourtessis, & Charitou, 2012) examined 54 five- and six-year old kindergarten children with developmental coordination disorder and 54 typical children matched for age. The assessments tested manual dexterity, and ball skills, along with static and dynamic balance. The Das Naglieri Cognitive Assessment System (Naglieri & Das, 1997) was used to determine the cognitive abilities of students in planning, attention, and simultaneous coding. Asonitou et al. (2012) found the performance of those with developmental coordination disorder was significantly poorer than the typically developing children on each task. After considering the findings of previous researchers indicating that planning, attention, and simultaneous processing are necessary for effective performance in mathematics (e.g., Kroesbergen, van Luit, Naglieri, Taddei, & Franchi, 2009) and reading other studies (e.g., Roebers, & Jäger, 2014), the researchers (Asonitou et al., 2012) suggested systematic intervention to improve the mental processing of children with developmental coordination disorder.

Four different approaches have been used to treat developmental coordination disorder: (1) process-oriented approaches that seek to develop or strengthen body functions needed to perform the motor activities; (2) task-oriented approaches that involve learning specific motor skills with particular attention to certain aspects of performance during the task that might be improved; (3) physical and occupational therapy; and (4) chemical treatments. A meta-analysis was conducted to compare the efficacy of these approaches (Smits-Engelsman et al., 2013), finding that the effects of task-oriented interventions were greatest, followed fairly closely by physical and occupational therapies, but process-oriented approaches showed very small effects. Although chemical treatments with methylphenidate (commonly known by the trade name Ritalin) showed fairly strong positive effects in three studies (Bart, Podoly, & Bar-Haim, 2010; Flapper & Schoemaker, 2008; Flapper, Houwen, & Schoemaker, 2006), the authors of the meta-analysis concluded that there was insufficient evidence to provide a recommendation (Smits-Engelsman et al., 2013).

Researchers (Smits-Engelsman et al., 2013) investigated the efficacy of different fine motor skill interventions with children who had developmental coordination disorder through a meta-analysis of the literature. They found that intervention was preferable to no intervention, but that task-oriented interventions and traditional motor-based skill training yielded significant effects greater than process-oriented interventions such as sensory integration, kinesthetic training, or perceptual training. A meta-analysis of studies conducted by other scholars (Logan, Robinson, Wilson, & Lucas, 2012) assessed fundamental motor skills of throwing, catching, dribbling, kicking, underhand rolling and striking in addition to running, hopping, skipping, galloping, sliding, and jumping. Although most of these skills tend toward gross, rather than fine motor skills, the findings of this meta-analysis showed that children demonstrated significant improvements in fundamental motor skill competence after intervention with a medium effect size. The lack of improvement in control groups (free play groups) indicated that motor skills do not develop naturally, but need to be taught and practiced.

Effective interventions to improve kindergarten children's fine motor skills have been documented in the literature. A pretest-posttest control group-experimental group study (Rule & Stewart, 2002) compared fine motor skills of kindergarten children from 13 public school classrooms, with 101 students in the eight experimental classes and 85 students in the five control classes. Students in the experimental classes used step-by-step directions with tongs, tweezers, or spoons to move and position small objects in themed sets based on Montessori's principles (Montessori, 1914/1965; Wentworth, 1998) for about 15 min a day for 6 months. Six new sets of materials were rotated into each experimental group classroom every 2 weeks. Students in the control groups spent the same amount of time each day using more traditional fine motor skill materials such as puzzles, snap-together building sets, markers and crayons, and dressing frames. The results of this study showed that kindergarten children in the experimental group improved their fine motor skills significantly more than students in the control groups. This difference was attributed to the step-by-step procedures of the experimental materials in which teachers demonstrated and narrated each step of the operation in a logical, orderly sequence, drawing attention to body motions and positions as objects were moved with the implements. The distance from the pincer grip of the fingers along the implement to the object being moved by tongs, tweezers or spoon required more control and allowed more fine motor challenge and practice during the exercise.

Attention Deficit Hyperactivity Disorder

First grader Marquis is completing a layout to match laminated word cards with pictures of the objects they represent. While sprawling on the carpet, he tilts a laminated card back and forth to watch the glossy reflection of ceiling lights roll up and down the card again and again. After the teacher reminds him to continue work, he agrees, and jumps up to obtain a pencil to copy the words into a notebook. He hops around the room, waving a fistful of pencils, stopping to interact with each student he encounters. The teacher asks him to go to his area and do his work. Very soon he becomes distracted by arranging the several different-length pencils he has brought with him, first by aligning the eraser ends, then by aligning the tips, and then again by aligning eraser ends. Nearby students arranging sets of materials on the carpet complain that Marquis is rolling about and bumping into their work. The teacher again asks Marquis to stay in his space and focus on doing his work….

Attention deficit hyperactivity disorder is the most pervasive behavioral disorder of children of school age, affecting 3–5% of American elementary students (American Psychiatric Association, 1994). Attention deficit hyperactivity disorder is a "neurodevelopmental condition which can persist throughout the lifespan. At its core is a persistent and pervasive pattern of inattention and/or hyperactivity and impulsiveness. Both genetic and environmental factors play an important role, leading to alterations of multiple circuits in the brain and creating various pathways to symptoms, different individual deficit profiles and resulting impairments" (Bolea-Alamañac et al., 2014, p. 3). The pattern of cortical brain development in children who have attention deficit hyperactivity disorder follows the same path as in typical children, but is delayed by an average of 2–3 years (Bolea-Alamañac et al., 2014).

Children with attention deficit hyperactivity disorder have poorer motor skills than more typically-developing children with more than half of children diagnosed with attention deficit hyperactivity disorder having difficulties with gross and fine motor skills (Kaiser, Schoemaker, Albaret, & Geuze, 2015). Researchers (Goulardins, Marques, Casella, Nascimento, & Oliveira, 2013) examined the motor performance of 34 children with attention deficit hyperactivity disorder compared to 32 age- and gender-matched, typically developing children of ages 7–11. Motor scores in all studied areas were lower for children with attention deficit hyperactivity disorder, although in general, the majority of subjects with attention deficit hyperactivity disorder scored in "normal medium" or "normal low" motor development ranges. The two groups showed statistically significant differences in general motor age and overall scores, balance, spatial organization, and fine and global motor abilities.

Researchers (Tseng, Henderson, Chow, & Yao, 2004) investigated the relationship between motor performance, attention deficit, impulsiveness, and hyperactivity in 42 children with attention deficit hyperactivity disorder, aged 6–11 years, compared to 42 typically-developing children matched for sex and age. They found that the best predictors of gross motor skills for children with attention deficit hyperactivity disorder were attention, impulse control, and parent ratings of activity level. In their study, the two best predictors of fine motor skills were attention and impulse control.

Other investigators (Schoemaker, Ketelaars, van Zonneveld, Minderaa, & Mulder, 2005) conducted an experiment to determine which motor control processes were impaired in children with attention deficit hyperactivity disorder. Sixteen children with attention deficit hyperactivity disorder and 16 typically developing children, matched for sex and age, participated. During all graphic tasks, children with attention deficit hyperactivity disorder held the pen so that it had a relatively high axial force and made slower, less accurate strokes than the control group, especially as accuracy demands increased, indicating deficits in parameter setting. These findings strongly support the need for early fine motor writing interventions, as previously mentioned in Part I of this chapter.

Concerns about medicalization and overuse of drug treatments have been raised in connection to attention deficit hyperactivity disorder (Singh and Wessely 2015). A review (Kaiser et al., 2015) of the 15 studies of the recent professional literature pertaining to the influence of medication on motor skills and motor control of subjects with attention deficit hyperactivity disorder found that between 28% and 76% of children improved their motor skills to the normal range with the use of medication. The British Association for Psychopharmacology (Bolea-Alamañac et al., 2014) issued recommendations concerning treatment for children and adults with attention deficit hyperactivity disorder. This professional organization recognized that the proportion of the population receiving treatment for ADHD in Western countries is still lower than the estimated population prevalence of the disorder. Untreated attention deficit hyperactivity disorder is costly to society because it produces poor academic outcomes; is associated with illicit drug use, alcohol addiction, and criminality; produces increased rates of unemployment; and is associated with higher rates of marital conflict.

The British Association for Psychopharmacology (Bolea-Alamañac et al., 2014) recommend that all children with severe attention deficit hyperactivity disorder (those children with all three components: inattention, hyperactivity, and impulsivity) be provided pharmacological treatment. In addition, children with moderate symptoms who have not responded to psychological interventions should also be given pharmacological treatment. Group parent training and/or individual psychological interventions may include cognitive training or behavioral intervention approaches. Scholars (Sonuga-Barke et al., 2013) conducting a meta-analysis of studies evaluating different non-drug interventions for attention deficit hyperactivity disorder found free fatty acid supplementation and exclusion of artificial food coloring had a beneficial effect on symptoms; neurofeedback, cognitive training, and restrictive diets potentially may have stronger, more positive effects, but more blinded assessments need to be conducted.

A study testing fine motor materials' effects on student attention (Stewart, Rule, & Giordano, 2007) examined the effects of using similar sets of materials with small objects moved by tongs, tweezers, or spoons to move and sort small objects. This pretest-posttest experimental group-control group design study involved 68 kindergarten children (36 in the experimental group and 32 in the control group). Both the experimental and control groups engaged in the fine motor activities for approximately 15 min a day for 6 months. Themed sets of materials for the experimental group involved, for example, using tweezers to move small tropical fish resin figures from a blue glass bowl to a board with multilevel painted spool pedestals. Each fish figure was carefully positioned on a spool until all had been placed. Then the fish were systematically returned to the glass bowl. In this study, instead of the teacher providing directions and modeling the activity, step-by-step directions were recorded on a cassette tape to which students listened through headphones. Control group students spent an equal amount of time engaged in typical fine motor activities (puzzles, building sets, marker and crayons, etc.) in their classrooms. Attention was measured using the attention subtests of the Standard Battery of the Cognitive Assessment System (Naglieri & Das, 1997). Results of the study indicated a group x sex interaction with females in the experimental group making significant gains in attention, while males did not. Classroom records showed that both boys and girls in the experimental group had used the materials with the same frequency; interviews with males indicated that they enjoyed and valued the activity sets. The authors of the study concluded that additional research into the gendered connection between fine motor skills development and attention is warranted.

Autism Spectrum Disorder

Kindergartner Roberta whispers to her teacher when she notices an unfamiliar adult in the classroom. She shyly approaches the visitor and, with encouragement from the teacher, quietly states her name. After doing so, she returns to the carpet. Her love for technology is apparent as she takes the lead on the iPad used for her lesson. During the lesson there are several questions posed by the teacher that show Roberta does not understand what is being asked. The teacher patiently asks if she needs help or needs thinking time. Roberta doesn't make eye contact and finally whispers that she was listening. Because she has few friends and lacks the skills to make friends, the topic of the lesson is social skills. As the lesson progresses Roberta's voice is quiet and her facial expressions rarely change. Most assessment throughout the lesson is verbal and when the time comes for a written assessment, the teacher writes for Roberta because of her limited fine motor skills and the frustration that results from her lack of ability in this area.

Although social impairments are used to define autism spectrum disorders, autism is often accompanied by abnormal motor functioning in children both with and without cognitive delays. In fact, motor delays in infancy are more strongly associated with children who develop autism than typically developing individuals and may be predictive of autism for children at risk for the disorder (Bhat, Galloway, & Landa, 2012). Research regarding autism spectrum disorders is important as these disorders are the most common pediatric diagnoses in the United States (Bhat, Landa, & Galloway, 2011). Impairments related to motor ability are often characteristic of those with autism spectrum disorders; fine motor delays are also common in siblings of children with autism spectrum disorders (Bhat et al., 2011). Issues with coordination and movement have social implications in the early years of schooling as some children may experience anxiety or refrain from participating in play (Bhat et al., 2011). Children with autism may exhibit basic fine and gross motor impairments along with more complex imitation and planning impairments (Bhat et al., 2011).

Several recent investigations have compared children with autism to other groups. Researchers (MacDonald, Lord, & Ulrich, 2014) conducted a study of 159 children: 136 with autism spectrum disorders and 23 without autism spectrum disorders. They found that fine motor and gross motor skills significantly predicted the severity of autism. These investigators also identified that children with weaker motor skills tend to have poorer social communication skills. Because fine motor skills appear to play a strong role in the severity of autism and because other research (Dawson et al., 2010) has indicated that early interventions from birth to 2 years can improve the autism diagnosis, fine motor skill interventions are needed (MacDonald et al., 2014). Another study (Hellendoorn et al., 2015) examined longitudinal relationships between fine motor skills and visuospatial cognition, exploration, and language development in two groups: 63 children with autism spectrum disorder and 46 children with other developmental delays/disorders. These researchers found that fine motor functioning was related to visuospatial cognition in both populations and connected to object exploration, spatial exploration, and social orientation only in the children with autism spectrum disorder. The results of this study support the theory that cognition emerges from bodily interaction with the environment as was previously noted in Part I of this chapter.

Autopsies of individuals with autism have shown that more than 90% of their cerebella displayed well-defined cerebellar anatomic abnormalities (Allen & Courchesne, 2003). Long-thought to be affecting motor control primarily, the cerebellum also may be responsible for behaviors in cognitive, affective, and sensory domains (Koziol et al., 2014). Researchers (Allen & Courchesne, 2003) studied eight subjects with autism compared to eight matched healthy subjects through magnetic resonance imaging during attention, motor, and sensory tasks involving use of a joystick with response button. These researchers found that activation of all regions of the cerebellum was greater in the healthy subjects for the attention tasks, but a greater, more diffuse pattern of activation was seen in the subjects with autism for the motor tasks. The overall volume of the cerebellum for autistic subjects was smaller than for healthy subjects and was correlated with the amount of attention activation (Allen & Courchesne, 2003). These results confirm the negative effects of a smaller cerebellum for individuals with autism.

A handwriting study (Fuentes, Mostofsky, & Bastian, 2010) provided evidence that children with autism spectrum disorder had poorer handwriting than peers with motor impairments predicting the quality of their handwriting while children, but with perceptual reasoning predicting handwriting quality for adolescents. Even though adolescents with autism still demonstrated motor impairments, they had learned strategies to compensate for their fine motor difficulties, thereby producing more legible handwriting. Because handwriting is so critical to academic success and communication in general, problems associated with writing may be an important factor for intervention in students diagnosed with autism spectrum disorders. Some of the interventions for fine motor handwriting skills discussed in Part I may be useful for these students.

Other Psychiatric Disorders and Toxicity Problems

Although the foregoing psychiatric disorders account for major populations experiencing fine motor difficulties, there are other populations with strong connections as well. A meta-analysis of studies of children evidencing cognitive and motor deficits in childhood, including individuals who later developed schizophrenia (Dickson, Laurens, Cullen, & Hodgins, 2012), showed that significant deficits in IQ and motor performance, but not general academic achievement or mathematics achievement, preceded the prodrome (set of early symptoms) of schizophrenia.

Exposure to toxins may affect motor and cognitive development of children. For example, the insecticide chlordecone, used extensively in the West Indies to control banana root borer, persists in the soil causing widespread human exposure. A study of the cognitive, visual, and motor development of 7-month-old infants from Guadeloupe exposed to this insecticide (Dallaire et al., 2012) showed that prenatal exposure resulted in lowered fine motor skills, while postnatal exposure was marginally associated with longer mental processing times and reduced preference for visual novelty.

Summary

Over 50 years ago, Piaget suggested that sensory and movement activities formed a foundation for cognitive abilities. More recent studies have confirmed that tactile exploration, depth perception, locomotion, postural control, and motor development have strong connections and predictive relationships to cognitive ability. Fine motor skill proficiency and academic achievement of children is also linked. Fine motor skill ability at kindergarten is predictive of later school achievement and attention with movement providing the types of interactions that result in cognitive advances. Lack of fine motor skills, in particular, related to use of a writing utensil, leads to a risk for low achievement in mathematics, reading, and science. These findings suggest that direct interventions should be given to students having difficulties with fine motor skills. Visual-spatial integration skills may be a driving force behind cognitive development throughout childhood and opportunities to practice these skills are needed. Executive function skills involving attention shifting, working memory, and inhibitory control are essential to school success. Children with effective mental manipulation of objects, attention to task, resistance of distraction, and control of impulses experience greater success in school. Inhibitory control not only predicts academic success, but also physical and mental health in adulthood. Mathematics, reading, and attention skills at school entry strongly predict later school achievement. Studies of children of a wide age range indicate that growth in executive function skills occurs early, while strategies are refined as children reach adolescence. Repeated practice and constant challenge in executive function skills have been shown to be most effective for improvement. Various programs have been developed that improve executive function skills.

Several widespread psychiatric disorders involve significant difficulties with fine motor skills. Developmental coordination disorder occurs in 6–13% of school-aged children who perform fine and gross motor tasks at a level below typical children of the same age and intelligence. Developmental coordination disorder often exists simultaneously with attention deficit disorder, dyslexia, and autism. Children with developmental coordination disorder perform more poorly than typical children in planning, attention, and simultaneous coding, indicating the need for interventions. Task-oriented interventions involving attention to specific aspects of the task that might be improved were found to be most helpful. Attention deficit hyperactivity disorder affects 3–5% of American elementary students, with more than half of these children having fine and gross motor skill difficulties. Focused attention and impulse control predicted fine motor skills in this population. Children with attention deficit hyperactivity disorder tend to have difficulty in handwriting, holding the writing implement with high axial force. A review of many recent studies indicates that medication helped improve motor skills for 28–76% of children with attention deficit hyperactivity disorder. Children diagnosed with autism spectrum disorder often have accompanying motor function difficulties. Motor delays in infancy predict autism for children at risk for the disorder. The severity of fine and gross motor impairment significantly predict the severity of autism, suggesting that early interventions are needed. Studies with children who have autism spectrum disorders connect object exploration, spatial exploration, and social orientation to better fine motor skills, supporting the theory that cognition emerges from bodily interaction with the surrounding world. Autopsy evidence indicates that individuals with autism tend to have abnormalities in the cerebellum. Live magnetic resonance studies of subjects with autism, compared to matched healthy subjects, showed a great reduction in cerebellum activity during attention tasks and a diffuse pattern of activation during motor tasks. Children with autism spectrum disorder have poorer handwriting than peers, but are able to learn strategies to improve their handwriting by adolescence. There are other psychiatric or toxicity-caused conditions that are linked to poor fine motor functioning. These include schizophrenia and exposure to the insecticide chlordecone.

Effective interventions are needed for children with poor fine motor skills. Two meta-analyses have shown that interventions are preferable to no intervention, as fine motor skills do not seem to develop entirely on their own. A controlled study of kindergarten children using tongs, tweezers and spoons to move and position small objects showed improvement in fine motor skills compared to a control group. Step-by-step coaching with reference to arm position and the distance between the fingertips and the object caused by the extended implement helped to challenge students and increase their fine motor skills. Another study of kindergarten children using similar sets of materials showed that girls, but not boys, increased their attention compared to control group students. Two action research studies by kindergarten teachers showcased some promising fine motor activities for increasing fine motor skills. These studies indicate the need for more exploration of fine motor skill interventions through controlled studies.

References

Allen, G., & Courchesne, E. (2003). Differential effects of developmental cerebellar abnormality on cognitive and motor functions in the cerebellum: An fMRI study of autism. *American Journal of Psychiatry, 160*(2), 262–273.

American Psychiatric Association. (1994). *Diagnostic and statistical manual of mental disorders* (4th ed.). Washington, DC: American Psychiatric Association.

American Psychiatric Association. (2000). *Diagnostic and statistical manual of mental disorders* (4th ed., text revision). Washington, DC: American Psychiatric Association.

Asonitou, K., Koutsouki, D., Kourtessis, T., & Charitou, S. (2012). Motor and cognitive performance differences between children with and without developmental coordination disorder (DCD). *Research in Developmental Disabilities, 33*(4), 996–1005.

Bart, O., Podoly, T., & Bar-Haim, Y. (2010). A preliminary study on the effect of methylphenidate on motor performance in children with comorbid DCD and ADHD. *Research in Developmental Disabilities, 31*(6), 1443–1447.

Berger, S. E. (2010). Locomotor expertise predicts infants' perseverative errors. *Developmental Psychology, 46*(2), 326–336.

Best, J. R., Miller, P. H., & Naglieri, J. A. (2011). Relations between executive function and academic achievement from ages 5–17 in a large, representative national sample. *Learning and Individual Differences, 21*(4), 327–336.

Bhat, A. N., Galloway, J. C., & Landa, R. J. (2012). Relation between early motor delay and later communication delay in infants at risk for autism. *Infant Behavior and Development, 35*(4), 838–846.

Bhat, A. N., Landa, R. J., & Galloway, J. C. (2011). Current perspectives on motor functioning in infants, children, and adult with autism spectrum disorders. *Physical Therapy, 91*(7), 1116–1129.

Bodrova, E., & Leong, D. J. (2007). *Tools of the mind: The Vygotskian approach to early childhood education* (2nd ed.). New York, NY: Merrill/Prentice Hall.

Bolea-Alamañac, B., Nutt, D. J., Adamou, M., Asherson, P., Bazire, S., Coghill, D., … Sayal, K. (2014). Evidence-based guidelines for the pharmacological management of attention deficit hyperactivity disorder: Update on recommendations from the British Association for Psychopharmacology. *Journal of Psychopharmacology, 28*(3), 179–203.

Brooks, R., & Goldstein, S. (2007). *Raising a self-disciplined child: Help your child become more responsible, confident, and resilient*. New York, NY: McGraw-Hill.

Brown, C. G. (2010). Improving fine motor skills in young children: An intervention study. *Educational Psychology in Practice, 26*(3), 269–278.

Bull, R., Espy, K. A., & Wiebe, S. A. (2008). Short-term memory, working memory, and executive functioning in preschoolers: Longitudinal predictors of mathematical achievement at age 7 years. *Developmental Neuropsychology, 33*(3), 205–228.

Burns, Y., O'Callaghan, M., McDonell, B., & Rogers, Y. (2004). Movement and motor development in ELBW infants at 1 year is related to cognitive and motor abilities at 4 years. *Early Human Development, 80*(1), 19–29.

Bushnell, E. W., & Boudreau, J. P. (1993). Motor development and the mind: The potential role of motor abilities as a determinant of aspects of perceptual development. *Child Development, 64*, 1005–1021.

Cameron, C. E., Brock, L. L., Murrah, W. M., Bell, L. H., Worzalla, S. L., Grissmer, D., & Morrison, F. J. (2012). Fine motor skills and executive function both contribute to kindergarten achievement. *Child Development, 83*(4), 1229–1244.

Campos, J. J., Anderson, D. I., Barbu-Roth, M. A., Hubbard, E. M., Hertenstein, M. J., & Witherington, D. (2000). Travel broadens the mind. *Infancy, 1*(2), 149–219.

Carlson, A. G., Rowe, E., & Curby, T. W. (2013). Disentangling fine motor skills' relations to academic achievement: The relative contributions of visual-spatial integration and visual-motor coordination. *The Journal of Genetic Psychology, 174*(5), 514–533.

Center on the Developing Child at Harvard University. (2014). *Activities guide: Enhancing and practicing executive function skills with children from infancy to adolescence*. Cambridge, MA: Harvard University. Retrieved from http://developingchild.harvard.edu/resourcetag/executive-function/

Dallaire, R., Muckle, G., Rouget, F., Kadhel, P., Bataille, H., Guldner, L., ... Thomé, J. P. (2012). Cognitive, visual, and motor development of 7-month-old Guadeloupean infants exposed to chlordecone. *Environmental Research, 118*, 79–85.

Dawson, G., Rogers, S., Munson, J., Smith, M., Winter, J., Greenson, J., ... Varley, J. (2010). Randomized, controlled trial of an intervention for toddlers with autism: The early start Denver model. *Pediatrics, 125*(1), e17–e23.

Dewey, D. (2002). Subtypes of developmental coordination disorder. In S. A. Cermak & D. Larkin (Eds.), *Developmental coordination disorder* (pp. 40–53). Albany, NY: Delmar Thomson Learning.

Diamond, A. (2000). Close interrelation of motor development and cognitive development and of the cerebellum and prefrontal cortex. *Child Development, 71*(1), 44–56.

Diamond, A. (2013). Executive functions. *Annual Review of Psychology, 64*, 135–168.

Diamond, A., & Lee, K. (2011). Interventions shown to aid executive function development in children 4–12 years old. *Science, 333*(6045), 959–964.

Dickson, H., Laurens, K. R., Cullen, A. E., & Hodgins, S. (2012). Meta-analyses of cognitive and motor function in youth aged 16 years and younger who subsequently develop schizophrenia. *Psychological Medicine, 42*(04), 743–755.

Dinehart, L., & Manfra, L. (2013). Associations between low-income children's fine motor skills in preschool and academic performance in second grade. *Early Education and Development, 24*, 138–161.

Duncan, G. J., Dowsett, C. J., Claessens, A., Magnuson, K., Huston, A. C., Klebanov, P., ... Japel, C. (2007). School readiness and later achievement. *Developmental Psychology, 43*(6), 1428.

Dunning, D. L., Holmes, J., & Gathercole, S. E. (2013). Does working memory training lead to generalized improvements in children with low working memory? A randomized controlled trial. *Developmental Science, 16*(6), 915–925.

Flapper, B. C., Houwen, S., & Schoemaker, M. M. (2006). Fine motor skills and effects of methylphenidate in children with attention-deficit–hyperactivity disorder and developmental coordination disorder. *Developmental Medicine and Child Neurology, 48*(03), 165–169.

Flapper, B. C., & Schoemaker, M. M. (2008). Effects of methylphenidate on quality of life in children with both developmental coordination disorder and ADHD. *Developmental Medicine and Child Neurology, 50*(4), 294–299.

Fuentes, C. T., Mostofsky, S. H., & Bastian, A. J. (2010). Perceptual reasoning predicts handwriting impairments in adolescents with autism. *Neurology, 75*, 1825–1829.

Goulardins, J. B., Marques, J. C. B., Casella, E. B., Nascimento, R. O., & Oliveira, J. A. (2013). Motor profile of children with attention deficit hyperactivity disorder, combined type. *Research in Developmental Disabilities, 34*(1), 40–45.

Grissmer, D., Grimm, K. J., Aiyer, S. M., Murrah, W. M., & Steele, J. S. (2010). Fine motor skills and early comprehension of the world: Two new school readiness indicators. *Developmental Psychology, 46*(5), 1008–1017.

Hadders-Algra, M. (2000). The neural group selection theory: Promising principles for understanding and treating developmental motor disorders. *Developmental Medicine and Child Neurology, 42*(10), 707–715.

Hellendoorn, A., Wijnroks, L., van Daalen, E., Dietz, C., Buitelaar, J. K., & Leseman, P. (2015). Motor functioning, exploration, visuospatial cognition and language development in preschool children with autism. *Research in Developmental Disabilities, 39*, 32–42.

Iversen, S., Berg, K., Ellertsen, B., & Tønnessen, F. E. (2005). Motor coordination difficulties in a municipality group and in a clinical sample of poor readers. *Dyslexia, 11*(3), 217–231.

Kaiser, M. L., Schoemaker, M. M., Albaret, J. M., & Geuze, R. H. (2015). What is the evidence of impaired motor skills and motor control among children with attention deficit hyperactivity disorder (ADHD)? Systematic review of the literature. *Research in Developmental Disabilities, 36*, 338–357.

Keifer, J. J. (2015). *Handwriting and fine motor skill development in the kindergarten classroom* (Masters thesis, Texas Christian University).

Koziol, L. F., Budding, D., Andreasen, N., D'Arrigo, S., Bulgheroni, S., Imamizu, H., … Pezzulo, G. (2014). Consensus paper: The cerebellum's role in movement and cognition. *The Cerebellum, 13*(1), 151–177.

Koziol, L. F., Budding, D. E., & Chidekel, D. (2012). From movement to thought: Executive function, embodied cognition, and the cerebellum. *The Cerebellum, 11*(2), 505–525.

Kroesbergen, E. H., Van Luit, J. E. H., Naglieri, J. A., Taddei, S., & Franchi, E. (2009). PASS processes and early mathematics skills in Dutch and Italian kindergartners. *Journal of Psychoeducational Assessment, 28*, 585–593.

Lawrence, V., Houghton, S., Tannock, R., Douglas, G., Durkin, K., & Whiting, K. (2002). ADHD outside the laboratory: Boys' executive function performance on tasks in videogame play and on a visit to the zoo. *Journal of Abnormal Child Psychology, 30*(5), 447–462.

Logan, S. W., Robinson, L. E., Wilson, A. E., & Lucas, W. A. (2012). Getting the fundamentals of movement: A meta-analysis of the effectiveness of motor skill interventions in children. *Child: Care, Health and Development, 38*(3), 305–315.

MacDonald, M., Lord, C., & Ulrich, D. A. (2014). Motor skills and calibrated autism severity in young children with autism spectrum disorder. *Adapted Physical Activity Quarterly, 31*, 95–105.

Marr, D., Cermak, S., Cohn, E. S., & Henderson, A. (2003). Fine motor activities in head start and kindergarten classrooms. *American Journal of Occupational Therapy, 57*(5), 550–557.

McPhillips, M., & Sheehy, N. (2004). Prevalence of persistent primary reflexes and motor problems in children with reading difficulties. *Dyslexia, 10*(4), 316–338.

Montessori, M. (1949). *Absorbent mind*. Oxford: ABC-CLIO.

Montessori, M. (1965). *Dr. Montessori's own handbook*. New York, NY: Schocken Books (Original work published in 1914).

Moreno, A. J., Shwayder, I., & Friedman, I. D. (2016). The function of executive function: Everyday manifestations of regulated thinking in preschool settings. *Early Childhood Education Journal Online First, 45*, 143–153.

Morrison, F. J., Ponitz, C. C., & McClelland, M. M. (2010). Self-regulation and academic achievement in the transition to school. In S. D. Calkins & M. A. Bell (Eds.), *Child development at the intersection of emotion and cognition* (pp. 203–224). Washington, DC: American Psychological Association.
Morrow, M. (2015). *Effectiveness of fine motor intervention in early childhood education* (Master's project, California State University at Channel Islands).
Murray, G. K., Veijola, J., Moilanen, K., Miettunen, J., Glahn, D. C., Cannon, T. D., ... Isohanni, M. (2006). Infant motor development is associated with adult cognitive categorisation in a longitudinal birth cohort study. *Journal of Child Psychology and Psychiatry, 47*(1), 25–29.
Naglieri, J. A., & Das, J. P. (1997). *Cognitive assessment system.* Austin, TX: ProEd.
O'Hare, A., & Khalid, S. (2002). The association of abnormal cerebellar function in children with developmental coordination disorder and reading difficulties. *Dyslexia, 8*(4), 234–248.
Oberauer, K., Süβ, H. M., Wilhelm, O., & Wittmann, W. W. (2008). Which working memory functions predict intelligence? *Intelligence, 36*(6), 641–652.
Piaget, J. (1953). *The origin of the intelligence in the child.* London, UK: Routledge.
Piek, J. P., Dawson, L., Smith, L. M., & Gasson, N. (2008). The role of early fine and gross motor development on later motor and cognitive ability. *Human Movement Science, 27*(5), 668–681.
Pienaar, A. E., Barhorst, R., & Twisk, J. W. R. (2013). Relationships between academic performance, SES school type and perceptual-motor skills in first grade South African learners: NW-CHILD study. *Child: Care, Health, and Development, 40*(3), 370–378.
Roebers, C. M., & Jäger, K. (2014). The relative importance of fine motor skills, intelligence, and executive functions for first graders' reading and spelling skills. *Perspectives on Language and Literacy, 40*(2), 13–17.
Romine, C. B., & Reynolds, C. R. (2005). A model of the development of frontal lobe function: Findings from a meta-analysis. *Applied Neuropsychology, 12*, 190–201. [PubMed: 16422660].
Rule, A. C., & Stewart, R. A. (2002). Effects of practical life materials on kindergartners' fine motor skills. *Early Childhood Education Journal, 30*(1), 9–13.
Schoemaker, M. M., Ketelaars, C. E., Van Zonneveld, M., Minderaa, R. B., & Mulder, T. (2005). Deficits in motor control processes involved in production of graphic movements of children with attention-deficit–hyperactivity disorder. *Developmental Medicine & Child Neurology, 47*(06), 390–395.
Singh, I., & Wessely, S. (2015). Childhood: A suitable case for treatment? *The Lancet Psychiatry, 2*(7), 661–666.
Smits-Engelsman, B. C. M., Blank, R., Van Der Kaay, A. C., Mosterd-Van der Meijs, R., Vlugt-Van Den Brand, E., Polatajko, H. J., & Wilson, P. H. (2013). Efficacy of interventions to improve motor performance in children with developmental coordination disorder: A combined systematic review and meta-analysis. *Developmental Medicine & Child Neurology, 55*(3), 229–237.
Sonuga-Barke, E. J., Brandeis, D., Cortese, S., Daley, D., Ferrin, M., Holtmann, M., ... Dittmann, R. W. (2013). Nonpharmacological interventions for ADHD: Systematic review and meta-analyses of randomized controlled trials of dietary and psychological treatments. *American Journal of Psychiatry, 170*, 275–289.
Stewart, R. A., Rule, A. C., & Giordano, D. A. (2007). The effect of fine motor skill activities on kindergarten student attention. *Early Childhood Education Journal, 35*(2), 103–109.
Tseng, M. H., Henderson, A., Chow, S. M., & Yao, G. (2004). Relationship between motor proficiency, attention, impulse, and activity in children with ADHD. *Developmental Medicine & Child Neurology, 46*(06), 381–388.
Wentworth, R. A. L. (1998). *Montessori for the new millennium.* Mahwah, NJ: Lawrence Erlbaum.
Wijnroks, L., & van Veldhoven, N. (2003). Individual differences in postural control and cognitive development in preterm infants. *Infant Behavior and Development, 26*(1), 14–26.

Audrey C. Rule is a former public elementary school teacher and Montessori teacher. She is currently a Professor of Elementary Science Education and Gifted Education in the Department of Curriculum and Instruction and a Fellow of the Center for Educational Transformation at the University of Northern Iowa in Cedar Falls, Iowa. Her research spans many areas connected to elementary education, including the connection between fine motor skills and attention.

Latisha L. Smith is a former Head Start teacher, family development specialist, and education coordinator. She is currently an Assistant Professor of Education at Upper Iowa University and a doctoral student at the University of Northern Iowa. Her research interests center on early childhood education as well as the effects of poverty in the educational setting.

Chapter 3
Early Childhood Education Environments: Affordances for Risk-Taking and Physical Activity in Play

Shirley Wyver and Helen Little

Introduction

Early Childhood Education (ECE) centres meet many needs, some of which are conflicting. US President Donald Trump's policy for child care reform emphasized workforce participation and affordability for middle- to low-income families (Trump, 2016). By contrast, the New Zealand Government set a 2016 target for 98% of children starting school to have attended ECE because of a belief in its important role in early learning and development (New Zealand Government Ministry of Education, 2016). Australia shares many similarities with New Zealand but its once high ECE standards were significantly eroded when government administration changed and ECE was "treated as little more than a commodity to be bought and sold – and, indeed, traded on the stock exchange" (Brennan, 2008). Governmental priorities and targets are important in determining factors such as staff-child ratios, staff qualifications and specifications for the environment. The broad political agenda may seem far removed from experiences within ECE centres, but these should always be kept in mind, particularly when a case is being made for more space, more contact with nature, better nutrition and more highly qualified staff in ECE centres. As discussed later in this chapter, New Zealand currently has a much higher 'grade' for children's physical activity than either the USA or Australia.

There is no systematic collection of data on physical activity or play in ECE centres. Nonetheless, the available evidence indicates serious inadequacies in many current contexts and that this is having an impact on children's health and development. In the US, there is concern that many centres are obesogenic (i.e. create

S. Wyver (✉) · H. Little
Department of Educational Studies, Macquarie University, Sydney, Australia
e-mail: shirley.wyver@mq.edu.au; helen.little@mq.edu.au

H. Brewer, M. R. Jalongo (eds.), *Physical Activity and Health Promotion in the Early Years*, Educating the Young Child 14,
https://doi.org/10.1007/978-3-319-76006-3_3

obesity) because they encourage sedentary behaviours and provide poor nutrition (McWilliams et al., 2009; Ward et al., 2008). In Australia, despite the requirement that children have a minimum of $7m^2$ outdoor space per child, some centres are in office blocks and have an area nominated as outdoors, but it is actually a built environment with unnatural surfaces, controlled temperature and artificial lighting. A recent survey of centres also found some to go below the required minimum of $7m^2$ (Little & Sweller, 2015).

Levels of Physical Activity in ECE Settings

With increasing numbers of children attending some type of Early Childhood Education (ECE) setting, these sites are recognised as being an important context for promoting physical activity (PA) through the provision of space and time for outdoor play with support from adults in the environment (Schneider & Lounsbery, 2008). Physical activity in ECE settings mainly occurs in the context of outdoor play, hence, an examination of levels of PA and the features of outdoor play environments that promote PA is warranted. A systematic review of research examining objectively measured levels of physical activity in early childhood services within the United States, Scotland, Belgium. Northern Ireland and Sweden, concluded that preschool children did not engage in the recommended 60 min of moderate-vigorous PA (Reilly, 2010). Not only are children not engaged in moderate-vigorous PA, other studies have found that children actually spend the majority of time outdoors engaged in sedentary activities (Brown et al., 2009; Cardon, Labarque, Smits, De Bourdeaudhuij, 2009; Dyment & Coleman, 2012).

Variations in levels of PA are associated with characteristics of the ECE setting such as available space, time spent outdoors, design elements within the environment, and centre policies and practices (Bower et al., 2008; Boldemann et al., 2006; Cardon, Van Cauwenberghe, Labarque, Haerens, & De Bourdeaudhuij, 2008; Coleman & Dyment, 2013; Trost, Ward, & Senso, 2010). Time spent outdoors is potentially limited due to weather conditions (i.e. spending more time indoors when it is either too sunny or raining) (Boldemann et al., 2006). Resources within the outdoor environment such as jumping equipment, fixed climbing structures, slides, tunnels, and structured tracks for cycling are associated with higher levels of activity. Conversely, resources such as sandboxes, portable slides and swings are associated with lower levels of activity (Gubbels, Van Kann, Jansen, 2012).

As well as variations in levels of physical activity being associated with the different types of resources provided within the preschool environment, variations in levels of physically active play have also been identified in comparisons of 'traditional' preschool environments and natural forest environments. Fjortoft (2001) found that the dynamic and rough topography of natural environments promoted higher levels of physical and motor fitness than standard playground equipment (swings, slide, seesaw etc.) provided within the ECE setting. This suggests that engagement with natural environments either within or beyond the ECE setting is likely to promote greater engagement in physically challenging active play.

A number of studies provide evidence that environmental factors such as space, playground design, access to natural environments and availability of sufficient quality equipment/resources influence children's physical activity (Boldemann et al., 2006; Cardon et al., 2008; Coleman & Dyment, 2013; Cosco, Moore, & Islam, 2010; Mygind, 2007; Trost et al., 2010; van Zandvoort et al., 2010) and opportunities for challenging, risky play (Fjørtoft, 2001; Little, 2015; Little, Wyver, & Gibson, 2011; Sandseter, 2009). Physically challenging play environments in ECE settings often involve higher levels of risk than is generally tolerated within the current climate of risk aversion (Waite, Huggins, & Wickett, 2014; Wyver et al., 2010). The Scandinavian countries have been recognised for exemplary provision of outdoor play environments, which is supported at all levels from ministerial policy through to pedagogical decision making (Sandseter, 2014). Nonetheless, recent evidence from Norway indicates that growing risk aversion is threatening to reduce what have been perceived as regular experiences for young children in ECE (Sandseter & Sando, 2016).

The Role of Adults in Supporting Physically Challenging Play

One of the issues that has been identified as influencing levels of PA in early childhood settings is the philosophy that underlies contemporary approaches to early childhood pedagogy. Within contemporary early childhood pedagogy, play-based learning is the means by which children organise and make sense of their worlds, as they actively engage with people and objects representations (DEEWR, 2009). A feature of this approach is that, whilst the educators provision the environment, children's play is unstructured and children freely engage with the space and equipment provided as they choose. There are opposing views on the role of unstructured play and PA. Tribolet (2016) argues that unstructured play is insufficient for effectively promoting PA and that educators need to be more involved in providing teacher-led structured activities in addition to free play. Tribolet's claim is consistent with physical activity guidelines, as discussed below.

Teacher knowledge and practices have also been identified in the research as potentially impacting on levels of PA (Dwyer, Higgs, Hardy, & Baur, 2008; Lanigan, 2014; van Zandvoort, Tucker, Irwin, & Burke, 2010). Even though teachers generally understand the value of PA, they are often unfamiliar with the physical activity guidelines for children (Dwyer et al., 2008). In addition, whilst teachers believe their outdoor environments promote physical activity, they also potentially overestimate the levels of physical activity that children engage in (Coleman & Dyment, 2013; Little, 2015) and often lack the knowledge and skills to promote children's physical activity and fundamental movement skills by implementing physical activity programs (Reithmuller, McKeen, Okely, Bell, & de Silva Sanigorski, 2009).

Issues related to safety have been identified as potentially limiting physically active play, especially play that provides opportunities for children to challenge themselves where there is a potential injury risk. Although parents and EC educators generally express positive beliefs about the benefits of some forms of risk-taking in children's play for children's learning and development, a number of factors have been identified that potentially limit the opportunities for children's engagement in physically challenging active play (Little et al., 2011). Teachers often raise issues related to safety concerns associated with risky play and the inclusion of natural elements within the environment, resulting in reduced opportunities for physical activity and believe their supervision duties often prevent them from actively engaging children in physical activity or setting up additional physical play opportunities for the children (Coleman & Dyment, 2013; Dyment & Coleman, 2012; Little, 2010). In addition, compliance with regulatory requirements also impact on the types of experiences provided (Little, 2010; van Zandvoort et al., 2010).

Physically Active Play in Childhood

Physical activity in childhood is important for many aspects of children's health, wellbeing and development. The World Health Organisation (WHO) defines "physical activity as any bodily movement produced by skeletal muscles that requires energy expenditure – including activities undertaken while working, playing, carrying out household chores, travelling, and engaging in recreational pursuits" (World Health Organisation, 2015). Physically active play during childhood contributes to individual patterns of physical activity and lifelong engagement in physical activity and the health benefits associated with being physically active and fit (Boldeman et al., 2006; Moore et al., 2003; Ortega, Ruiz, Castillo, & Sjöström, 2008; Strong et al., 2005).

Most countries have developed government recommendations for levels of physical activity to promote health and wellbeing for young children (e.g. Canadian Physical Activity Guidelines for Children [aged 5–11] and Youth [aged 12–17], 2010; Physical Activity Guidelines for Americans, 2008; UK Physical Activity Guidelines for Children and Young People [aged 5–18 years], 2010). Typically the guidelines specify the minimum amounts of structured and unstructured time with recognition that infants and young children do not accumulate daily physical activity in consolidated blocks but instead have smaller bouts of physical activity and therefore need a longer period than adults to accumulate their daily physical activity. Guidelines also include maximum amounts of sedentary time. For example, the National Association for Sport and Physical Education (NASPE) guidelines specify that each day pre-schoolers should have at least 60 min of structured physical activity, at least 60 min and up to several hours of unstructured physical activity and no more than 60 consecutive minutes of sedentary time, except when sleeping (2006). The Australian Government Department of Health (2014) physical activity guidelines recommend that children aged one to 5 years should be physically active every day for at least 3 h, spread throughout the day. These guidelines for younger children are particularly important as adults typically believe that young children are generally active throughout the day and their natural physical activity is adequate (Brown, Googe, McIver, & Rathel, 2009; Tremblay, Boudreau-Larivière, & Cimon-Lambert, 2012); however, a number of studies have found that young children often engage in low levels of physical activity (Boldemann et al., 2006; Cardon et al., 2008; Coleman & Dyment, 2013; Okely, Trost, Steele, Cliff, & Mickle, 2009; Tribolet, 2016; Trost et al., 2010) with only 50% of preschool aged children meeting the recommended physical activity level on weekdays, compared to 80% on weekends (Okely et al., 2009).

The Active Healthy Kids Global Alliance was established in 2014 and completed report cards on physical activity of children in 38 countries. The grades include an overall score on physical activity and scores on organized sport participation, active play, active transportation, sedentary behaviours, family and peers, school, community and built environment, government strategies and investments. USA, Canada and Australia all received a D- for the overall score which indicates less than half of the children in these countries are meeting recommended requirements. Grades could not be assigned for active play in these countries as there were insufficient data. This is in contrast to New Zealand which received a B- overall as well as in active play. A grade of B indicates the country is succeeding with 60–79% of children (Active Healthy Kids Global Alliance, 2016). A strong score in active play was not necessarily indicative of a strong overall score. For example, Slovenia had an overall score of A-, but an active play score of D. The Netherlands has an overall score of D but an active play score of B. The only other countries to score as well as the Netherlands on active play were Ghana and Kenya, but as noted, most countries had insufficient data to be scored on this category.

Physical Activity and Risk-Taking

The unstructured, flexible, open-ended and dynamic nature of outdoor play provides an ideal context for children's engagement in challenging, physically active play. At the same time, the unpredictability of the outdoor environment and children's engagement with it inherently involves a certain element of risk or uncertainty. Through exploratory, challenging and risky play children become familiar with their environment, its possibilities and boundaries as well as their own capabilities. This type of risk-taking behaviour as an integral part of children's play has been the focus of recent research. In an effort to describe the characteristics of this type of play, Sandseter (2007) identified six categories of risky play: (1) play involving great heights; (2) play involving great speed; (3) play with dangerous tools; (4) play near dangerous elements; (5) rough and tumble play; and, (6) play where children can 'disappear/get lost'. Risk-taking in play, such as that described by Sandseter, allows children to try new skills, test their limits, learn about their bodies and their capabilities, and in doing so, acquire and eventually master a wide range of fundamental motor skills. The increased motor competence and confidence that children gain through these experiences are likely to contribute to physical fitness and ongoing engagement in physical activity (Robinson, Wadsworth, & Peoples, 2012).

Amongst the difficulties in ECE with the provision of this type of play is that educators may be working from theoretical perspectives that value higher order cognitive processes over perceptual-motor engagement and/or come from a maturationist tradition. We recently contrasted the main developmental influences for Australian and Norwegian ECE because Australian educators have, in our research, been shown to value outdoor play and physical activity but have had difficulty incorporating these values into their pedagogy. This is in contrast to Norwegian educators who clearly incorporated outdoor play including risk and physical activity into their pedagogical decision making. We found that the Norwegian preservice teaching program had a greater emphasis on Gibsonian (affordance) theory and dynamic systems approaches (Sandseter, Little, & Wyver, 2012).

Affordance Theory

Affordance theory is one of many ways to understand the interaction between children's playfulness and environmental features. Affordance theory has been influential in areas such as early childhood (Mawson, 2014) human geography (Kyttä, 2004) and psychology (Bahrick & Lickliter, 2012; Franchak & Adolph, 2014; Heft, 1988). There have been numerous extensions and applications of affordance theory, most notably by Heft (1988) and Kytta (2006). While these revisions have been theoretically rigorous and supported by empirical work, Waters (2017) warns that there can be a tendency to simplify the complexity of the concepts and when this is done, implications of the theory for children's environments are lost.

Eleanor and James Gibson

Affordance theory originated in the work of James J. Gibson (1977) and Eleanor J. Gibson (1994) as a theory of perception. It contrasts with most theories of cognition that assume knowledge to be a representation of the external world. Gibsonian theory is one of 'direct realism' which contends that "cognition is a direct *relation* between the knower (an organism) and the known (an objective situation) and that it is not mediated by cognitive representations internal to the mind or brain" (Michell, 1988, p.228). Important within Gibsonian theory is the concept of differentiation. Perceptual learning is not a pattern of associations, such as touching a rock in the sun and associating it with heat. Rather, it is a process of *differentiation* which involves "specification of significant information" (E.J. Gibson, 2000, p. 296). Certain information is considered to be of more or less importance to each species and differentiation is the process through which this information is obtained. For example, for humans, facial expressions and face recognition is far more important than knowing about another person's arm or leg morphology and movements. Environmental exploration and repetition is important for differentiation. "Human perceptual systems are not designed for momentary exposure to stimulation but for bouts that include cycles of perception and action. Thus, an opportunity is provided for observation of the play-by-play cycles of whatever activity is being performed by the organism and what follows as a consequence" (E.J. Gibson, 2000, p.297–298). This suggests, therefore, that regular exposure to interesting environments is important. For example, young children are often interested in animals, in climbing and a range of experiences that are, if available at all, not part of their regular experience.

Often overlooked is the focus on amodal information (Bahrlick & Lickliter, 2012). Much of the information that is important to humans does not belong to a single modality. An obvious example is human speech which is detected through hearing and vision. Most cognitive theories assume the infant learns associations between hearing and vision. However, in Gibsonian theory amodal information is originally detected as a unified whole and even newborns appear to seek out this information by, for example, looking towards the source of a sound (Bahrick, 1992). Through experience infants learn to differentiate one speaker from another. Research on amodality has emphasised hearing and vision, but Eleanor Gibson also supported her results with experiments in which infants examined the relationship between tactile exploration and vision (Gibson & Walker, 1984).

The approach came to be known as *the ecological approach to perceptual learning and development* because of its emphasis on both the reciprocity and complementarity of specific species and their environments. The relational aspect of affordance theory is particularly interesting when consideration is given to young children in outdoor environments, particularly in natural environments. During a 12 month period, children's body height, weight, centre of pressure, use of peripheral vision and a range of other developmental changes (Assaiante & Amblard, 1992; Austad & van der Meer, 2007) result in rapid modifications in balance and walking. A risky manoeuvre over a rock at 36 months may be a regular step at 48 months. Outdoor environments also change over the period of a year. What starts as a hard ground surface in summer, may be slippery and require more postural control in winter.

Heft's Taxonomy

Heft has continued to advance Gibsonian theory, particularly with contributions to understanding its role in perception and cognitive psychology (Heft, 2003). His contribution to affordance theory is substantial, but he is possibly best known for his functional taxonomy of outdoor environments. Heft (1988) identified ten superordinate categories for classification of outdoor environments: Flat, relatively smooth surface; Relatively smooth slope; Graspable/detached object; Attached object; Non-rigid, attached object; Climbable feature; Aperture; Shelter; Moldable material such as dirt and sand; Water. Under each of these categories is a range of affordances, e.g. water affords splashing. Natural elements and play spaces that potentially afford both PA and risk-taking include trees, rocks, grass, uneven ground and slopes, flat areas, digging patches, large open spaces, and areas for gross motor equipment and secluded spaces. Resources provided within the environment that afford risk-taking include equipment for balancing and climbing, trampolines, swings, slides, trees for climbing, and bikes. Importantly, given that affordances are relational, it is essential to have an individual or type of individual in mind when making claims about what is afforded. A young tree might afford climbing for a young child but not for a large adult, for example (Heft, 1988). Likewise, a tree may afford shelter in summer but not in winter when its branches are bare.

Heft's taxonomy can be used effectively for research or practice to examine affordances (Kyttä, 2002). For example, a Norwegian study of used the taxonomy effectively to examine differences between a traditional and natural playground (Storli & Hagen, 2010). A recent Danish study with preschoolers found the taxonomy to have important features for use in practice including that it works from the child's point of view and it is relatively easy to use (Lerstrup & Konijnendijk van den Bosch, 2016).

In her review of research on affordances, Kernan (2014) notes that exploration of nature for adults can be as a scenery whereas for children the experience is direct, hands on, potentially dirty and potentially risky. Adults often design environments with regularities and uniformities that are appealing as the type of scenery Kernan discusses, but are not sufficiently challenging for children, and are less appealing when analysed using Heft's taxonomy which allows the observer to take the viewpoint of the child. An example comes from two studies from a group of researchers in the Netherlands who have been interested in uniformities introduced into playgrounds by adult designers. They noted that stepping stones in playgrounds and ECE contexts are often uniformly spaced and were interested to find out how children would organise stepping stones if given the opportunity. Children varied spaces between the stones potentially to afford a wider range of movements by a wider range of individuals with different motor skills (Jongeneel, Withagen, & Zaal, 2015). They also created a contrived playscape that involved jumping across polystyrene blocks. Children could select different distances to jump from one block to another and could stay with the same distance between blocks or select a variation. They found that children mainly selected affordances within their capabilities, but sometimes selected affordances that offered more challenge (Prieske, Withagen, Smith, & Zaal, 2015). Children also selected variations in gaps between blocks rather than selecting the same gaps. In other words, the children selected variation rather than uniformity. The authors argue that this type of variation provides better opportunities for development of motor skills than repetition of the same movements.

Kyttä Bullerby Model

The Bullerby Model uses Heft's work on affordances and Gibsonian theory to describe four environment types. The four types are determined by the degree of independent mobility (high or low) and the degree of actualised affordances (high or low) (Kyttä, 2006) (see Table 3.1). The term Bullerby comes from a novel by Astrid Lindgren that describes the adventures of six children. Within Kyttä's model, Bullerby refers to contexts in which children have high levels of independent mobility and high levels of actualised affordances. This creates a positive cycle where children experience a high level of actualised affordances which motivates them to continue to explore. Children with low independent mobility and low actualised affordances on the other hand are in a negative cycle (the Cell – see Table 3.1) (Broberg, Kyttä, & Fagerholm, 2013). According to this model, Bullerby is where children are most likely to be engaged and physically active, Cell is where children are most likely to disengage and become sedentary. As can be seen from Table 3.1, both the actualised affordances and independent mobility need to be present to motivate optimal exploration.

The Bullerby model is empirically testable and while it has been influential in some, mainly European, areas of research, the significance of this model is yet to be recognised. The Bullerby model can be extended to a wide range of environments that infants, children, adolescents and perhaps even some adults occupy. The categorisation lends itself well to both qualitative and quantitative research and it has potential as a diagnostic tool for children's environments. For example, a school might change their outdoor play time to include loose parts play as a way of promoting physical activity (Bundy et al., 2009; Engelen et al., 2013; Hyndman & Leanne Lester, 2015), but find there is no change and this may be because there continue to be real or perceived restrictions placed on children's autonomous access to the new equipment. It is therefore important to consider both the opportunities available on the playground and the beliefs, attitudes and concerns of adults with a duty of care for the children (van Rooijen & Newstead, 2016). The Sydney Playground Project has developed protocols for this type of approach to playground change (Bundy et al., 2011, 2015).

Table 3.1 Kytta's four types of environments

Number of actualised affordances			
Degree of independent mobility		*Low*	*High*
	High	Wasteland	Bullerby
		Exploration reveals a barren environment with limited opportunities.	Positive cycle: Exploration motivates more engagement and exploration.
	Low	Cell	Glasshouse
		Negative cycle: Limited or no opportunity to form a relationship with the environment.	The environment has ample affordances and the child may be aware of these opportunities but is unable to autonomously access these affordances.

Storli and Hagen (2010) compared physical activity of children when they were in a traditional playground and natural playground. Although it would be expected that children would be more active in the natural playground which had greater diversity and a higher number of affordances, this was not found. Nonetheless, if the results are examined in the context of the Bullerby model, it is possible that the children in this study were on a positive cycle which supported physical activity even when in a less interesting environment. This is an area in which there should be further research as it suggests a means of supporting movement from Wasteland, Glasshouse or Cell to the positive cycle of Bullerby.

Assumptions About Environment

The results of Storli and Hagen are also interesting in terms of variation in physical activity within and between children. Researchers have noted that there is more variation in an individual child's physical activity across different contexts than a group of children within the same context (Ward Thompson, 2013). This understanding has underscored much of the consideration of the importance of environment for physical activity. Storli and Hagen found the opposite. They found that children's physical activity levels were somewhat independent of the environment and there was more variation between children than variation of individual children across contexts. Few studies report within and between child variations in physical activity across contexts and this is an essential area to for future research as it may be that individual variation is more important than currently considered. In particular, interventions that examine group changes in physical activity related to the environment may be overlooking important individual characteristics of children that predict change.

Affordances in ECE, Future Directions

Affordances are widely discussed in scholarly articles relating to ECE but are yet to become part of mainstream practitioner thinking (Sandseter et al., 2012). Affordance theory has become more accessible in recent years, especially through works of authors such as Kernan (2014) and Waters (2017) coupled with accessible tools such as Heft's taxonomy and the Bullerby model that can be used to analyse any outdoor play context. Affordance theory can be used with an individual ECE context and it can also be used to address the larger issue of low grades on the global report card of physical activity.

References

Active Healthy Kids Global Alliance. (2016). http://www.activehealthykids.org/. Accessed 18 Dec 2016.

Assaiante, C., & Amblard, B. (1992). Peripheral vision and age-related differences in dynamic balance. *Human Movement Science, 11*(5), 533–548.

Austad, H., & van der Meer, A. L. (2007). Prospective dynamic balance control in healthy children and adults. *Experimental Brain Research, 181*(2), 289–295.

Australian Government Department of Health. (2014). *National physical activity guidelines for Australians. Physical activity recommendations for children 0–5years*. http://www.health.gov.au/internet/main/publishing.nsf/content/health-pubhlth-strateg-phys-act-guidelines#npa05. Accessed 4 Jan 2016.

Bahrick, L. E. (1992). Infants' perceptual differentiation of amodal and modality-specific audio-visual relations. *Journal of Experimental Child Psychology, 53*(2), 180–199.

Bahrick, L. E., & Lickliter, R. (2012). The role of intersensory redundancy in early perceptual, cognitive, and social development. In *Multisensory development* (pp. 183–205). New York, NY: Oxford University Press.

Boldemann, C., Blennow, M., Dal, H., Mårtensson, F., Raustorp, A., Yuen, K., & Wester, U. (2006). Impact of preschool environment upon children's physical activity and sun exposure. *Preventive Medicine, 42*(4), 301–308. https://doi.org/10.1016/j.ypmed.2005.12.006

Bower, J. K., Hales, D. P., Tate, D. F., Rubin, D. A., Benjamin, S. E., & Ward, D. S. (2008). The childcare environment and children's physical activity. *American Journal of Preventive Medicine, 34*(1), 23–29.

Brennan, D. (2008). Reassembling the childcare business. *Inside Story*. http://insidestory.org.au/reassembling-the-childcare-business. Accessed 18 Dec 2016.

Broberg, A., Kyttä, M., & Fagerholm, N. (2013). Child-friendly urban structures: Bullerby revisited. *Journal of Environmental Psychology, 35*, 110–120. https://doi.org/10.1016/j.jenvp.2013.06.001

Brown, W., Googe, H., McIver, K., & Rathel, J. (2009). Effects of teacher-encouraged physical activity on preschool playgrounds. *Journal of Early Intervention, 31*(2), 126–145. https://doi.org/10.1177/1053815109331858

Brown, W., Pfeiffer, K., McIver, K., Dowda, M., Addy, C., & Pate, R. (2009). Social and environmental factors associated with preschoolers' nonsedentary physical activity. *Child Development, 80*(1), 45–58.

Bundy, A. C., Luckett, T., Tranter, P. J., Naughton, G. A., Wyver, S. R., Ragen, J., & Spies, G. (2009). The risk is that there is "no risk": A simple, innovative intervention to increase children's activity levels. *International Journal of Early Years Education, 17*(1), 33–45.

Bundy, A. C., Naughton, G., Tranter, P., Wyver, S., Baur, L., Schiller, W., … Charmaz, K. (2011). The sydney playground project: Popping the bubblewrap – Unleashing the power of play: A cluster randomized controlled trial of a primary school playground-based intervention aiming to increase children's physical activity and social skills. *BMC Public Health, 11*(1), 680.

Bundy, A. C., Wyver, S., Beetham, K. S., Ragen, J., Naughton, G., Tranter, P., … Sterman, J. (2015). The Sydney playground project- levelling the playing field: A cluster trial of a primary school-based intervention aiming to promote manageable risk-taking in children with disability. *BMC Public Health, 15*(1), 1125. http://www.pubmedcentral.nih.gov/articlerender.fcgi?artid=4647495&tool=pmcentrez&rendertype=abstract

Cardon, G., Labarque, V., Smits, D., & De Bourdeaudhuij, I. (2009). Promoting physical activity at the pre-school playground. The effects of providing markings and play equipment. *Preventive Medicine, 48*, 335–340.

Cardon, G., Van Cauwenberghe, E., Labarque, V., Haerens, L., & De Bourdeaudhuij, I. (2008). The contribution of preschool playground factors in explaining children's physical activity during recess. *International Journal of Behavioral Nutrition and Physical Activity, 5*(1), 11–11. https://doi.org/10.1186/1479-5868-5-11

Coleman, B., & Dyment, J. (2013). Factors that limit and enable preschool-aged children's physical activity on child care centre playgrounds. *Journal of Early Childhood Research, 11*(3), 203–221.

Cosco, N., Moore, R., & Islam, M. (2010). Behavior mapping: A method for linking preschool physical activity and outdoor design. *Medicine & Sciencein Sports & Exercise, 42*(3), 513–519. https://doi.org/10.1249/MSS.0b013e3181cea27a

Department of Education, Employment and Workplace Relations. (2009). Early years learning framework. Retrieved from https://www.education.gov.au/early-years-learning-framework-0

Dwyer, G., Higgs, J., Hardy, L., & Baur, L. (2008). What do parents and preschool staff tell us about young children's physical activity: A qualitative study. *International Journal of Behavioral Nutrition and Physical Activity, 5*(1), 66–66. https://doi.org/10.1186/1479-5868-5-66

Dyment, J., & Coleman, B. (2012). The intersection of physical activity opportunities and the role of early childhood educators during outdoor play: Perceptions and reality. *Australasian Journal of Early Childhood, 37*(1), 90–98.

Engelen, L., Bundy, A. C., Naughton, G., Simpson, J. M., Bauman, A., Ragen, J., … van der Ploeg, H. P. (2013). Increasing physical activity in young primary school children – It's child's play: A cluster randomised controlled trial. *Preventive Medicine, 56*(5), 319–325.

Fjørtoft, I. (2001). The natural environment as a playground for children: The impact of outdoor play activities in pre-primary school children. *Early Childhood Education Journal, 29*(2), 111–117.

Franchak, J., & Adolph, K. (2014). Affordances as probabilistic functions: Implications for development, perception, and decisions for action. *Ecological Psychology, 26*(1–2), 109–124.

Gibson, E. J. (1994). *An odyssey in learning and perception*. Cambridge, MA: MIT Press.

Gibson, E. J. (2000). Perceptual learning in development: Some basic concepts. *Ecological Psychology, 12*(4), 295–302.

Gibson, E. J., & Walker, A. S. (1984). Development of knowledge of visual-tactual affordances of substance. *Child Development, 55*(2), 453–460. https://doi.org/10.1111/j.1467-8624.1984.tb00305.x

Gibson, J. J. (1977). The theory of affordances. In *Perceiving, acting, and knowing: Toward an ecological psychology* (pp. 67–82). Hillsdale, NJ: Erlbaum.

Gubbels, J., Van Kann, D., & Jansen, M. (2012). Play equipment, physical activity opportunities, and children's activity levels at childcare. *Journal of Environmental and Public Health,* Article ID 326520, 1–8.

Heft, H. (1988). Affordances of children's environments: A functional approach to environmental description. *Children's Environments Quarterly, 5*(1), 29–37.

Heft, H. (2003). Affordances, dynamic experience, and the challenge of reification. *Ecological Psychology, 15*(2), 149–180.

Hyndman, B. P., & Lester, L. (2015). The effect of an emerging school playground strategy to encourage Children's physical activity: The accelerometer intensities from movable playground and lunchtime activities in youth (AIM-PLAY) study. *Children, Youth and Environments, 25*(3), 109–128. https://doi.org/10.7721/chilyoutenvi.25.3.0109

Jongeneel, D., Withagen, R., & Zaal, F. T. (2015). Do children create standardized playgrounds? A study on the gap-crossing affordances of jumping stones. *Journal of Environmental Psychology, 44*, 45–52.

Kernan, M. (2014). Opportunities and affordances in outdoor play. In *The SAGE handbook of play and learning in early childhood* (pp. 391–402). London, UK: Sage.

Kyttä, M. (2002). Affordances of children's environments in the context of cities, small towns, suburbs and rural villages in Finland and Belarus. *Journal of Environmental Psychology, 22*(1), 109–123.

Kyttä, M. (2004). The extent of children's independent mobility and the number of actualized affordances as criteria for child-friendly environments. *Journal of Environmental Psychology, 24*(2), 179–198.

Kyttä, M. (2006). Environmental child-friendliness in the light of the Bullerby Model. In *Children and their environments: Learning, using and designing spaces* (pp. 141–158). Cambridge, MA: Cambridge University Press.
Lanigan, J. (2014). Physical activity for young children: A quantitative study of child care providers' knowledge, attitudes, and health promotion practices. *Early Childhood Education Journal, 14*(1), 11–18.
Lerstrup, I., & Konijnendijk van den Bosch, C. (2016). Affordances of outdoor settings for children in preschool: Revisiting heft's functional taxonomy. *Landscape Research, 42*(1), 47. https://doi.org/10.1080/01426397.2016.1252039
Little, H. (2010). Risk, challenge and safety in outdoor play: Pedagogical and regulatory tensions. *Asia Pacific Journal of Research in Early Childhood Education, 4*(1), 3–24.
Little, H. (2015). Promoting risk-taking and physically challenging play in Australian early childhood settings in a changing regulatory environment. *Journal of Early Childhood Research,* online first. doi: https://doi.org/10.1177/1476718X15579743.
Little, H., & Sweller, N. (2015). Affordances for risk-taking and physical activity in Australian early childhood education settings. *Early Childhood Education Journal, 42*, 337–345. https://doi.org/10.1007/s10643-014-0667-0
Little, H., Wyver, S., & Gibson, F. (2011). The influence of play context and adult attitudes on young children's physical risk-taking during outdoor play. *European Early Childhood Education Research Journal, 19*(1), 113–131.
Mawson, W. B. (2014). Experiencing the "wild woods": The impact of pedagogy on children's experience of a natural environment. *European Early Childhood Education Research Journal, 22*(4), 513–524.
McWilliams, C., Ball, S. C., Benjamin, S. E., Hales, D., Vaughn, A., & Ward, D. S. (2009). Best-practice guidelines for physical activity at child care. *Pediatrics, 124*(6), 1650.
Michell, J. (1988). Maze's direct realism and the character of cognition. *Australian Journal of Psychology, 40*(3), 227–249.
Moore, L. L., Di Gao, A. S., Bradlee, M. L., Cupples, L. A., Sundarajan-Ramamurti, A., Proctor, M. H., … Ellison, R. C. (2003). Does early physical activity predict body fat change throughout childhood? *Preventive Medicine, 37*(1), 10–17.
Mygind, E. (2007). A comparison between children's physical activity levels at school and learning in an outdoor environment. *Journal of Adventure Education and Outdoor Learning, 7*(2), 161–176.
NASPE. (2006). *Active start – Physical activity guidelines for children birth to five years*. http://journal.naeyc.org/btj/200605/NASPEGuidelinesBTJ.pdf
New Zealand Government Ministry of Education. (2016). *Current Ministry priorities in early childhood education*. http://www.education.govt.nz/early-childhood/ministry-priorities/. Accessed 13 Dec 2016.
Okely, A., Trost, S., Steele, J., Cliff, D., & Mickle, K. (2009). Adherence to physical activity and electronic media guidelines in Australian pre-school children. *Journal of Paediatrics and Child Health, 45*, 5–8.
Ortega, F. B., Ruiz, J. R., Castillo, M. J., & Sjöström, M. (2008). Physical fitness in childhood and adolescence: A powerful marker for health. *International Journal of Obesity, 32*(1), 1–11.
Prieske, B., Withagen, R., Smith, J., & Zaal, F. T. J. M. (2015). Affordances in a simple playscape: Are children attracted to challenging affordances? *Journal of Environmental Psychology, 41*, 101–111.
Reilly, J. (2010). Low levels of objectively measured physical activity in preschoolers in child care. *Medicine & Science in Sports & Exercise, 42*(3), 502–507.
Reithmuller, A., McKeen, K., Okely, A., Bell, C., & deSilva Sanigorski, A. (2009). Developing and active play resource for a range of Australian early childhood settings: Formative findings and recommendations. *Australasian Journal of Early Childhood, 34*(1), 43–52.
Robinson, L. E., Wadsworth, D. D., & Peoples, C. M. (2012). Correlates of school-day physical activity in preschool students. *Research Quarterly for Exercise and Sport, 83*(1), 20–26.

Sandseter, E. B. H. (2007). Categorising risky play – How can we identify risk-taking in children's play? *European Early Childhood Education Research Journal, 15*(2), 237–252.
Sandseter, E. B. H. (2009). Affordances for risky play in preschool: The importance of features in the play environment. *Early Childhood Education Journal, 36*(5), 439–446.
Sandseter, E. B. H. (2014). Early years outdoor play in Scandinavia. In T. Maynard & J. Waters (Eds.), *Exploring outdoor play in the early years*. Berkshire, UK: Oxford University Press.
Sandseter, E. B. H., Little, H., & Wyver, S. (2012). Do theory and pedagogy have an impact on provisions for outdoor learning? A comparison of approaches in Australia and Norway. *Journal of Adventure Education & Outdoor Learning, 12*(3), 167–182.
Sandseter, E. B. H., & Sando, O. J. (2016). "We don't allow children to climb trees": How a focus on safety affects Norwegian children's play in early-childhood education and care settings. *American Journal of Play, 8*(2), 178–200.
Schneider, H., & Lounsbery, M. (2008). Setting the stage for lifetime physical activity in early childhood. *Journal of Physical Education, Recreation & Dance, 79*(6), 19–23.
Storli, R., & Hagen, T. L. (2010). Affordances in outdoor environments and children's physically active play in pre-school. *European Early Childhood Education Research Journal, 18*(4), 445–456.
Strong, W., Malina, R., Bumke, C., Daniels, S., Dishman, R., Gution, B., … Trudeau, F. (2005). Evidence based physical activity for school-age youth. *Journal of Pediatrics, 146*(6), 732–737.
Tremblay, L., Boudreau-Larivière, C., & Cimon-Lambert, K. (2012). Promoting physical activity in preschoolers: A review of the guidelines, barriers, and facilitators for implementation of policies and practices. *Canadian Psychology, 53*(4), 280–290.
Tribolet, K. (2016). Outdoor play: Friend or foe to early childhood physical activity? Challenging the context of unstructured outdoor play for encouraging physical activity. In T. Brabazon (Ed.), *Play: A theory of learning and change*. Basel, Switzerland: Springer.
Trost, S., Ward, D., & Senso, M. (2010). Effects of child care policy and environment on physical activity. *Medicine & Science in Sports & Exercise, 42*(3), 502–507.
Trump, D. J. (2016). *Child care*. Retrieved December 13, 2016 from: https://www.donaldjtrump.com/policies/child-care
van Rooijen, M., & Newstead, S. (2016). Influencing factors on professional attitudes towards risk-taking in children's play: A narrative review. *Early Child Development and Care, 187*, 1–12. https://doi.org/10.1080/03004430.2016.1204607
Van Zandvoort, M., Tucker, P., Irwin, J., & Burke, S. (2010). Physical activity at daycare: Issues, challenges and perspectives. *Early Years, 30*(2), 175–188.
Waite, S., Huggins, V., & Wickett, K. (2014). Risky outdoor play: Embracing uncertainty in pursuit of learning. In *Exploring outdoor play in the early years* (pp. 71–85). Maidenhead, UK: Open University Press.
Ward, D., Hales, D., Haverly, K., Marks, J., Benjamin, S., Ball, S., & Trost, S. (2008). An instrument to assess the obesogenic environment of child care centers. *American Journal of Health Behavior, 32*(4), 380–386.
Ward Thompson, C. (2013). Activity, exercise and the planning and design of outdoor spaces. *Journal of Environmental Psychology, 34*, 79–96.
Waters, J. (2017). Affordance theory. In Waller, E. Ärlemalm-Hagsér, E. B. H. Sandseter, L. Lee-Hammond, K. Lekies, & S. Wyver (Eds.), *The SAGE handbook of outdoor play and learning*. London, UK: SAGE.
World Health Organisation [WHO]. (2015). Physical activity. *Fact Sheet N°385.* http://www.who.int/mediacentre/factsheets/fs385/en/. Accessed 4 Jan 2016.
Wyver, S., Tranter, P., Naughton, G., Little, H., Sandseter, E. B. H., & Bundy, A. (2010). Ten ways to restrict children's freedom to play: The problem of surplus safety. *Contemporary Issues in Early Childhood, 11*(3), 263–277.

Shirley Wyver is a Senior Lecturer in child development in the Department of Educational Studies, Macquarie University, Australia. Her research interests are in early play and cognitive/social development. She also conducts research in the area of blindness/low vision and development.

Helen Little is a Senior Lecturer in the Department of Educational Studies, Macquarie University, Australia. Prior to this she was an early childhood teacher with experience teaching in preschools and primary schools in Sydney. Her research interest focuses on individual, social and environmental factors influencing children's engagement in risk-taking behaviour in outdoor play. Her current focus relates to how the physical features of the outdoor environment and pedagogical practices relating to outdoor play provision in Early Childhood settings impact on children's experiences of risk-taking in play.

Chapter 4
Viewing Children's Movement Through an Ecological Lens: Using the Interaction of Constraints to Design Positive Movement Experiences

Linda M. Gagen and Nancy Getchell

Ecological Perspective

For many years, conventional wisdom posited that young children developed motor skills 'naturally', as a by-product of unstructured play at home and in preschool. To a certain extent, this viewpoint still prevails today. In the United States, although 39 states mandate that preschool facilities include undefined "gross motor activity" in their daily activities, only eight states specify that the intensity levels should be high enough to noticeably raise children's heart rates (Kaphingst & Story, 2009), and only Alaska, Delaware, and Massachusetts provide specific time requirements (e.g. 20 min every 3 h). In Europe, Canada and Australia, gross motor development through free play has much greater value and is prescribed as a major learning experience in the early childhood years. The most common recommendation is for at least two free play periods every day (or one period every 3 h) and one additional gross motor play which is teacher-led (Butcher & Eaton, 1989; Dyment & Coleman, 2012; Singer, Singer, D'Agostino & DeLong, 2009; Soini et al., 2014). The early childhood models in Eastern Europe are more similar to those in Asia. Free play is considered to be the main vehicle by which children learn and is included in most learning experiences in the early childhood curriculum. However, there is some difference between state-run programs and privately-owned ones. Most state-run curricula, available to many but not all government workers and others with status, required daily outdoor play from 30 to 45 min. Private curricula required up to 2 h

L. M. Gagen (✉) (retired)
Norfolk State University, Norfolk, VA, USA
e-mail: lmgagen@nsu.edu

N. Getchell
University of Delaware, Newark, DE, USA
e-mail: getchell@udel.edu

H. Brewer, M. R. Jalongo (eds.), *Physical Activity and Health Promotion in the Early Years*, Educating the Young Child 14,
https://doi.org/10.1007/978-3-319-76006-3_4

of daily free play and many call for additional physical education periods that are teacher-led. The Chinese curricula are also very specific about the equipment and facilities that should be available to children during these play times (Graves and Gargiulo, 1994; Wong & Huang, 1999). In all these curricula, neither intensity of exercise nor prescription of movement are addressed.

The assumption made in preschool movement curricula, implicit in their minimalist requirements, is that children acquire fundamental motor skills naturally as a function of the maturing of the central nervous system and that these skills emerge within free play, with no need for consistent, structured practice experiences. Fundamental motor skills are those lower level, basic skills that are the underpinnings for later participation in sport and physical play. These would include ballistic skills like throwing and dribbling, locomotor skills like skipping or hopping, and non-locomotor skills like balance. To assume that the acquisition of these skills may be genetically driven denies the effects of appropriate instruction and practice.

From a theoretical perspective, this viewpoint comes from a maturational perspective that gained popularity early in the twentieth century with researchers Arnold Gesell and Myrtle McGraw (McGraw, 1946; Thelen, 1986). According to this perspective, maturation drove motor development; until children were developmentally ready, experience or practice would not substantially improve motor proficiency. During the latter half of the twentieth century, both theorists and researchers began to challenge the notion that maturation alone explained developmental changes in motor skill. Since the mid-1980's, a fundamental shift in our assumptions has been underway that has radically changed the way we think about motor development. A major part of this shift comes from a move away from a maturational perspective to an ecological approach or perspective.

This ecological perspective stems from the works of J.J. Gibson, an experimental psychologist, whose empirical work and philosophical writings on organism-environment relationships began as a rebuttal to popular behaviorist and cognitivist theory of the early twentieth century. The ecological perspective looks at the interaction of two entities, one of them the person who is moving and the other the environment in which they are moving. It is important to understand that many things exist within a person to create or change movements but that the environment also has an influence on the movement ultimately produced. A young child's walking pattern would be influenced by changes in the environment in which they walked. The underfoot surface of sand at the beach, grass in the park, or snow and ice would make their walking look much different from the walking pattern they would produce in an uncluttered room. In these cases, the environment interacts to produce a more difficult walking task.

Applying the ecological perspective to motor development, changes in movement occur due to interactions among different systems within and outside the human body (hence, "organism-environment relationship"). A generally accepted definition of 'environment' includes our physical surroundings; within this perspective, environment is viewed more broadly so that it includes not only physical conditions but also social and cultural ones. For example, within our bodies, we have multiple systems (e.g. cardiorespiratory, skeletal, metabolic) that perform interrelated roles so that we can function as one system (i.e. a person). Similarly, individuals interact with various groups (family, friends, teachers) that constitute larger social environments. When examining an individual's motor development, therefore, we must consider how these many systems interact over the movement time. As movement practitioners, we can also learn to manipulate some aspects of the environment to improve motor proficiency.

Applying an Ecological Lens: Constraints

Application of the ecological perspective to a motor development context requires practitioners to consider the entire human organism within a context when designing movement experiences. Given the complexity of the human body and the number of interacting systems along with multiple environments, it would be easy to feel overwhelmed trying to determine where to begin. Fortunately, motor development researchers have interpreted some of the more salient parts of the ecological perspective and described these in a way that is easy to understand and apply. One such interpretation is Karl Newell's model of constraints on action (1986), which we will briefly review here. The model of constraints provides the rare occasion where theory fits almost seamlessly with practice, making application to educational and sport contexts for children relatively easy. Newell began by defining movement as resulting from the interaction of an individual performing a movement task within an environment. This provides three unique entities (individual, task, and environment) which he termed 'constraints'. Constraints are characteristics of the individual, task or environment that simultaneously encourage or permit – make more likely to occur – or discourage or delimit specific movement patterns, much like the banks of a river channel the flow of water. Keep in mind that constraints, in this context, are not necessarily negative. They can be positive enablers of movement as well as inhibitors. Therefore, in understanding developmental change, we must look at individual, environmental and task constraints. Within each category of constraint, we can further sub-divide into more specific systems of interest. In terms of individual constraints, a mover has both structural constraints (related to physical systems, such as skeletal, cardiovascular, muscular, etc.) and functional constraints (related to psychological or behavioral constructs, such as motivation, attention, memory, etc.) that interact with each other.

The relevant elements of the environment that encourage or discourage the development of motor proficiency can be categorized as physical, such as terrain, temperature, light, humidity and even gravity. They can also be social, such as gender role stereotypes or cultural norms, influencing sport or game preferences. Finally, specifics of the movement task also serve to encourage or discourage certain movements. For example, movements occurring in a sport context frequently must fall within a narrow range specified by either the goals or rules of the task. The equipment used also encourages or discourages specific movements. Consider this: In soccer, most players may not touch the ball with their hands and would be penalized for doing so. The shape and length of the field hockey stick encourages movements that keep an individual's center of gravity low. However, a large bat, too long and too heavy for a child, does not encourage a good striking movement.

It's important to note that identifying constraints as 'individual', 'task' or 'environment' is not particularly useful in and of itself. Where the concept of constraints really aids practitioners is through an examination of the influence of different constraints on each other, i.e. how they interact, within a movement context. A child's shoes (a task constraint) with rubber toe caps that keep them from wearing out so quickly often interact with carpeting or grass (an environmental constraint) to cause the child to trip and fall (because gravity is an environmental constraint that is always present). Toys (task constraints) that are too large for a child's hand size (a structural constraint) are difficult to manage, as well as toys that are too heavy for their hand and arm strength. In choosing appropriate equipment and environments for children, it is necessary to consider how these interactions may affect a child's ability to perform desired movements appropriate for their motor development (Diagram 4.1).

Interactions are not limited to changing the nature of a movement. Interactions can also elicit movements from small children. Favored adults in a child's social circle (environmental constraints) or a favorite or interesting toy (task constraint) can often elicit movements by motivating a child to walk or creep toward them (motivation is a functional constraint). A new colorful or interesting toy or book might elicit a particular movement response of excitement from young children. As these interactions occur, the movement will cause the body to self-organize to produce a movement with a particular flow.

Thus, the model demonstrates a system whose resultant movement arises from the relationship of many elements, and if one or two change, the resultant movement might change. The individual, the environment, and the specific task at hand are always dynamically interacting, and characteristics of each change can be influenced by other changes that are taking place, as seen in Newell's triangle (See Fig. 4.1). When considering developmental change, two concepts related to Newell's constraint model are of particular importance to the movement practitioner when trying to facilitate motor proficiency. First is the notion of 'rate limiters', which are individual constraints that hold back the emergence of certain motor skills. In our walking example above, the individual's strength and ability to balance both acted as rate limiters. Second, 'body scaling' evaluates individual constraints in relation to environmental or task constraints where in some instances, ideal relative proportions exist. As in our example above, body scaling occurs when we choose toys that are an appropriate relative size for children's hands and a weight that can be accommodated by their relative strength to grasp and hold them. We will discuss each concept in greater detail below.

Identifying Interactions			
Task: Beginning walking	**Individual Constraints:** Leg and arm strength, core strength, weight, balance, fear, motivation	**Environmental Constraints:** Surface (carpet, slippery tile, grass), gravity, social interaction	**Task Constraints:** Socks, shoes, furniture to pull up on
Possible Interactions	Socks or shoes ⟺ surface ⟺ balance and core strength Fear of falling ⟺ balance and gravity Strength ⟺ weight Motivation ⟺ social interaction Strength ⟺ available furniture to pull up on		
Task: Throwing a ball at a wall	**Individual Constraints:** Hand size and strength, arm length and strength, balance, motivation	**Environmental Constraints:** Underfoot surface, gravity, social interaction	**Task Constraints:** Choice of ball, size of wall, distance to wall, shoes
Possible Interactions	Hand size and strength ⟺ ball size and weight and gravity Arm length and strength ⟺ ball weight Shoes ⟺ underfoot surface Strength ⟺ size of wall and distance to wall Motivation ⟺ social encouragement		

Diagram 4.1 Identifying interactions

Rate Limiters

Certain individual constraints can serve to slow the rate at which individuals can acquire motor skills (Thelen, Ulrich, & Wolff, 1991). If an individual cannot produce a particular movement until a rate limiter changes, then the rate limiter acts to control when the new pattern can emerge. It may be the slowest-developing element or subsystem in multiple subsystems that interact to give rise to the movement. If the movement that arises from the interaction of subsystems is considered a developmental marker, that is, an indicator of the rate of development, then the rate-limiting system influences the rate of development. For example, balance and

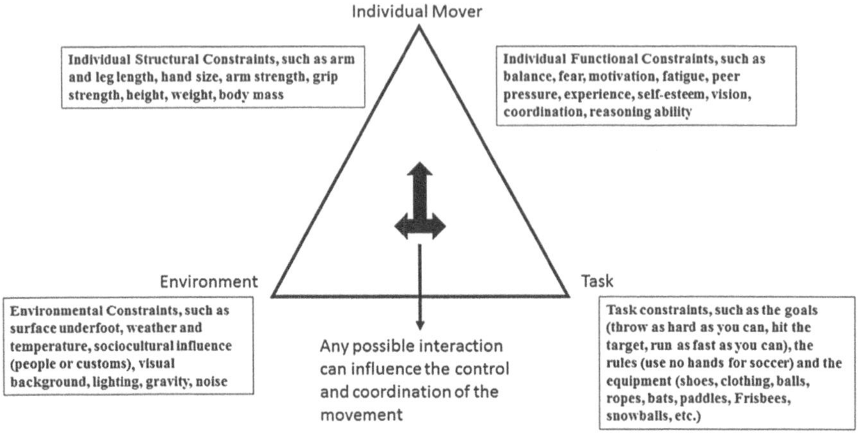

Fig. 4.1 Newell's constraints

strength are often early rate limiters to walking. Both must be developed enough for children to maintain upright posture and move ahead. If children are strong enough to stand but do not have sufficient balance to take steps and remain upright, walking will be limited until balance catches up. In this case, balance would be the rate limiter. Note, though, that the new behavior is still emerging from the interaction of elemental subsystems rather than a directive from genetic code or stored instructions. The change in a subsystem has brought about a change in the relationship of the components so that a new movement can emerge.

The cause of developmental advancement does not have to be a single, same system for every advancement or developmental marker. One subsystem is not always the most important subsystem (Abraham, Abraham, & Shaw, 1992; Kelso, 1997; Newell, 1984; Smith & Thelen, 2003). An example of this is watching a child learn to jump rope. There is a wide range of ages in which children acquire the ability to jump. Often children's first jumps only raise one of their feet off the floor, even though jumping needs both feet in flight. Strength on the non-dominant side of the body must develop to a threshold to allow both feet to leave the floor at the same time. So strength would be one rate limiter for jumping. In order to jump, children also need to have some level of dynamic balance (balance while moving). So strength and balance would also be the rate limiters for jumping but with greater demands than would be needed to just walk. If we add a rope, timing and coordination become additional requirements. If any of these is lagging behind, the child may be motivated to jump a single rope but will not be able to produce an appropriate movement. Since there are many different coordinated elements to jumping rope, the rate limiters cause this to be a later emerging skill. As soon as all of these rate limiters move to the required levels, jumping will be achieved and jumping with a rope will follow. These subsystems are rate limiters for jumping but also may be rate limiters for other movements. It should be no surprise that researchers adopting a systems perspective are interested in identifying the subsystem or combination of subsystems that have an impact on the emergence of new behaviors, that is, the rate-limiting systems.

Practitioners designing active play experiences for children must determine the rate limiters that may be holding back movers. Do they need more strength, perhaps only on one side of the body, or are balance and coordination holding back the desired movement? When early childhood educators seek appropriate activities for their preschoolers, rate limiters for some children may be evident and influence the choice of activity. The three-year-old who cannot yet jump with both feet off the ground at the same time will not be able to jump rope, even if the adult turns the rope. Children who are still developing equal strength on both sides of the body or bilateral coordination will not yet be able to skip. These are not developmental deficits but rather the evidence of different rates of development within different subsystems. Practitioners will see children struggling with certain tasks, often because one or more of the rate limiters are not well developed, but children will magically acquire the skill with little more effort when that system develops to the rate limit threshold. This accounts for the wide age range at which children acquire motor skills since those rate limiting systems develop on very individual time lines.

Body Scaling

Understanding the nature of interactions among constraints can be useful to practitioners such as physical educators, early childhood educators, or physical therapists. Although individual constraints may be difficult to change at any one point in time (i.e in one play period), a practitioner can help change the way in which an individual develops motor skills with repeated manipulation of the environment or task. One way to illustrate this is through the notion of body scaling. Individuals 'body scale' when they adjust their actions or movements based on the relationship between their individual characteristics and those of the environment (Gagen, Haywood, & Spaner, 2005). For example, if an adult reaches for a cup of coffee on a desk, he or she scales the opening of hand and fingers to the size of the handle based on the relative size of the fingers to the handle. This allows for grasping the cup easily and efficiently without spilling its contents. However, if a toddler reaches for the same cup, he or she will most likely use two hands. This occurs when this movement is scaled to the size of the cup; because a toddler's hands are much smaller than the adult's, this adjustment in grip provides the most efficient and effective grasp of the cup for this particular child. How a task is accomplished therefore differs depending on the body scaling of the individual to the environment. If we as adults wanted to make this task easier, we would provide a cup that is already scaled to the hand size of the child.

Different researchers have found empirical support for body scaling in a variety of tasks. One of the most well-known studies comes from Newell and his colleagues in a 1989 study of grasping (Newell, Scully, Tenenbaum, & Hardiman, 1989). Prior to this study, the research of Halverson (1931) suggested that children progressed through an invariant sequence of grasps, from a primitive squeeze to a precision, pincher grasp; Halverson believed these were genetically determined stages. Newell and his colleagues replicated the Halverson study with children aged 3–5 years old, and rather than giving the children the same object, they systematically changed the size of the object to be grasped. They determined that, by scaling the size of the object to be grasped, individuals changed their grasp when the object reached a relative size of 40% of their hand width. That is, change in grasp was not in a predetermined, maturational sequence, but occurred as a result of the interaction between the size of the child's hand and the size of the object to be grasped (Newell et al., 1989).

Another study looked at body scaling and choice of tennis racquets in children aged 4–10 years of age (Gagen et al., 2005). Children were provided with 4 differently-sized racquets and asked to swing at a target with each one. Racquet speed and the accuracy of the strike were measured for swings with each racquet. Unlike Newell et al.'s, 1989 study, no systematic relationship existed between individual characteristics and performance outcomes (allowing selection of the best racquet for each child). However, each child had one specific racquet that provided him or her with the best performance, suggesting that all of the individual's constraints (grip strength, hand size, body dimensions, etc.) interacted in a way that one racquet 'scaled' best for the particular child. This study and the Newell et al. (1989) study exemplify how movements change as the relationship between the mover and the environment changes and this has implications for designing movement experiences for children.

Providing Active Movement Experiences

Early childhood educators should not be passive in providing play experiences. Training and successful planning is needed to provide valuable learning experiences. Breslin, Morton, & Rudisill, (2008) concluded in their study of preschool movement programs that "the teachers needed more guidance in implementing an age-appropriate physical activity program." (p. 430). Education and staff development for early childhood educators should include specific training in providing positive movement activities since recess and free play, while valuable for young children, do not provide enough attention to developing skills that children need. "Informal and random opportunities for physical activity (recess, before- and after-school games, and occasional classroom-based physical activities) do indeed contribute to physical development, they are far from sufficient as the basis for meeting all of the young child's needs." (Stork & Sanders, 2008, p. 200).

As early childhood educators, we must become educated in ways to provide active play that is attuned to practicing emerging skills and designed to introduce variations that will expand the child's movement knowledge and vocabulary

(Martyniuk & Tucker, 2014; Wright & Stork, 2013). This is where we can utilize the principles from the theory of constraints to help design the most effective experiences for each child by taking into account the interactions of the child's individual constraints with the environment and the task (Gagen & Getchell, 2006).

Stodden and his team of researchers speak to the effects of acquiring motor skill competence in developing active movers (Stodden et al., 2008). If our mission is to help children develop in ways that promote engagement in physical activities throughout the lifespan, we must begin in the early childhood years, when behaviors are developing and children are willing to engage in play of all kinds. Training for teachers is needed in how to present organized, appropriate activities in addition to free play.

Three Areas of Movement

All fundamental movements can be categorized into locomotor, manipulative, and non-manipulative movements (Graham, Holt-Hale & Parker, 2010). Locomotor movements are any movement that moves you across the floor, such as walking or skipping. Manipulative movements involve using a piece of equipment that is manipulated as part of the movement, such as a ball or a paddle. Non-manipulative movements are movements that don't involve the other two areas and tend to be more stationary in nature, such as balancing, twisting and turning, or bending and stretching. Within these three categories, a consideration of constraints would assist with planning appropriate and useful activity lessons.

Locomotor Movements

Locomotor movements result in travel across space (See Diagram 4.2). How do developmental readiness and the interaction of constraints suggest when and how these movements might be most easily learned? If we look at some typically emerging locomotion in early childhood, we can examine the constraints needed for them. We know that some children achieve these movements earlier than others and that many of them emerge naturally. Babies do get up and walk without being taught but we also know that there is a wide range of ages at which that happens. We can identify constraints that might affect the emergence of locomotion such as the development of balance and leg strength, but consider also that the functional constraints of fear and motivation may have some bearing on when children are ready and willing to explore upright stance and leave the safety of holding on. Children typically spend some upright movement time cruising - walking around furniture safely holding on - before they walk independently. Cruising allows the further development of balance and leg strength that will be needed for independent walking. Running follow close behind as stimuli motivate children to explore their environment.

Locomotor Movements	Manipulative Movements	Non-locomotor Movements
Walking, running or marching	Throwing (overhand or underhand, bowling or rolling)	Balancing
Galloping or sliding	Catching or trapping (hands or feet)	Twisting and turning
Jumping, leaping or hopping	Dribbling (hands or feet)	Pushing and pulling
Skipping	Striking (hands, paddles, rackets, sticks, bats)	Bending and stretching
Creeping or crawling	Kicking and punting	Curling and reaching
Rolling	Jumping single ropes	Shifting your weight

Diagram 4.2 Common fundamental movements

Jumping happens soon after walking and running are achieved. Early jumping requires a flight phase but the child is propelled by using both feet. Typical early jumping attempts might involve jumping on one foot that is strong enough to come completely off the ground (with the other foot maintaining contact in some way) but repeated attempts will eventually result in enough strength on both sides to achieve a full flight phase with both feet. Hopping would emerge much later since the strength required to propel the full weight of the body into a flight phase must come from one foot. Even hopping on the dominant or preferred foot requires greater strength and balance development than jumping. It makes sense that it would be more difficult due to these individual constraints. Since both jumping and hopping require a flight phase, the risk of losing balance may have something to do with the level of fear that a child will tolerate and their motivation to try new things, both functional constraints. Some children are content with moving slower through these processes and may not be so comfortable with flight until much later than others. This accounts for the wide range in ages over which these movements are accomplished.

Consider why children typically gallop before they achieve skipping. Galloping is a one-sided movement. While it does use uneven rhythm (long-timed step, short-timed backward leap), it does not require children to have the strength to achieve flight from both the dominant and the non-dominant foot, nor does it require them to coordinate the changing of the movement from one side of the body to the other. Skipping would require strength to achieve flight on both sides of the body, the capability to coordinate the uneven rhythm (long-timed step, short-timed hop) and the capability to switch sides of the body on each repetition. Skipping remains the most difficult of the locomotor movements of early childhood and it can be quite late in development before a child achieves this. If a child is not skipping well in the early childhood years, this is not yet a mark of developmental delay but rather just an example of diversity in the timetable of the development of subsystems and the interaction of constraints. Another constraint, considered an environmental constraint, might be that skipping is an activity that is not always considered culturally acceptable for boys (not a "manly" activity) so practice in this movement might be discouraged for some young boys. In this case, skipping might not be learned until the child reaches school and can be introduced to it there.

In order to move a child across space, the locomotor movement must follow some pathway. This might be an open pathway, which would look like wandering in any direction but soon we can prescribe more closed pathways that encourage vocabulary development. Pathways can be straight, curved or a combination of both. Straight pathways can move in one direction or change directions by turning corners. From here we get to concepts of right and left, eventually forming shapes like squares and rectangles. Soon we can move these forward and backward. We can walk straight ahead or on a diagonal. Once we have a diagonal, we can walk in the shape of a triangle. Curved pathways can be arcs or whole circles. Following increasingly complex pathways requires the use of logical reasoning and experience, both functional constraints. More complex pathways, with more than one change of direction, support the skill of sequencing or remembering the moves in order. A complex pathway with a sequencing requirement would sound something like "walk straight ahead on the red line, walk in a circle around the green square and walk back to the blue line." The development of logical reasoning skills also happens over a wide time span. Practicing moving to and remembering sequences may support music education and also play a part in the development of math and language skills (Gordon, 2003).

Locomotor movements often require patterning for repetitive movement. Visual patterning could involve a "map" of footprints on the floor for the child to follow, involving changes of direction and encouraging different locomotor movements by their placement. In other activities, hand signals given by the teacher could signal those changes of direction to follow. Interpreting the hand signals adds another, more advanced, dimension to the activity. Learning vocabulary words such as over, under, around, through, behind, and between give children new ideas for pathways relative to objects in the room.

We might also provide an auditory pattern with which to move, such as clapping, a drum beat or music. Moving exactly to the beat will be a more advanced, learned skill but often very young children can move their feet and clap at the same time. This promotes the idea that the patterning connects the upper and lower body. Young children do love to clap and to stamp their feet and incorporating these into other movements will extend their capabilities as they develop cognitive skills in conjunction with new movement skills.

Manipulative Movements

Manipulative movements require the use of the body to manipulate play objects during a movement. These might be balls or other throwing, catching and dribbling objects, hoops, ropes for jumping, or paddles, racquets and sticks for managing balls or pucks. Equipment like this can often be manipulated in different ways using a variety of body parts. In this case, the choice of equipment, as a task constraint which interacts with the individual constraints of each child, can be influential in encouraging a particular movement or making it more difficult.

Consider the scaling of a 22″ playground ball, often a standard purchase for early childhood venues. Relative to the size of the children, what can you do with a 22″ ball? It is too large for the size of the child's arms and hands so you can't really handle it like a ball. Attempting to throw this ball causes the throwing motion to be significantly altered since children can't manage this ball with one hand, or even attempt to balance it on one hand to throw with a pushing motion. They can't throw with two hands because the ball is too large to move it to one side past their body. It's too heavy to throw with two hands over their heads and it's too large and heavy to even throw it underhand from between their knees. So throwing this ball is not really an option. A ball that would support the development of good throwing technique needs to be sized to the hand of the child so they can grip it properly and it needs to be light so their arm movement is not influenced by the weight of the ball. Therefore, something more like a tennis ball would be in order for throwing. The interaction of constraints with this large 22″ ball prohibits one-handed throwing as a developmental task.

Rolling the ball is a form of underhand throwing. While this 22″ ball could be pushed with two hands on the ground to roll it between children, this pushing movement needed to move it and the position of the body with the hands high on the ball's surface would not approximate underhand throwing. So this activity would only be pushing. Since it doesn't provide a basis for improving throwing of any kind, this activity would not be very useful in developing appropriate motor skills.

Likewise, this ball would inhibit catching. The ball is too large to fit comfortably in a child's hands or be scooped into the chest with the arms. The ball would not fit well in that small area between hands, arms and chest so the child would likely be hit with the ball when trying to catch. When children are hit with a ball during catching, they often develop the functional constraint of fear and this would certainly interfere with learning to catch in the future, even with a more appropriately sized ball. In one of the first signs of fear in catching, the child's head turns to the side, often with the eyes closed, and this interrupts eye-tracking of the ball. That would make catching much more difficult without having the ability to track the ball's movement. A ball for catching should be a size to easily fit into a two hand grasp, so that would be around 5–7 inches in diameter for these small hands. It should be light-weight and of a material that would not introduce fear into the process. Another consideration is the color of the ball, which should not blend into the background so that it remains very visible in flight for visual tracking. Compare the size of the ball best for catching with the size of the ball best for throwing and you can easily see that these two skills cannot be used together in early practice. Catching the same ball you can throw is a much more advanced skill.

Kicking is another ball skill that this 22″ ball would not support. The size of the ball relative to the size of the legs of the child is much too large. Contacting the ball at the center back of the ball, an appropriate position for kicking, would require the child to raise their kicking leg quite high and alter the kicking motion. The ball is also too heavy for the leg strength of a beginning kicker so it would be a difficult task to move the ball very far and may actually injure the kicking foot if the ball were contacted incorrectly with the toes.

So what activities could we do with this ball that would promote positive physical development? Children could be encouraged to run by chasing the ball. The ball would provide a focus for the running activity. The ball could be pushed and then chased, to encourage directional knowledge and the concepts in Newton's Laws of Motion (Gagen & Getchell, 2008). In which direction should it be pushed to get it to go where we intend? This type of exploration gives a child the benefit of experiencing sensory and cognitive knowledge while at play (Vidoni, Lorenz, & de Paleville, 2014). If the ball were very large, 24 inches or larger, it would be possible to use the ball to lie on but what skills, other than an unusually positioned balance skill, would we be promoting? Additionally, are we introducing a safety issue into this activity?

If a program thinks about investing in a piece of equipment like a 22″ (or larger) playground ball, and this equipment is not useful for helping to develop a number of appropriate motor skills, wouldn't it be more prudent to invest whatever limited resources are available in equipment that is useful in allowing children to have appropriate practice in multiple skills? Equipment that matches the child's individual constraints and provides good practice in correct skill processes is more valuable in developing skills that will later be useful in participating in sport and physical activity with others. Balls that fit into one hand, perhaps the size of a tennis ball, allow better throwing. Balls that fit into two hands that can easily encompass most of the girth of the ball allow for better catching. Balls to kick should be low enough to the ground that the foot can contact the ball slightly below the middle back of the ball while keeping the foot close to the ground. Using equipment that matches the constraints of the child allows the body to self-organize into correct movement patterns. Allowing a child to learn the movement correctly from an early age promotes success in movement later in childhood. Trying to correct poor movement patterns that were learned early will hold children back from participation or interfere with their ability to participate at all.

This is true for various pieces of equipment children might use for active play. Breslin et al. (2008) suggest that children need a wide range of implements with which to development movement skills. These implements, aside from balls, might include jump ropes, paddles, other throwing implements like bean bags or interesting shaped implements, and props that might encourage movements such as hoops or foam noodles. When gathering these implements, the theory of constraints should again be the guiding principle.

Perhaps you've seen children try to jump an individual rope that is too long for their height or made of a material that is too heavy for them to move easily. This results in frustration when the rope cannot be easily turned over the head. Changing the rope to a lighter one that is an appropriate length solves many of those problems and allows the child to focus on the task and the timing, unencumbered by the equipment. This is an example of the benefit of using the interaction of constraints to allow children to learn movement tasks appropriately.

Young children can easily learn to strike with paddles. Remember that the individual constraints of hand size and strength, arm strength, visual acuity and the ability to perceive the object to be struck all factor into this task. The first, most basic, paddle should be the hand. Getting the idea of the contact of striking is the first step. The hand can be extended into a paddle by cutting two slits across a paper plate and slipping it onto the hand, providing a wider surface than the palm. This can easily be used to strike a balloon, a small light ball (perhaps made of rolled up socks) or a small cut piece of a foam noodle. From here, moving to a paddle which is light, has a reasonably-sized striking surface and a short handle for control might be the next step. The surface of the paddle should be close to the hand because the perception of matching the striking surface with something to strike is more difficult when the length of the handle causes the object to be farther away from the control of the striking object in the hand. Even if the striking object is stationary, such as on a batting tee or cone, if the striking surface is far from the hands, perceiving how far away to stand is very difficult, something that takes experience and practice. This is definitely a more advanced striking task.

In throwing tasks, the implement thrown does not have to be a ball. Bean bags toss well and can be adapted to many other activities so they are a valuable asset. They are flexible and mold well to the configuration of the child's hand so they are easy to grasp and control. Other objects that could be throwing-appropriate might be small stuffed animals, because of the weight and the texture. Fleece balls made of yarn are a good size and weight for throwing in the early childhood. Beach balls of smaller than traditional sizes, which are available from physical education vendors, are good striking implements and can be used for catching in the 7.5 and 10 inch sizes where they can be grasped in two hands. Be aware that the light weight of beach balls makes them very vulnerable to wind (an environmental constraint) if children are playing outside.

Foam noodles, also called swim noodles are long cylinders of light foam, around 2 m in length. They are very flexible and often have a small hole running down the center. They began as a swim product but are now used in many other ways. They are called water woggles in the UK, schwimmnudeln in Germany, Yóuyǒng miàntiáo in China, nouilles de natation in French and fideos de natación in Spanish. They seem to exist in every country's swimming pools and are inexpensive resources that can function to encourage development of a number of motor skills. They can be cut into short chunks to provide throwing implements. Longer chunks of about 12″ might make a light, easy to swing striking implement, although the diameter is quite large for small hands. They can also be used full size as boundaries to design tracks or pathways to move around or through because they are light and will move easily out of the way without becoming a hazard.

The choice of appropriately scaled equipment is important but the design of the task is equally important. A well-chosen task with a poorly designed outcome goal will not attain the desired result (Langendorfer, 1990). Take the task of early throwing. While it seems intuitive to many adults that throwing and catching are connected as related tasks, they are two different tasks and early movers do not have the skill to connect these skills into one exercise. Throwing and catching with a partner is a very advanced activity, not appropriate for very young children. Throwing at the early levels should be simply throwing. Propelling the ball forward from the body would be a good first outcome. Throwing at a target would need the target to be carefully chosen. The initial target might be chosen as a large space such as a wall. The capability of hitting the wall with some consistency might then allow limiting the target to some part of the wall. As accuracy increases, other tasks can be included, such as tossing bean bags into hoops. Correctly designing the outcome of the task allows the task design to be developmentally appropriate for the beginning thrower.

Task design is equally important in all tasks. If we think about catching, the ball must be an appropriate size for the hands and a color that does not blend with the background so it can be easily seen. Yet, how does it arrive to be caught? The first catching task would involve a short lob of low velocity almost assuredly landing in the hands. The arc of the ball, the ball speed and the distance from the catcher will all eventually be altered but should be very controlled in a beginning task. This is equally true of kicking and striking, where a beginning task would have the object stationary and in a position to be easily accessed by the striker such as sitting on a beanbag for kicking or propped on a cone or a ball tee for striking. Again, the first goal is contact and propelling it forward. Well-designed tasks, taking into account the theory of constraints, allow for better skill development.

Non-manipulative Movements

Non-manipulative movements, also sometimes called non-locomotor or stationary movements in literature, involve all the movements that don't provide locomotion or object manipulation. The common ones in this group are bending, stretching, twisting, turning, pushing, pulling, and reaching. All movement skills require balance to perform them effectively, but balance is placed in this category because many balance tasks involve non-manipulative movements. Success with these movements is directly tied to functional constraints and the development of the central nervous system. As with all skills, some children will have enough balance to be successful early and some will develop much later, but active play that is both fun and challenging will allow practice and mastery at whatever level is possible for each individual child.

Non-manipulative skills encourage children to utilize different levels in movement, a concept that will come into specific sports skills much later in childhood. Creative story activities that involve imagining and moving help children to relate movement to everyday situations. A story might include things like "reach as high as you can to pick the highest apple on the tree" or "bend down and pick the prettiest flower." These encourage children to leave their normal mid-level orientation and work at more unfamiliar high and low levels. It also requires them to use dynamic balance (balancing while moving). They can paint the walls of their imaginary house from the very top to the bottom. They can stretch to be as tall as they can or bend to be as small as possible. An imaginary task can provide many different movements while satisfying the imagination and even introducing additional language development in the process.

The concept of moving at different levels can also be combined with locomotor movements. Children can learn to move at high levels like a giraffe, using their arms as the long neck. They can move on all fours at a low level like a bear or a turtle or slither like a snake. There are many possibilities and children love to emulate not only animals but other familiar objects. How do trees look when the wind is blowing and the storm is coming? A young friend of mine always knew when it was going to rain when she "saw the trees dancing." Using movement to bend and stretch many different muscle groups promotes flexibility as well as stimulates the imagination and practices dynamic balance.

Practicing balance should be an on-going objective in our movement program, since balance is involved in almost every movement. Remember that balance is different under different movement and positional demands. Balance on one foot is much more difficult than on both feet. Children should be encouraged to explore the elements of balance through well-designed movement tasks. Consider challenging students to explore what movements can they do while balancing on both feet. Did they find some more difficult than others? Does the alignment of their feet make the task easier or more difficult? What happens when they switch to balancing on one foot only? Is it easier or more difficult to balance when squatting down or when stretching up high? If they reach for something in different directions at different levels, how does that influence balance? Does the movement change when a beanbag is on your head, on your shoulder, or balanced on your hand, knee or elbow? All of these concepts can be incorporated into either the locomotor or non-locomotor activities. Be sure that you account for occasional falling by using a mat or safety surface when engaging in the more difficult of these tasks.

Conclusion

Designers of developmental movement experiences for young children should consider the constraints of the children to enhance planning and to assist in choosing equipment or designing tasks for this purpose. Equipment must match (be scaled to) the physical size and strength capabilities of children but also the balance and perceptual abilities. Equipment should never introduce negative constraints like fear, which would inhibit the development of movements for future play. Considering the theory of constraints when planning activities and choosing equipment will provide the most appropriate experiences and allow each child more opportunity to succeed in developing motor skill competence. Since we know that motor skill competence is a necessary part of future involvement in physical activity (Stodden et al., 2008), this important part of the early education of our children must be knowledgeably and intentionally included in our curricula and applied in our daily lessons.

References

Abraham, F. D., Abraham, R. H., & Shaw, C. D. (1992). Basic principles of dynamical systems. *Analysis of dynamic psychological systems, 1*, 35–143.

Breslin, C. M., Morton, J. R., & Rudisill, M. E. (2008). Implementing a physical activity curriculum into the school day: Helping early childhood teachers meet the challenge. *Early Childhood Education Journal, 35*(5), 429–437.

Butcher, J. E., & Eaton, W. O. (1989). Gross and fine motor proficiency in preschoolers: Relationships with free play behavior and activity level. *Journal of Human Movement Studies, 16*, 27–36.

Dyment, J. E., & Coleman, B. (2012). The intersection of physical activity opportunities and the role of early childhood educators during outdoor play: Perceptions and reality. *Australasian Journal of Early Childhood, 37*(1), 90–98.

Gagen, L., & Getchell, N. (2008). Applying Newton's apple to elementary physical education: An interdisciplinary approach. *Journal of Physical Education, Recreation & Dance, 79*(8), 43–51.

Gagen, L. M., & Getchell, N. (2006). Using 'constraints' to design developmentally appropriate movement activities for early childhood education. *Early Childhood Education Journal, 34*(3), 227–232.

Gagen, L. M., Haywood, K. M., & Spaner, S. D. (2005). Predicting the scale of tennis rackets for optimal striking from body dimensions. *Pediatric Exercise Science, 17*, 190–200.

Gordon, E. (2003). *Learning sequences in music: Skill, content, and patterns: A music learning theory*. Chicago: GIA Publications.

Graham, G., Holt-Hale, S. A., & Parker, M. (2010). *Children moving: A reflective approach to teaching physical education*. New York: McGraw-Hill.

Graves, S. B., & Gargiulo, R. M. (1994). Early childhood education in three eastern European countries. *Childhood Education, 70*(4), 205–209.

Halverson, H. M. (1931). An experimental study of prehension in infants by means of systematic cinema records. In *Genetic psychology monographs*. Provincetown, MA: Journal Press.

Kaphingst, K. M., & Story, M. (2009). Child care as an untapped setting for obesity prevention: State child care licensing regulations related to nutrition, physical activity, and media use for preschool-aged children in the United States. *Preventing Chronic Disease, 6*(1), A11.

Kelso, J. A. S. (1997). Relative timing in brain and behavior: Some observations about the generalized motor program and self-organized coordination dynamics. *Human Movement Science, 16*(4), 453–460.

Langendorfer, S. (1990). Motor-task goal as a constraint on developmental status. *Advances in Motor Development Research, 3*, 16–28.

Martyniuk, O. J., & Tucker, P. (2014). An exploration of early childhood education students' knowledge and preparation to facilitate physical activity for preschoolers: A cross-sectional study. *BMC Public Health, 14*(1), 727.

McGraw, M. B. (1946). Maturation of behavior. In L. Carmichael & J. E. Anderson (Eds.), *Manual of child psychology* (pp. 332–369). Hoboken, NJ: Wiley. https://doi.org/10.1037/10756-007

Newell, K. M. (1984). Physical constraints to development of motor skills. In J. R. Thomas (Ed.), *Motor development during childhood and adolescence* (pp. 105–120). Minneapolis, MN: Burgess Publishing.

Newell, K. M., Scully, D. M., Tenenbaum, F., & Hardiman, S. (1989). Body scale and the development of prehension. *Developmental Psychobiology, 22*(1), 1–13.

Singer, D. G., Singer, J. L., D'Agostino, H., & DeLong, R. (2009). Children's pastimes and play in sixteen nations. Is free play declining? *American Journal of Play, 4*, 283–312.

Smith, L. B., & Thelen, E. (2003). Development as a dynamic system. *Trends in Cognitive Sciences, 7*(8), 343–348.

Soini, A., Villberg, J., Saakslahti, A., Gubbels, J., Mehtala, A., Kettunen, T., & Poskiparta, M. (2014). Directly observed physical activity among 3-year-olds in Finnish childcare. *International Journal of Early Childhood, 46*, 253–269.

Stodden, D. F., Goodway, J. D., Langendorfer, S. J., Roberton, M. A., Rudisill, M. E., Garcia, C., & Garcia, L. E. (2008). A developmental perspective on the role of motor skill competence in physical activity. *Quest, 60*(2), 290–306.

Stork, S., & Sanders, S. W. (2008). Physical education in early childhood. *The Elementary School Journal, 108*(3), 197–206.

Thelen, E. (1986). Development of coordinated movement: Implications for early human development. In M. G. Wade & H. T. A. Whiting (Eds.), *Motor skills acquisition* (pp. 107–124). Dordrecht: Nijhoff.

Thelen, E., Ulrich, B. D., & Wolff, P. H. (1991). Hidden skills: A dynamic systems analysis of treadmill stepping during the first year. *Monographs of the Society for Research in Child Development, 56*(1), i–103. https://doi.org/10.2307/1166099

Vidoni, C., Lorenz, D. J., & de Paleville, D. T. (2014). Incorporating a movement skill programme into a preschool daily schedule. *Early Child Development and Care, 184*(8), 1211–1222.

Wong, P. S. S., & Huang, S. (1999). A comparative study on the preschool physical education curriculum in Zhuhai, China and Macau government kindergartens. *New Horizons in Education, 40*(11), 58–70.

Wright, P. M., & Stork, S. (2013). Recommended practices for promoting physical activity in early childhood education settings. *Journal of Physical Education, Recreation & Dance, 84*(5), 40–43.

Linda M. Gagen has been teaching for over 35 years in both P-12 education and higher education. She began her career in elementary school by teaching health and physical education for children in grades K-5 and was recognized as Outstanding Teacher for the St. Louis region. She has conducted research on preschool and elementary movement patterns, which she has published in peer reviewed journals and presented at national conference.

Nancy Getchell is currently a professor in the Department of Kinesiology and Applied Physiology at the University of Delaware. During her academic career, she has focused her research on the development of neuromotor control and coordination in typical and atypical populations, specifically children with autism, learning disabilities, and developmental coordination disorder. She also studies the relationship among motor proficiency, physical activity, and health related fitness in typically and atypically developing young children. Besides numerous scholarly publications, she is also the co-author of the textbook *Life Span Motor Development*.

Chapter 5
The Importance of Physical Literacy and Addressing Academic Learning Through Planned Physical Activity

David A. Wachob

Barriers to Learning

In a small kindergarten classroom, laughter and noise rings through the room as the students work through stations in small groups. They learn how to work as a team to complete each task as they progress through the lesson. There are students (1) throwing a damp sponge at numbers drawn on the chalkboard, (2) hopping on numbers scattered around the floor, (3) rolling large foam dice, and a few (4) working quietly at the reading table. The teacher is moving around the room interacting with the students and checking their work. Every few minutes she turns the lights off, and within seconds, the students stop working and move to another station. When the lesson is complete, the groups turn in their completed packets that they have been working on while at each stations.

In this example, the teacher is using planned physical activity to practice math concepts that the students have been learning. At first glance, an outside observer might quickly assume that the students are just playing and there is no teaching or learning. The reality of this scenario is that the students are learning how to add single digit numbers, the same content they would be completing at their seats on practice worksheets. The main difference between this example and typical seat work is that the students in this example are also practicing problem solving, gross motor skills, balance, teamwork, and touch processing skills, to name a few.

Although this example is educational and engaging, many teachers avoid this type of experience (Goodlad, 2004; McDermott, Mordell, & Stoltzfus, 2001). Instead of allowing the students to move around the room and work through their own practice problems, many teachers assign worksheets for the students to complete at their seats. This highly regulated and controlled atmosphere is part of the traditional classroom system that has been in practice, mostly unchanged, for over

D. A. Wachob (✉)
Department of Kinesiology, Health, and Sport Science, Indiana University of Pennsylvania, Indiana, PA, USA
e-mail: d.wachob@iup.edu

H. Brewer, M. R. Jalongo (eds.), *Physical Activity and Health Promotion in the Early Years*, Educating the Young Child 14,
https://doi.org/10.1007/978-3-319-76006-3_5

a century (Hirsh-Pasek, Golinkoff, Berk, & Singer, 2008; Yair, 2000). Part of the reason this system continues to dominate classrooms is because teachers fear a loss of control over the children's behavior (Wachob, 2015).

This traditional model has littered the education system with mounds of teaching tools designed to improve test scores. This narrow focus on learning often leads to lower than expected results and an even lower level of student engagement (Yazzie-Mintz, 2010). These sedentary teacher-controlled activities, commonly referred to as seatwork, oftentimes create unintentional barriers to learning.

A fundamental principle of quality instruction is identifying and minimizing barriers to learning (Fitzsimmons & Lanphar, 2011). Common barriers that often hinder a student's performance include the inability to organize, store, and retrieve information; generalize and transfer learned knowledge to new and unknown tasks; show adequate use of strategies for solving tasks; and engage in appropriate social interactions essential for school connectedness (Hay, Elias, & Booker, 2006). Although certain learning challenges are internal to each student and are based on cognitive abilities, many barriers to learning can be minimized by expanding the way literacy skills are taught and practiced in the classroom.

Physical Literacy

The term literacy goes well beyond being able to read and write. According to the United Nations Educational, Scientific and Cultural Organization (UNESCO, 2004), "Literacy involves a continuum of learning that enables an individual to achieve his or her goals, [and] to develop his or her knowledge and potential" (pp. 12–13). This multifaceted concept involves using a variety of means (e.g. listening, speaking, and writing) to exchange information across a range of social contexts (Hay et al., 2006). One branch of literacy that is effective when teaching young children is known as physical literacy. Physical literacy involves expanding the student's ability to (1) interpret and respond to the environment and to others through interaction, (2) use the body as an instrument of expression and communication, (3) and demonstrate knowledge, skills, and understanding through movement (Daggett, 2010).

Being literate involves having the ability to "exchange" information; which occurs in many ways. How information is exchanged directly impacts how much learning will occur (Ratey & Hagerman, 2008). A key to having strong literacy skills is through the process of metacognition. Metacognition is the ability to focus on the actions needed to complete a task (Curwen, Miller, White-Smith, & Calfee, 2010). Simply stated, it is the process of thinking about thinking. Students who develop metagconitive skills are focused on the process of problem solving and not just coming up with a basic answer. By incorporating movement opportunities, physically literate students are better able to work through problems and govern their own steps needed to complete a task (Almond & Whitehead, 2012).

Movement and Learning

Early years are not only optimal for children to learn through movement, but also a critical developmental period. If children are not given enough natural movement and play experiences, they start their academic careers at a disadvantage (Diamond, & Lee, 2011). They oftentimes have difficulty with paying attention, controlling their emotions, utilizing problem-solving skills, and demonstrating difficulties with social interactions (Ratey & Hagerman, 2008). The Alliance for Childhood's *Defending the Early Years* Project advocates that, "Active, play-based experiences in language rich environments help children develop their ideas about symbols, oral language and the printed word — all vital components of reading" (Carlsson-Paige, McLaughlin, & Almon, 2015).

Research on neuroscience and the relationship between movement and cognition is well established (Ratey & Hagerman, 2008). Incorporating movement into the school day has been shown to improve academic performance (Mahar et al., 2006; Ratey & Hagerman, 2008). Brain scans have shown that children who engage in movement appear to have more neural activity in the frontal areas of their brains, an important area for executive function, or the ability to complete complex tasks (Davis et al., 2007). Furthermore, physical activity has been shown to increase blood flow to the brain, which has several positive effects. Blood vessels are stimulated to grow which increases the brain's access to energy and oxygen, improving cognitive function (Ratey & Hagerman, 2008).

Another benefit to incorporating movement into the classroom is the social aspect. When children are engaged in physical activity, they practice interacting with both the environment, as well as other children. This reciprocal interaction directly assists in expression, communication, and understanding; all major components literacy (Carlsson-Paige et al., 2015). When students are proficient in different movement types they are more engaged in the physical activity (Diamond, & Lee, 2011) and this leads to quality interaction and development of key learning skills.

Movement Categories

Understanding the key aspects of movement categories helps to ensure a well-rounded approach to regularly incorporating physical activities into lessons. Movement proficiency for developing children can be grouped into four main categories.

Motor Skills

Also known as fundamental movement, motor skills include basic movements that allow children to move efficiently within their environment (Darst, Pangrazi, Brusseau, & Erwin, 2014). Most basic motor skills are identified by single verbs such as running, jumping, crawling, and twisting. Children who fully develop motor skills often have positive feelings about performing activities and gravitate towards an active lifestyle (Allender, Cowburn, & Foster, 2006).

Manipulative Skills

Often considered one of the most difficult set of movement skills to learn, manipulative activities involve the use of an implement to create movement. This category of movement is where children really develop hand-eye and foot-eye coordination and dexterity; skills that are crucial to everyday function (Darst et al., 2014). Some basic manipulative movements include catching, throwing and kicking.

Body Management Skills

In order to move efficiently, children must have adequate body management skills. Efficient movement requires a combination of agility, coordination, balance, flexibility, strength, and spatial awareness. Moving around objects or others, jumping on or off an object, chasing or fleeing are important body management skills.

Rhythmic Movement Skills

Movement tends to be rhythmic and is particularly important for young children. Rhythmic movement skills involve the ability to move gracefully and expressively. Locomotor skills are inherently rhythmic in execution, and by adding rhythm can enhance the child's ability to develop these skills (Darst et al., 2014). Rhythmic movement can be seen in everything from skipping and dribbling a ball, to creative movements such as dances and musical games.

Student-Centered Classroom

Incorporating movement during learning tasks is a natural process of learning that is often neglected in the traditional classroom (Brown, 2009; Goodlad, 2004; Hirsh-Pasek et al., 2008). The teacher-centered approach operates with the belief that a well-managed classroom includes students sitting at their seats working quietly (Stuart & Thurlow, 2000; Wright, 2011). In this setting, the teacher is constantly working against nature and students' natural desire to move (Ratey & Hagerman, 2008). Common examples that illustrate students' need to move include ongoing requests to sharpen a pencil, throw away trash, get a tissue, or use the restroom. Once one student is successful in his or her attempt at getting up to move, the teacher is often faced with several more students wanting to complete the same task. When children see an opportunity to get up and move, they will take it.

It has been well established that most students are kinesthetic learners (Jensen, 2008), or learn best by doing. In the opening example, the students are able to physically work through the activity by coming up with ways to solve the problems.

The group of students in the 'Cross the River' station must hop across the rocks (e.g. piece of paper with a number written on it) using a number flash card they grab from a pile sitting on the table. The other group members help by counting out load with the student who is hopping across the rocks. When all of the group members get across the river using correct addition, they have completed the challenge.

Teachers want to feel in control of their classrooms; which is a natural and appropriate expectation. The problem is how this control is achieved. Researchers have repeatedly found that students respond better to hands-on lessons and show increased achievement results with student-centered activities (Carlsson-Paige et al., 2015: Favre, 2007). When students are engaged in the learning process, behavior problems decrease (Favre, 2007; Nussbaum, 2010). Engagement in a lesson also means that more information is reaching the students' brains; resulting in optimal learning (Willis, 2007). Having an understanding of key concepts and considerations can make incorporating movement into the classroom a manageable and rewarding process.

Integrating Movement into the Classroom

The process of including movement should be thoroughly understood in order for it to be successful. First, the primary reason to include physical activity into a lesson is to enhance learning, and not having fun. Though having fun is important for optimal engagement, it is not the main reason for the inclusion. An activity that is fun but has little or no educational component lacks focus and meaning. Giving the students a break from learning to play a fun game is important, but is not the focus of this chapter.

The activity selected should be directly related to the content of the lesson. Having this strong connection between the content and the activity makes it easier to keep students focused on learning and allows for a more seamless integration of the activity component. When students can experience what they are being taught, they are better able to retain that information (Jensen, 2008).

The students at the 'Target Practice' game must stand behind a line marked on the floor and throw a slightly damp sponge at a numbered target drawn on the chalkboard. When the sponge hits the board, it makes a wet mark inside a numbered ring (i.e. 1, 2, 3, 4) on the target. Every time a student hits the target, the group adds that number to their score. They must write down each number that is hit as well as the final sum score. They record their work station packets that the teacher will collect at the end of the lesson. The students are assessed on their completed packets to determine their understanding of counting and adding single-digit numbers.

Organizational Considerations

In order to be successful, organizational considerations need to be considered before integrating physical activities into a lesson. Prior planning is essential to the success of any activity. An attempt to include a physical activity component into a lesson without prior planning often results in a poor learning experience, off-task students, and a very frustrated teacher. When this happens, teachers are more reluctant to include physical activity into their class (Williams, & Coles, 2007). Taking time for proper planning and considerations can make integrating movement a natural part of the classroom environment.

Instructional Cues

One of the most important factors to consider with any lesson is how to transition the students into and out of an activity as efficiently as possible. Transitioning to and from a physical activity can be challenging due to the multiple steps involved and the fact that students are out of their seats and moving around the room.

An effective strategy that helps get students to start and stop naturally is through the use of environmental cues (i.e. starting and stopping music, ringing a small bell, etc.…). Environmental cues are very effective when they are used consistently and for the same purpose (Fisher, & Frey, 2013). The teacher can also give verbal cues, however environmental cues are distinctly different than the teacher's voice, that the students hear all day, and may be more effective at gaining students' attention.

Table 5.1 Instructional cues using "*When Before the What*" statements

"Alright class, **when** I say rabbit, [**what**] get up and hop by your desk. **When** I say fox, [**what**] sit back down at your seat. Everyone ready...rabbit."
"**When** the music starts, you may [**what**] stand up and start dancing in your own space. **When** the music stops, quietly [**what**] go back to your seats."
"**When** the lights turn off, [**what**] move to the carpet like your favorite animal. **When** the lights turn on, [**what**] sit criss-cross applesauce on your assigned spot."
"**When** I ring the bell on my desk, quietly [**what**] walk around the room and find a word or object that begins with the letter 'S' and point at it."

Using instructional cues requires less energy to incorporate when compared to the teacher using verbal cues (e.g. constantly repeating the cues, yelling, etc....).

When the lights turn off, the students know that it is time to quietly move on to the next station. They also know that this is a time when they are not to be talking. The students are really good with following this expectation because they are interested in the game and do not want to miss out on the activity. The teacher doesn't have to say a single word during this time; the light switch does it for her.

As illustrated in the above example, the use of established starting and stopping cues is essential for proper movement integration. An effective strategy for developing strong instructional cues is by stating the *"when before the what"*. This approach lets the students know the starting and stopping cue before being told the activity. The *when* tells the students to start and stop the activity. The *what* is the activity that will occur in between the starting and stopping cues. Students are given the instructional cue before hearing about the activity. Using the scenario above, the teacher gave the instructions that included, "When I turn the lights off, quietly move to the next station".

If the instructions in the example were reversed and the activity explained before the instructional cues, "your group will go to the next station, when I turn the lights off", it is very likely that some students would have started going to the activities before the teacher even finished her sentence. Table 5.1 provides several examples of explaining the *'when before the what'* strategy.

Grouping Strategies

Another important component necessary to effectively integrate a physical activity into the lesson involves grouping strategies. Grouping strategies involve the process of assembling students into teams that are equal in size and, ideally, skill level. Depending on the activity, students may need to be with a partner or in small groups. Grouping strategies should be quick and efficient to implement; requiring little down time to complete.

One effective grouping strategy involves setting the desks or tables in a way that groups the students before they even arrive to the classroom. If an activity requires students to be in small groups, arrange the desks so the grouping is done without taking time away from instruction. If a group is not working out due to behavior issues or skill level, the teacher can just switch a desk or two amongst the groups. The biggest consideration to this strategy is the prior planning and effort from the teacher before the students arrive.

For a quick grouping strategy that does not require much preparation involves the use of tangible items. Using different colored popsicle sticks or a deck of playing cards are examples of tangible items that can be used. The teacher just needs to ensure that the items being passed out matches the intended number of groups that need to be formed. For instance, if the activity requires groups of four, use a deck of cards and pass out the face cards (i.e. king, queen, jack), giving each student one card. All of the students who have similar cards are assigned to a group.

Prior to the start of the station activity, the teacher handed each student a colored popsicle stick. She then instructed each student with a blue stick to start working at station #1, red at station #2, green at station #3, and orange at station #4. This resulted in there being 3–4 students grouped at each station. While calling each color, the teacher stood at the assigned station to collect the popsicle sticks. This ensured that each student was in the correct spot and it removed the sticks from the students since they were no longer needed.

The biggest consideration to this method is counting out the required items ahead of time. It is crucial that the items being passed out equals the grouping needs. For example, if using a deck of cards to place students into groups of four, only pass out enough cards- with four-of-a-kind matches- that equal the total number of students in the class.

There is one last type of grouping strategy that is quick, easy, and gets the students up and moving. This strategy uses starting and stopping cues (i.e. music, lights on/off, etc.…) and is similar to musical chairs. When the teacher gives the starting cue, the students move around the room. When the teacher gives the stopping cue, the students quickly stand by other peers; making a quick group. To change it up, have the students stand touching body parts (i.e. elbows, shoulders, feet, etc.…) with their peers.

The instructional cues for this grouping strategy might include the teacher saying; "When the music starts, [what] quietly walk around the room not touching anyone or anything. When the music stops, you will [what] touch toes with two students near you. Ready, begin…". Once the music stops and the groups appear like they will work, move on to the activity. If certain groups will not work well due to behavior or ability concerns, play another round instructing the students to touch toes with two different peers.

When grouping students, prior planning is crucial. Not only to ensure that the correct number of groups are formed, but also to ensure the groups are even. One potential challenge is when there are uneven numbers of students. For instance, if the teacher wants to include a relay race during the lesson, the teams need to be even in numbers. If one team has five students and the rest of the teams have four, the group with five in it would struggle to ever win the race due to having an extra student. A simple fix would be to make the first person in each of the four student teams go twice; evening out the relay.

Most classroom activities can be easily adapted, or are unaffected, to meet the challenge of uneven groups. However, since every activity is different and the outcomes vary based on the task, prior planning in the area of grouping strategies is important to help manage the success of integrating a physical activity into the lesson.

Space and Body Awareness

Another planning strategy that can help with the successful integration of an activity is space and body awareness. Young children are continuing to learn about their body movement, making it more difficult to travel around in a confined space. Students run into each other or tripping over the corner of a rug are common examples that illustrate this point. To minimize these situations, a teacher should plan accordingly based on the number of students and the amount of available space.

If space is limited or there are numerous objects throughout the area (i.e. desks and chairs) several options can be considered. If available, students can be taken to a larger, more open space such as outside, in the hallway, or to a multipurpose room. Furthermore, the classroom can be reconfigured to include an open space for movement activities. When the above options have been exhausted, the teacher can control movement by restricting the number of students who move at a time and by selecting appropriate movements for the space.

If there is not enough room for all the students to move at the same time, limiting how many students move at once is an option. For example, if the space has enough room to accommodate half of the students moving, the teacher can split the class in half and allow only one group to complete the activity at a time. Or if less than half of the class can be accommodated by the limited space, use small groups of students; only allowing one group to complete the activity at a time. Instructional cues for limiting the number of students who move might include the teacher saying, "When I say GO, if you are wearing a blue I want you to skip up to the board and grab a lowercase letter and bring it to your seat." This structure limits the number of students who are moving in a confined space at the same time. Having to restrict the movement to only a few students at a time does require extra time, but is important to ensure that the activity is safely completed.

The stations used during the activity were spaced around the room to spread the students out. The 'Cross the River' station needed the most physical space so it was set up on the large circle carpet area. The 'Target Practice' station used the chalkboard so it was in the front of the room at the board. The 'Roll the Dice' station was set up in the area where the students hang their coats and bags. This was plenty of space since the students were just standing and rolling two large foam dice and adding those numbers. Since there was no more space for another movement activity, the last station was at the reading table. Here, students sat and completed a worksheet that was part of their station packets.

Assessment

As outlined earlier in this chapter, the primary reason for incorporating physical activity is to enhance learning. In order to determine if an activity was educational or not, student knowledge needs to be assessed. Assessment through physical activity can be tangible (i.e. gathering items that start with the 'I' sound), observational (i.e. all of the students acted out the main character's feelings when hearing the word "outraged" during the text read aloud), or both.

One of the easiest ways to assess student knowledge is through the outcome of an activity. Having the students physically demonstrate their knowledge is a major component of physical literacy. In the traditional classroom, assessment is conducted primarily through written work such as worksheets and quizzes; making assessment very concrete, and easy to manage. Assessing students through physical literacy skills can be just as easy if proper planning is invested.

The key to managing assessment during a physical activity starts with a well written, measurable objective. A strong objective spells out both the content being assessed, as well as the criteria that determine student success.

At the end of the station activity, the student's turn in their completed packets. The packets are basically math worksheets that they would normally complete at their seats. The only real change is that the students generated their own numbers to practice instead of using the ones on a typical worksheet [see Fig. 5.1 for an example station sheet]. *The packets are graded the same as standard practice worksheets. The students are assessed on how many addition problems they answered correctly.*

Assessing the product of an activity is a convenient way to measure student learning. Collecting a tangible artifact as part of a physical activity is very similar to grading worksheets and exams. Table 5.2 provides physical activities that have measurable outcomes and are aligned to Common Core academic standards. In these examples, the students either complete the components correctly or not; making assessment of physical activities more concrete and manageable.

Summary

With any well implemented lesson, prior planning is imperative for success. This includes selecting developmentally appropriate content, transitioning efficiently throughout the lesson, and assessing student knowledge of the content. When these components of a lesson are addressed, the inclusion of physical activity can easily become part of the daily routine.

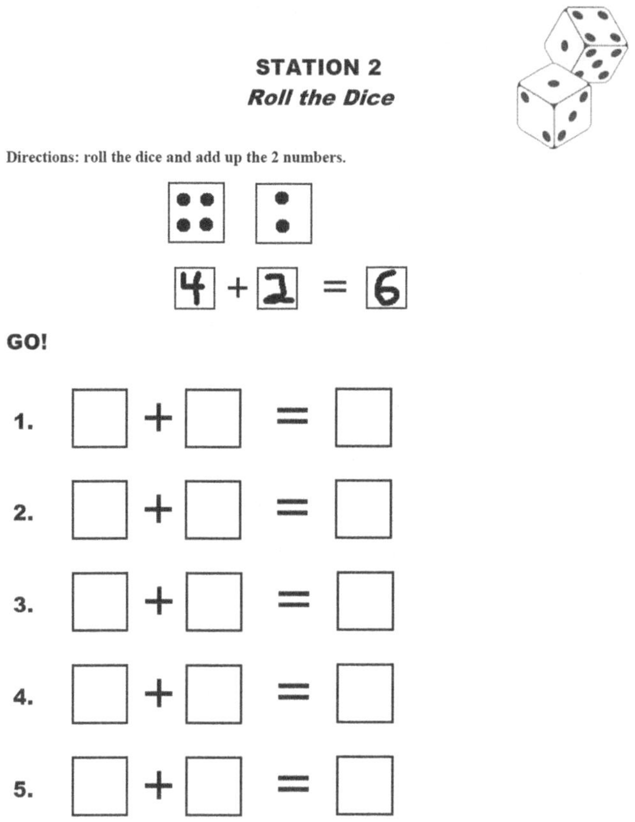
STATION 2
Roll the Dice

Directions: roll the dice and add up the 2 numbers.

4 + 2 = 6

GO!

1. □ + □ = □
2. □ + □ = □
3. □ + □ = □
4. □ + □ = □
5. □ + □ = □

Fig. 5.1 Activity station sheet where students roll two large foam dice to generate addition problems to solve

In the opening scenario, the students are provided with the opportunity to express themselves and interact with one another through planned physical activity; allowing them to demonstrate knowledge, skills, and understanding through movement. The students were provided with (1) clear expectations and instructional cues, (2) the resources necessary to be successful, and (3) measurable learning outcomes. When lessons include those elements, and learning becomes more transparent to the students, they are better able to reach their fullest potential. Teachers who create this type of atmosphere have highly motivated students who are fully engaged in the learning process.

Table 5.2 Sample activities aligned to common core standards

Activity	Objective and Assessment	Common Core Academic Standard
Spelling dash: Place the students into small groups of 3–4 students. Give each group a set of letter flash cards (one letter per card). Verbally assign each group 5 different spelling words they are learning.	**Objective**: In small groups, the students will be able to correctly spell all 5 of their assigned spelling words with no assistance from the teacher.	**CCSS.ELA-Literacy.RF.K.1.c** Understand that words are separated by spaces in print.
One group member at a time takes a letter from their assigned word and sticks it on a wall (bulletin board, sticky board, etc.…). This continues until each group has spelled all 5 of their assigned words.	**Assessment**: Looking at the board of student spelled words, all groups spelled their words correctly (including the use of correct spacing between the words) except one group who miss-spelled one of their words (4 out of 5 correct).	**CCSS.ELA-Literacy.RF.K.1.d** Recognize and name all upper- and lowercase letters of the alphabet.
At the end of the activity, all of the weekly vocabulary words will be displayed in the classroom.	Complete this activity each day, assigning different vocabulary words to each group; ensuring that each group attempts all of the words.	
Word detectives: Group students in pairs and assign a simple rhyming word (i.e. cat, dog, bee). Using stickers (post-it notes with their names on it), the students must go around the classroom (or school if appropriate) looking for items that rhyme with their assigned word.	**Objective**: The students will be able to correctly identify two words that rhyme when given an assigned word from the teacher.	**CCSS.ELA-Literacy.RF.K.2.a** Recognize and produce rhyming words.
The teacher must ensure that each assigned word has different rhyming options available to the students. This can be as simple as placing pictures or objects around the room. For example, if assigning the word *bee*, have pictures placed around the room of items such as tea, knee, flea, etc.…	**Assessment**: Comparing the each groups assigned word with their selected objects (indicated by their post-it notes), the teacher identified that all but 2 groups were able to find two words that rhymed with their assigned word. Those 2 groups could only find one word each.	**CCSS.ELA-Literacy.RF.K.2** Demonstrate understanding of spoken words, syllables, and sounds (phonemes).
	Have the rest of the class see if they can help those two groups find another rhyming word.	

Stepping into the story: During storytime, have students act out parts of a story they are reading (i.e. main characters, settings, emotions, etc.…). The easiest way to incorporate this activity is by choose stories that encourage movement.	**Objective**: The students will be able to answer questions about the main characters by physically demonstrating actions and emotions as presented during the text read aloud with 100% accuracy.	**CCSS.ELA-Literacy.RL.1.3** describe characters, settings, and major events in a story, using key details.
	Assessment: During the text read aloud, all of the students were able to identify words that suggest feelings and actions of select characters 100% of the time they were asked by the teacher.	**CCSS.ELA-Literacy.RL.1.4** identify words and phrases in stories or poems that suggest feelings or appeal to the senses.
Suggested titles include:	For older students, wait until after reading several pages or the entire story before having students identify parts of the story to encourage reading comprehension skills and memory recall.	**CCSS.ELA-Literacy.SL.K.2** Confirm understanding of a text read aloud…by asking and answering questions about key details.
From Head to Toe by Eric Carle		
Fast and Slow: An Animal Opposites by Lisa Bullard and Gail Smith		

References

Allender, S., Cowburn, G., & Foster, C. (2006). Understanding participation in sport and physical activity among children and adults: A re-view of qualitative studies. *Health Education Research, 21*(6), 826–835.

Almond, L., & Whitehead, M. E. (2012). Physical literacy: Clarifying the nature of the concept. *Physical Education Matters, 7*(1), 68–71.

Brown, S. L. (2009). *Play: How it shapes the brain, opens the imagination, and invigorates the soul*. New York: Penguin Books.

Carlsson-Paige, N., McLaughlin, G. B., & Almon, J. W. (2015). *Reading instruction in kindergarten: Little to gain and much to lose*. Retrieved from www.allianceforchildhood.org/sites/allianceforchildhood.org/files/file/Reading_Instruction_in_Kindergarten.pdf

Curwen, M., Miller, R., White-Smith, K. A., & Calfee, R. C. (2010). Increasing teachers' metacognition develops students' higher learning during content area literacy instruction: Findings from the read-write cycle project. *Issues in Teacher Education, 19*(2), 127–151.

Daggett, S. (2010). Physical education and literacy: The odd couple or a match made in heaven. *Educator's Voice, 3*, 42–49.

Darst, P. W., Pangrazi, R. P., Brusseau, T., Jr., & Erwin, H. (2014). *Dynamic physical education for secondary school students*. San Francisco: Benjamin Cummings.

Davis, C., Tomporowski, P., Boyle, C., Waller, J., Miller, P., Naglieri, J., & Gregoski, M. (2007). Effects of aerobic exercise on overweight children's cognitive functioning: A randomized controlled trial. *Research Quarterly of Exercise and Sport, 78*(5), 510–519.

Diamond, A., & Lee, K. (2011). Interventions shown to aid executive function development in children 4–12 years old. *Science, 333*(6045), 959–964.

Favre, L. R. (2007). Analysis of the transformation of a low socioeconomic status African-American, New Orleans elementary facility into a demonstration learning-style school of excellence. *Journal of Urban Education: Focus on Enrichment, 4*(1), 79–90.

Fisher, D., & Frey, N. (2013). *Better learning through structured teaching: A framework for the gradual release of responsibility*. ASCD: Aexandria, VA.

Fitzsimmons, P., & Lanphar, E. (2011). When there's love inside there's a reason why: Emotion as the core of authentic learning in one middle school classroom. Australian Journal of Language & Literacy, 34(2), 35–40.

Goodlad, J. I. (2004). *A place called school: Prospects for the future*. McGraw-Hil: New York.

Hay, I., Elias, G., & Booker, G. (2006). Students with learning difficulties in relation to literacy and numeracy. *The Australian Government Department of Education, Science and Training*. Retrieved from www.dest.gov.au/sectors/school_education/publications_resources/schooling_issues_digest/schooling_issues_digest_learning_difficulties.htm#1

Hirsh-Pasek, K., Golinkoff, R. M., Berk, L. E., & Singer, D. (2008). *A mandate for playful learning in preschool: Applying the scientific evidence*. New York: Oxford University Press.

Jensen, E. (2008). A fresh look at brain based education. *Phi Delta Kappan, 89*(6), 408–417.

Mahar, M. T., Murphy, S. K., Rowe, D. A., Golden, J., Shields, A. T., & Raedeke, T. D. (2006). Effects of a classroom-based program on physical activity and on-task behavior. *Medicine & Science in Sports Exercise, 38*(12), 2086–2094.

McDermott, P. A., Mordell, M., & Stoltzfus, J. C. (2001). The organization of student performance in American schools: Discipline, motivation, verbal, learning, nonverbal learning. *Journal of Educational Psychology, 93*, 65–76.

Nussbaum, S. S. (2010). *The effects of "Brain Gym" as a general education intervention: Improving academic performance and behaviors*. (Doctoral dissertation). Available from ProQuest Dissertations and Thesis database. (UMI No. 3411166).

Ratey, J. J., & Hagerman, E. (2008). *Spark – The revolutionary new science of exercise and the brain*. Little Brown and Company: New York.

Stuart, C., & Thurlow, D. (2000). Making it their own: Pre-service teachers' experiences, beliefs and classroom practices. *Journal of Teacher Education, 51*, 113–121.

UNESCO Education Sector. (2004). *The plurality of literacy and its implications for policies and programs: Position paper*. Paris: United National Educational, Scientific and Cultural Organization.

Wachob, D. (2015). Teacher beliefs about learning and their instructional practices: Discrepancies in the classroom. *The International Journal of Pedagogy and Curriculum.*, *22*(3), 27–36.

Williams, D., & Coles, L. (2007). Teachers' approaches to finding and using research evidence: An information literacy perspective. *Educational Research, 49*(2), 185–206.

Willis, J. (2007). Cooperative learning is a brain turn-on. *Middle School Journal, 38*(4), 4–13.

Wright, G. B. (2011). Student-centered learning in higher education. *International Journal of Teaching and Learning in Higher Education, 23*(1), 92–97.

Yair, G. (2000). Reforming motivation: How the structure of instruction affects students' learning experiences. *British Educational Journal, 26*, 191–210.

Yazzie-Mintz, E. (2010). *Charting the path from engagement to achievement: A Report on the 2009 high school survey of student engagement*. Retrieved from http://ceep.indiana.edu/hssse

David A. Wachob has been teaching for over 10 years and has taught physical education at all levels. He has conducted research and workshops on promoting physical activity in traditional classrooms. He has also published in peer-reviewed journals and presented at national conferences on topics related to physical literacy.

Part II
Evidence-Based Teaching Strategies that Promote Physical Activity and Health During Early Childhood

Chapter 6
Using Interactive Video Games to Enhance Physical Activity Among Children

Jennifer L. Rudella and Jennifer V. Butz

Introduction

Currently, children spend an average of seven hours every day on entertainment media including televisions, computers, and other electronic devices (American Academy of Pediatrics, 2015). Specifically, children between the ages of two and eight spend an average of two hours a day with screen media, such as video games (Common Sense Media, 2013). It is recommended that children engage in less than two hours of leisure screen time daily (American Academy of Pediatrics, 2013; National Heart, Lung, and Blood Institute, 2012). Furthermore, children should engage in at least 60 minutes of moderate to vigorous physical activity every day (World Health Organization, 2016). If children do not meet this recommendation, they are at a greater risk for chronic diseases including high blood pressure, high cholesterol, and obesity (Centers for Disease Control and Prevention, 2012). Nonsedentary activities associated with screen time are one way of addressing such concerns. Gaming consoles, such as the Nintendo Wii and Xbox, created a way to help children utilize their use of screen time to be more engaging through physical activity and can now be used in home and school settings.

Interactive video games, referred to as exergames, require physical movement to participate in the game. There are a variety of game play movements such as dancing, aerobics, and virtual personal trainer exercises. Actions are recorded using

J. L. Rudella (✉)
Department of Health Science, Lock Haven University of Pennsylvania,
Lock Haven, PA, USA
e-mail: jlr1147@lockhaven.edu

J. V. Butz
Department of Health and Physical Education, Northern Lehigh School District,
Slatington, PA, USA
e-mail: jbutz@nlsd.org

H. Brewer, M. R. Jalongo (eds.), *Physical Activity and Health Promotion in the Early Years*, Educating the Young Child 14,
https://doi.org/10.1007/978-3-319-76006-3_6

a device that is connected to the video game console which provides individual feedback and scores. Some examples of how physical movements are recognized include a hand held device, dance pads, and cameras but vary based on the game and console. Exergames have been around for over a decade and the history of exergames began as an arcade game.

One of the first exergames, *Dance Dance Revolution*, started out in arcades. The popularity of this game showed that individuals were interested in playing video games that required whole body movement. The transfer of these games into home and school settings seemed expected, but not a first. The hefty price of the consoles made it nearly impossible to incorporate the concept of exergaming anywhere else except arcades. For many, it was not until more affordable versions were created that exergaming became popular outside of arcades, particularly for children.

Children can participate in exergames while increasing enjoyment, motivation, physical activity, gross motor skill ability, and academic performance. Children are motivated because they enjoy participating in the variety of activities exergames provide (Gao, Chen, & Stodden, 2015; Sun, 2012, 2013). The Just Dance series consists of at least 25 songs per game, including popular songs in which children are familiar. The Nintendo *Wii Fit* consists of four categories, such as yoga, and each category offers several activities to select. Furthermore, children are motivated because they can create a personalized avatar (Li, Lwin, & Jung, 2014). These avatars can look like the player or whomever the player wishes their avatar to look like. Interactive video games have the potential to increase heart rate levels up to a moderate to vigorous physical activity workout (Adkins et al., 2013; Gao, Zhang, & Podlog, 2014; George, Rohr, & Byrne, 2016). One study found that children spent more time participating in exergames than physical education (Gao et al., 2015). Even though exergames increase physical activity, children also have the potential to gain motor skill improvement. Recently, a study concluded that early elementary students in Greece experienced object control skill improvement after participating in Xbox Kinect exergames (Vernadakis, Papastergiou, Zetou, & Antoniou, 2015). Children also have health-related fitness and academic performance benefits. Gao (2013) suggested that children's one mile run, math standardized testing, and body mass index scores improved after participating in *Dance Dance Revolution*. In short, when children participate in exergames, they may experience physical and cognitive improvements.

Educators can choose appropriate exergames for their classroom and create a safe environment where students enjoy participating in physical activity. There are an abundance of exergames and gaming consoles at a variety of prices on the market, many of which are more affordable than the initial high prices from a decade ago. Selecting the best game and gaming console can be overwhelming. Once this decision has been made, the next challenge is how to effectively implement exergames and increase physical activity. Specifically, a holistic manner is an effective methods for implementation to meet objectives (Hong, Tsai, Ho, Hwang, & Wu, 2013). Strategies for creating a safe environment while implementing a holistic approach to exergames need to be considered to meet the needs of the children. It is important to find the exergame or exergames that are suitable for leaners and determine the best practices for an enjoyable experience while meeting classroom objectives.

This chapter explains the benefits of using exergames including enjoyment, motivation, increasing physical activity, and implementation of exergames. The exergames that will be discussed are *Dance Dance Revolution, Nintendo Wii Fit, Just Dance,* and *Zumba*. Each exergame section includes instruction, classroom setup, assessment, and cost. Heart rate monitors and pedometers can be utilized in each of these exergames which will also be presented. By the end of this chapter, educators can make decisions for effective implementation of exergames to increase physical activity within their own setting.

Dance Dance Revolution

Dance Dance Revolution is often thought of as the foundation of exergaming in the physical education setting. This is mainly because of the increased interest in the dance vision that began in the early millennium. The idea of moving the entire body to control a video game was a welcome and refreshing change.

Dance Dance Revolution is a dance-based exergame where the player matches their movements to the arrows on the screen that correspond with the beat of the song. Arrows scroll up the screen so players can see upcoming movements. The player is to perform the arrow movement when the arrow reaches the highlighted part of the screen. Their movements are recorded using a connected mat that calculates if the player not only placed their foot at the correct time but on the correct arrows on the mat. The difficulty levels can be changed according to ability. The beginner versions may simply use two different arrow movements. The more advanced setting uses eight different arrows with some arrows needing to be activated simultaneously. Music varies from songs made specifically for *Dance Dance Revolution*, to that of popular culture, to Disney songs depending of the game version being played. While participating in *Dance Dance Revolution*, children can engage in a moderate to vigorous level of physical activity (Adkins et al., 2013; Gao, Huang, Liu, & Xiong, 2012; Graf, Pratt, Hester, & Short, 2009). Not only do children increase physical activity, but the amount of sedentary screen time significantly decreases (Maloney et al., 2008). *Dance Dance Revolution* is available on the Wii and Wii U systems from Nintendo, Kinect for Xbox 360 and Xbox One, and PlayStation Move for PlayStation 3 and PlayStation 4. There are also computer-based versions as well as television plug and play systems.

Classroom Setup

Most of the arcade version game consoles allow only two dance pads to be connected at once, while several of the home versions allows for up to four dance pads to be connected simultaneously. Since between two to four students can dance at a time, a station format works best for upper elementary students and working in groups provides a more holistic environment (Rudella & Butz, 2015; Hong et al., 2013). Depending on equipment, children can break into groups of four if using the two pad version, and groups no larger than eight for the four pad version. Some students will use the dance pads connected to the console, while the others practice on the unconnected pads. Once the song is over, students on connected dance pads can record their scores and move to the practice pad. If students are too young to record their own scores, adult assistance can be offered as needed. Students on the practice pads will then move to the scoring pads. This activity allows for students to be physically active and engaged while other assessments, such as fitness testing, can be conducted (Rudella & Butz, 2015). This is a great mobile activity that can easily be moved into a classroom or small space. The difficulty level of each song can also be changed to accommodate ability level by choosing settings from "beginner" through "challenge," allowing all students to participate (Rudella & Butz, 2015).

Instruction

Dance Dance Revolution instruction is dependent on the age group. Primary students should begin practicing the rhythm of the dance movements. This can be done by marching and clapping with the beat of a "beginner" level song (Rudella & Butz, 2015). Arrow movements can be explained followed by having children perform a stomp in accordance to the arrows on the screen (Rudella & Butz, 2015). When the students appear to be ready to move forward, they can begin using the dance pad arrows to move along with the song (Rudella & Butz, 2015). Children need to tap the correct arrows on the pad in accordance to the arrows on the screen. With continued practice pads, the difficulty level can be increased as experience and familiarity increases. As children continue to be more comfortable with the dances, students can become the leaders of the class. The leaders will be on the connected dance pads to demonstrate the dance. It is important to be mindful and allow all students the chance to be leaders. Children can lead the song from beginning to end, or they can rotate during the song being sure to pause the game if there is a large class size. The game also incorporates arm movements, however, it is recommended to provide this as a challenge to the students as their coordination is still developing and it may be difficult to focus on their feet and arms simultaneously.

Assessment

Student performance can be assessed by documenting the dance difficulty level, final score, pedometers, and heart rate monitors. These scores could be used as a form of formative and summative assessment. It is important to note that the score given at the end of the dance does not assess student's ability to dance, and therefore, should be used as formative assessment (Rudella & Butz, 2015). Summative assessment can include keeping track of pedometer and heart rate scores as these results are an effective tool for measuring physical activity (Rudella & Butz, 2015). To maintain student interest and motivation, a tournament dance off can be implemented where teams of students compete against others for the highest scores from the game, pedometer, and heart rate monitor. This could be done as a collective team score where the sum of the teammates is the score for the team. Or, it could simply be the person that scores the highest would advance. Teams with higher scores would continue advancing through the tournament with one team being eliminated at the completion of each song. Remind students that it is a friendly competition and reiterate good sportsmanship.

Cost

The game itself averages approximately $20, with the each new dance pad averaging about $30. Used versions of the dance pads can be purchased online. In some cases, additional dance pads need to be purchased to have four players dancing at once. These vary depending on if the home version or arcade versions of the pads are purchased. Practice pads come at an additional cost of $22. Practice pads do not necessarily have to be the costly ones from the manufacturer. They can be anything from old or unattached dance pads to old linoleum samples. New technology allows for an entire class to play the game at once using wireless dance pads. Each pad keeps score and at the end of the song, tops scorers are visually announced. This comes at a cost of $47,850 for a set 24 (US Games, 2016). However, in many situations, this price is not a feasible option without the assistance of grants or outside funding. A big cost saving measure that some schools have utilized involves a *Dance Dance Revolution* PowerPoint. Students would dance on practice pads while a PowerPoint presentation with arrows appear on a screen along with music. This is another cost saving measure but does not keep track of movement and scores like traditional exergames.

Wii Fit

The Nintendo *Wii Fit* consists of a variety of different games and incorporates all five components of health-related fitness; flexibility, body composition, muscular strength, muscular endurance, and cardiovascular endurance. Versions of Wii Fit include *Wii Fit*, *Wii Fit Plus*, *Nickelodeon Fi*t, and *Wii Fit U*. The *Nickelodeon Fit* includes characters children are familiar with including Dora, Diego, Kai-lan and The Backyardigans and consists of 30 exercise games. Children who participate in the *Wii Fit* activities can achieve a moderate intensity level and have positive benefits including an increased heart rate, accelerometer counts, and perceived exertion (Gao et al., 2015; O'Donovan, Roche, & Hussey, 2014; Perron, Graham, Feldman, Moffett, & Hall, 2011). For example, children from Dublin participated in the Nintendo *Wii Fit Free Jogging* activity and achieved a moderate intensity physical activity level (O'Donovan et al., 2014). Yoga, balance games, strength training, and aerobics are the categories to choose from and each includes an array of activities so children can stay motivated. Student enjoyment also increases because of the video game components and variety of activities (Gao et al., 2014). Furthermore, Sheehan and Katz (2012) found that third grade children from Canada improve postural stability when participating in the gymnastics and dance segments of the *Wii Fit* games. Profiles can be created to set goals, test balance, and track progress making it more appealing for assessment and tracking progress. With a variety of *Wii Fit* games, educators can choose the version that best fits their student's age and interests without affecting the positive benefits of exergaming.

A recent Nintendo *Wii Fit* game, called the *Wii Fit Plus,* is an extension of the *Wii Fit* and can be played on the Nintendo Wii console. This game also has a website dedicated to keeping track of the players progress, including routines and trainers, which can be visually documented on a graph using the color coded fit credits (Nintendo, 2015). There are 15 new activities added to train and increase physical activity, including Bird-Eye, Bulls-Eye, and Obstacle Course (Nintendo, 2015). These additional games maintain the interest of children by providing a variety of games in which the player can participate.

The most recent game, *Wii Fit U*, is for the Nintendo Wii U game console and has additional features including a Fit Meter device, Personal Trainer Mode, Virtual Gym Communities, and Dance Category. The Fit Meter device uses an acceleration sensor and atmospheric pressure to more accurately determine and document physical activity progress and calories burned (Ubisoft, 2015c). Each device is designed for up to 12 individual profiles so children can share the device. The Personal Training Mode allows users to customize their routines and get workout recommendations based on goal preferences (Ubisoft, 2015c). The Gym Communities is a social networking site that allows a personal gym and can be shared with other Gym Community members (Ubisoft, 2015c). The Dance Categories include salsa, hip-hop, and jazz dances (Ubisoft, 2015c). Also, children will be exposed to dances of other cultures, such as salsa, to incorporate a cross-curricular component within the lesson.

The *Wii Fit Plus* has similar options as the *Wii Fit U* include personalized exercise routines while keeping track of calories burned and performance. Recently, a Training Plus mode was added that consists of 15 new activities including obstacle courses, driving range, and island cycling (Ubisoft, 2015a, 2015b, 2015c). These activities provide children with more activity choices to increase motivation and enjoyment. The equipment needed for *Wii Fit* includes a balance board and if using the *Wii Fit U*, the balance board is essential but the Fit Meters are optional. The *Wii Fit* series is exclusively for Nintendo Wii consoles.

Classroom Setup

Since the Nintendo Wii and *Wii Fit* accessories can be costly (further explained in this chapter), one console will most likely be purchased. Therefore, a station format is a more effective classroom setting, as only one person can use the balance board at a time (Rudella & Butz, 2015). Students can be divided into small groups and allow one person to virtually play while the others follow along with the movements on the screen. Students will take turns using the balance board to track their progress, which is at the discretion of the educator. One student will use the balance board and the remaining students follow accordingly. Other stations need to be created to allow the entire class to take turns at the Nintendo *Wii Fit* station. These stations can include fitness-based exercises that utilize the health-related fitness components (Rudella & Btuz, 2015). For example, in a class of 20 students, there will be five groups of four. Stations consist of the Nintendo *Wii Fit* station, upper body exercises, lower body exercises, exercise video for cardiovascular endurance, and stretching exercises. These stations provide the opportunity for each student to utilize all health-related fitness components by the end of class.

Instruction

It is important that students understand how to use the Nintendo *Wii Fit* before using the equipment. First, the educator will explain and demonstrate how to use the *Wii Fit* including the purpose of the game, proper use of the balance board, and how to incorporate the additional purchased accessories, such as the fit meter. Children can get acclimated to the balance board and the game by taking fitness assessments that measure balance, body mass index, and body control that are quick and easy. These tests can be used to determine base levels and students retest periodically, such as every marking period to document improvement. Profiles can be created on the *Wii Fit* by grouping children of similar heights and weights. These students can share the same profile while the educator helps children keep track of their individual results separately. Children will then follow along to a chosen game, such as a *Nickelodeon Wii Fit* exercise game, while the educator uses the balance board. A simulated balance board can be added for students to use, utilizing equipment of their choice, such as aerobic steps, or they can follow along the game without using any equipment. Learners can begin participating by using lower body movements, and then add arm movements as they get better at the games. While participating in the activities, some of the moves might be difficult. To reduce this difficulty, children can focus on lower body movements. Children who are familiar with the Nintendo *Wii Fit* can volunteer to lead and can be grouped with children who are unfamiliar. By doing this, the classroom environment includes socialization and leadership opportunities.

As students become more familiar participating in the fitness activities, educators can introduce other games. Since each Nintendo *Wii Fit* game can incorporate on one or more of the five components of health-related fitness, children can participate in activities to meet specific objectives. For example, to improve flexibility, children can engage in one of the balance games for *Wii Fit Plus* or to increase cardiovascular endurance, educators can choose dance activities from the *Wii Fit U*. To meet muscular strength objectives, children can participate in the training sessions. Since there are a variety of training sessions to choose from, educators can select the sessions for the children to introduce them to the exercise. As learners become more familar, they can choose the sessions thus increasing motivation. It is important to note that only one balance board is purchased with the *Wii Fit* game which means that only one student can use it at a time. As mentioned earlier, a station format is recommended and it is important to be mindful of time and ensure each student gets an opportunity to use the balance board. Children can take turns during an activity session if there are time constraints, however, the results given at the end of the activity will not be an accurate portrayal of the individual student performance. Therefore, pedometer or heart rate monitors are recommended for individual assessment. When transitioning to the next station, music can be played and children can march or free dance on a poly spot to maintain safe distances to increase activity. Lastly, the educator should be in charge of the controller to increase activity time.

Children may find the *Wii Fit* challenging, as their gross motor skills are continuing to develop. To help children have a positive experience, some of the games need to be modified along with choosing age appropriate activities. Educators should use the controller while children participate in the activities. This allows children to focus on executing the movement rather than quality of the performed movement. First, children can imitate some of the more basic yoga poses from *Wii Fit*. The bridge, half moon, downward facing dog, and palm tree are all great poses that should not require movement modifications. Each pose can take up to five minutes to complete so students should try each pose for around 10 seconds due to short attention spans. Other yoga poses can be performed with some adjustments. The standing knee pose can be modified by having children practice lifting one leg off the ground for approximately one to two seconds. Educators can provide a folded mat or tumbling wedge to assist children with balance as needed. The chair pose can be modified by having students practice sitting onto an actual chair and return to a standing position. Rather than focusing on balance, children can count the number of times they stand and sit while maintaining balance. Educators can provide a ballet bar or small table for children to hold onto to help balance as well.

The *Wii Fit U* dance segments help children with rhythm and movement while being exposed to many styles of music. The activities introduce a variety of different dances such as hula, jazz, and salsa. Educators should use the controller while children perform the modified dance movements. To introduce children to how the game is played, educators can choose the beginner dance activity. Then, children can either clap or march when introducing new dances. As children become more familiar with the tempo, educators can have them focus on upper or lower body modified movements during each dance at one time, rather than both as the dance requires. For example, children can tap their foot forward for the jazz dance and move their hips side to side for the hula dance. Dancing can be a suitable activity for children of all ages and abilities and *Wii Fit U* dance helps provide a visual of dance movements. Educators can have students focus on upper and lower body movements separately as well. Another modification would be to allow the older children to use the controller while participating in the activity; however, the educator needs to ensure they are well versed in the movements and comfortable with the music tempo. Overall, if a child has difficulty at any time, the educator can go back to the beginner dance activity which is the least challenging setting.

Assessment

When children become exposed to the *Wii Fit* games and balance board, they can participate in the fitness tests for baseline testing and utilize the Personal Training Mode to create goals. When retesting, throughout the school year, these results can be used as formative assessment. Children can be formally graded or the educator can provide informal feedback to help children understand physical activity and how their bodies respond to exercise. The Personal Training mode can be used as a form of assessment by having children set and achieve goals and revise as needed to improve their fitness. However, these goals need to be age-appropriate and realistic which may require educators to take on more of an integral role in this process. Children can be assessed on setting, achieving, and revising goals.

The *Wii Fit* games can be used to keep track of student performance. The *Wii Fit Plus* website has a section called My Wii Fit Plus that customizes and personalizes routines while recording calories and fit credits (Nintendo, 2015). As another form of assessment, children can participate in the *Wii Fit Plus* activities focusing on calorie expenditure. This will also introduce young children to numbers for a cross-curricular lesson. Children will need adult assistance logging in the calories burned for the day. Educators can assign this as an in class activity or homework. If there are large class sizes, it may be time consuming to allow every student to participate in an activity from start to finish and log scores, therefore, pedometers and heart rate monitors are highly recommended for assessment. Students can keep track of these scores as opposed to the activity scores received in the game. A step by step instruction list is recommended to send home along with the amount of calories the child expended if assigned for homework.

Cost

Cost should be considered when deciding whether to purchase new or used equipment. If purchasing the equipment brand new, the *Wii Fit* and balance board price is around $40 while the *Wii Fit U*, balance board, and Fit Meter is around $55. The Fit Meter costs around $10 each if purchased separated. To decrease this cost, equipment can be purchased on other websites, such as Amazon. The *Wii Fit U* balance board and accessories used equipment rate is around $28. The *Wii Fit Plus* with balance board used equipment price is around $25. The Nintendo Wii used starts at $36 and the Nintendo Wii U costs around $130 used which is significantly more expensive. A more cost-effective approach is for educators to bring their own Nintendo *Wii Fit* equipment from home to use at their discretion. This also allows the educator to preview the effectiveness of that specific product with their students before adding it to their budget to purchase. However, it is recommended that educators be aware their personal equipement may become damaged.

Just Dance

The premise behind the *Just Dance* Series is very similar to that of aerobic dance videos. Currently, games include *Just Dance Disney* and *Just Dance for Kids* with approximately 25 songs per game (Ubisoft Entertainment, 2015a). There are physical and emotional benefits including improvement of motor skills, particularly manual dexterity, achieving moderate to vigorous activity, and increasing motivation and enjoyment (Adkins et al., 2013; Gao et al., 2015; George et al., 2016). To play the game, the player mirrors the choreographed dance movements on the screen produced by the hologram dancer. The exergaming technology embedded in the game is what differentiates it from an instructional video. The gaming system keeps track of the number of occurrences each player performs the movements on cue. Dance level difficulty can also be altered by allowing players to choose their own level of play while moving to the same song. Some dances are group dances, which allow the students to interact with each other while performing a choreographed dance number providing a holistic experience. Songs vary from those in popular culture to songs made specifically for the game. The *Just Dance* series is compatible with the Wii and Wii U systems from Nintendo, Nintendo Switch, Kinect for Xbox 360 and Xbox One, and PlayStation Move for PlayStation 3 and PlayStation 4.

Classroom Setup

Most platforms allow for a maximum of four players dancing simultaneously. In some cases, such as with the Nintendo and PlayStation systems, players are required to hold a hand held remote. Other systems like the Xbox Kinect do not require hand held controllers, instead the players must be in visual sight of the Xbox Kinect camera. Because only four players can be connected for synced play, a station format is recommended.

It is recommended to begin separating children into groups no larger than eight per group. All students at the station, even those not synced for that song may participate in the dancing. To make this possible, all students at that station need to see the screen so unsynced players can practice the dance moves until it is their turn. Once the song is over, students who were synced can document their score and the next four students can participate. These stations keep students active and engaged during a fitness testing lesson or on a cardiovascular fitness day (Rudella & Butz, 2015).

Instruction

Instruction of the *Just Dance* activities depends on the grade level. For students at the early childhood elementary level, it would be best to start using this activity simply as a warmup to help familiarize children with the concepts (Rudella & Butz, 2015). Have students learn the dance moves in a teacher-directed chunking format (Rudella & Butz, 2015). Students will then dance along with the visual cues on the screen while the educator provides individualized support (Rudella & Butz, 2015). Students will learn how to sync up with the game console, handle the remotes, and select a song. Students can be selected to dance while synced up to the game, while other students practice the moves with their classmates. It is important to ensure proper safety and handling of the controllers and console is thoroughly explained followed by how to sync up, select difficulty levels, and appropriate songs. Once students become more familiar with the use the equipment and participation components of the game, students can volunteer to use the controllers and lead the class (Rudella & Butz, 2015). Students without controllers will dance along with the movements on the screen. Finally, educators need to allow students to select songs which increases enjoyment and ultimately increases physical activity (Rudella & Butz, 2015).

There are a few techniques that can assist in creating a positive dance experience. First, the toddler songs need to be selected in the *Just Dance Kids* series along with modifying and practicing dance moves. Then, the educator needs to use the controller and participate the dances with the children while demonstrating modifications along with verbal cues. *The Freeze Game* (*Just Dance Kids 2014*) is one great way to introduce children to imitating dance moves which can be followed by *Five Little Monkeys* (*Just Dance Kids 2*). *YMCA* would also be a great introductory dance from *Just Dance Kids 2*. When practicing the dance with children, focus on one to three movements at a time. To modify dance moves, focus on the upper or lower body movements. To keep children interested during the entire length of the dance, which are approximately two to four minutes in length, students can march, clap, or freestyle dance until the practiced dance moves are performed. Educators need to give verbal cues and demonstrate as needed to help children prepare and perform the dance moves. As children become more comfortable, additional dance movements can be added. The older children can use the controller while playing the game once they are comfortable performing the dance moves to the song. *Despicable Me* (*Just Dance Kids 2*) and *Give Your Heart A Break* (*Just Dance Kids 2014*) are popular dances and appropriate for the older children. If a child gets frustrated at any time, have them march, clap, or freestyle dance to the music and practice the corresponding dance moves without the music once again.

Assessment

Assessment can take place in a variety of ways. In the traditional sense, students can document the song, difficulty level and score. An increased difficulty level and higher gameplay score would indicate overall dancing improvement. To help encourage students, a motivational board could be put in place to help the educator note each child's achievement. Children who cannot write can receive a sticker or some type of object that can stick to the motivational board. Table 6.1 is a visual representation of the motivational tool using *Just Dance* scores.

Or, a chart can be created consisting of each student's name and colored stickers can be placed beside their name depending on how they scored. The Xbox 360 version has a "just create" feature which allows the user to create a dance challenge that other players play. This allows for assessment in a different form. By creating a rubric with required components, students can create a dance rhythm and input the created dance into Xbox 360 console Kinect. It is important students are assessed on the created dance and not their ability to follow this dance. Furthermore, the created dance assessment works best in small groups and needs an age-appropriate dance rhythm to increase the chance of success.

Table 6.1 Keeping track of student results using a motivational board

Just Dance Score – A	*Just Dance* Score – B	*Just Dance* Score – C
Students sign names or put stickers here when they score an A.	Students sign names or put stickers here when they score a B.	Students sign names or put stickers here when they score a C.

Cost

The system consoles vary in price based on memory, they range from $169 for the Xbox 4GB version to $240 for Xbox 500GB. Used and refurbished versions could always be purchased online. In some cases, additional accessories need to be purchased to have four players dancing at once. The average cost of the wireless hand held controllers is $34. The Kinect is purchased separately from the Xbox for $164. The games vary depending on the console. For example, the *Just Dance Kids 2* games for PlayStation 3 costs about $35. If these prices are too expensive for the annual budget, educators can use the internet and locate other means to utilize these exergames in their classrooms.

Cost saving measures include an internet search or sharing the equipment with other faculty. For example, YouTube allows free access to some songs including, but not limited to, *Gummy Bear, Despicable Me*, and *Five Little Monkeys (YouTube, 2015)*. This would allow the teacher to see how children respond and become more familiar with implementing the technology. These videos can introduce the *Just Dance* series to increase the amount of students who can participate in the dances at the same time. While educators would lose the exergaming scoring capability, large groups of students could dance along to the videos online. Therefore, heart rate monitors and pedometers can be used to track individual physical activity and as assessment, depending upon the teacher-created objectives. For international students, there are YouTube songs from other countries including *International Love, Loba,* and *Run the Show* available in languages other than English, such as Spanish and French. *Just Dance* has Japan and China exclusive games available to purchase as well. Another cost saving measure would be to purchase one console and exergame or exergames for the district and rotate the materials around every building. This would provide the opportunity for other faculty to try the console and see how the children respond to the games before adding it into their budget. Also, student teachers could borrow the console, with school district permission, for their classrooms.

Just Dance Now App

Just Dance Now app is from the *Just Dance* series and has many advantages to increasing physical activity in the classroom through the use of technology devices. The *Just Dance Now* app offers the *Just Dance* dances but only requires a mobile device, such as a cell phone, and a computer device, such as a laptop. Once the free app is downloaded, users need to open the app on their device and access the website on their computer device (Ubisoft Entertainment, 2015b). The connection of the website with the app is almost instantaneous, thus increasing the amount of time students spend being physically active. Educators can then project the dance from the computer for children to mimic. The app uses a mobile device instead of a controller to participate in the dances. One of the best features this app has to offer is that it has unlimited players. Therefore, as long as one mobile device has the VIP access, there is no limit to the amount of additional players as long as they have the app downloaded onto their mobile device. Students can play with each other in the classroom or users from all over the world. The connection of multiple players to the dance game is instant as well, which ultimately increases physical activity time. Educators can organize their classrooms throughout the school so students can play with or against other students from fellow classrooms of the same school or even other schools.

Instruction

A few steps can be taken to make the *Just Dance Now* app more effective in their classroom. First, the dances should be projected from the website onto a larger surface, like a smartboard, for optimum viewing. Most school districts have mobile smart boards or projectors that can easily be hooked up with a computer or laptop. Second, the cell phones are the controllers which are not safety attached to the user's wrist. It is important to ensure that children have a firm grip on their cell phones when participating in the dances. It is recommended that educators use the mobile device themselves while the children follow along to create a safer environment as children may struggle keeping the mobile device secure while performing dance movements. However, using a phone arm band may assist in keeping mobile devices secure. Secondly, educators need to make sure students have enough space in the classroom and from each other to safely participate. Poly spots are a great way for students to maintain this space or floor tape can be used to write "X"s. Finally, the app does not include dance level difficulty so educators need to participate in the dances and create a list of songs to match the ability-level of the children. A list can be created in the favorites section of the app to organize and easily access the songs, increasing the amount of time students are physically active. Age appropriate songs for younger children include *Alphabet Song, The Lion Sleeps Tonight,* and *Mary Had A Little Lamb. Jingle Bells, Hickory Dickory Dock, I Like to Move It,* and *We Go Well Together* may be more age appropriate for children later in early childhood. The *Just Dance Now* App website contains a list of *Just Dance Kids* songs and explains how some of the moves are performed. Educators can utilize the same methods for teaching dance movements in the *Just Dance* instruction section including modifying dance movements, teaching one to three dance moves at a time, demonstrations, and verbal cues.

Assessment

This app can be used as various forms of assessment. Children are able to sync their scores after each dance to their own health apps. For example, if a student has an iPhone, the app has the option of sending the activity to the health app which tracks physical activity. This would be an effective form of personal assessment although a barrier to this approach is that it would require the child to have his or her own iPhone. Another form of assessment requires students to wear a pedometer and keep track of the number of steps taken after each song. Children can also wear a heart rate monitor to track heart rate levels from each dance which can be taken before, in the middle, and at the end of the dance to show the different heart rate levels. Children can learn which dances increase their heart rates and begin to understand the concept of exercise intensity. It is important to be aware that even though the dance app gives a score at the end of the dance, it should not be used as a formal assessment because the score does not reflect the user's ability to dance effectively. However, educators can use student scores to increase motivation by having students write their names, or place stickers, on the motivational board for their scores using the same method mentioned in the Just Dance assessment section.

Cost

The *Just Dance Now* app is a less expensive avenue when compared to the cost of purchasing game consoles, such as the Nintendo Wii, and the *Just Dance* games. Downloading the app is free, however, only one free song is available. There are over 300 available songs currently, this number continues to increase with each update of the app. These songs can be purchased "in app", with the option of purchasing access to all songs or purchasing songs individually. The price for VIP access is $29.99 per year which includes all songs without advertisements. If this price is too expensive, a monthly pass can be purchased for $4.99. Another alternative is to purchase the songs for 3 months, which costs $12.99. This price is still less expensive when compared to purchasing a Nintendo Wii console and *Just Dance* games. In order to participate in the dances, the mobile device is synced with a computer device. A computer device is most likely located in every classroom and educators can choose a mobile device to download the app. Therefore, the cost is only for the downloading of a 1 year, 1 month, or 1 week subscription depending upon funding and discretion of the educator. Regardless of which avenue is chosen to purchase the game console and accessories or the app, children can participate in multiple dances to increase physical activity in the classroom.

Zumba

Zumba is a dance workout that has influences from many different cultures and dance styles. *Zumba Fitness* is an exergaming dance series that consists of actual choreographed *Zumba* dances, without needing to attend a face-to-face class. The Latin music can motivate students and larger classes can participate as students do not need equipment to participate (Toscano, Ladda, & Bednarz, 2014). Physical activity level increases to enhance cardiovascular fitness while increasing physical competence in the practice mode (Martin, Ameluxen-Coleman, & Heinrichs, 2015). Like other traditional exergames, the player follows along with the movement of the hologram on the screen. The system keeps track of the movements that were performed correctly and at the appropriate time. Many of the movements and songs are simular to those included in a traditional *Zumba* class. Difficulty levels for this game cannot be customized. Instead, different songs are rated at different difficulty levels. All players can dance to the same difficulty level assigned to that song. *Zumba Fitness* is available on many consoles including the Wii, Kinect for Xbox 360 and PlayStation Move Motion Controller. There are also iPad versions of the game available.

Classroom Setup

The classroom setup is similar to *Just Dance*. Between two and four players can sync at a time depending on the game console. With *Zumba Fitness*, larger groups could play this game together because of the nature of the dancing. Children can be divided into groups of up to 12. Have students sync to the game while the other students are in a place where they can visually see the screen. After the song is over, children switch positions so another group of students can be synced to the game. Students at other stations could be participating in other cardiovascular activities, such as jogging or jumping rope. Another station idea would consist of students engaging in step aerobics or yoga. This would also work great for fitness assessment activities.

Instruction

Educators need to practice the *Zumba* dances before implementing them in the classroom and slowly introduce the *Zumba* dance moves to children for effective implementation. The educator would first introduce the dance movement combinations to the class. After some practice, the educator would lead the class through the whole dance by connecting segmented movement combinations. Students will then practice dancing along to the song by matching their movements to the images on the screen. This will be completed on the beginner level but at a regular tempo. After children are familiar with the dances, they can take turns leading the class by using the Quick Play option. This allows only one song to be played at a time, rather than having a block of songs play for a specific period of time like during Full Party play. As students improve on the dances, the difficulty level of the song choice can be increased. One way of differentiating instruction is by selecting student leaders to dance at different levels; beginner, intermediate, and advance. Children can then be placed based on their ability level while providing an opportunity for individual instruction as needed. Eventually, children will be able to practice with their other classmates with minimal remediation and enrichment instruction.

Some caution needs used when selecting an appropriate *Zumba* game version for the elementary age group. Not all version of the game are rated "E", which is appropriate rating for students age six and over. *Zumba Fitness: Join the Party, Zumba Fitness: World Party*, and *Zumba Kids* were all awarded the "E" rating. This rating ensures that the music will be age appropriate and dance movement patterns are acceptable for younger students.

Assessment

Student performance based assessment can be done through a variety of assessment means. By simply documenting the child's dance score and difficulty" level for the selected song, improvement can be monitored. The scores and difficulty levels can also serve as a form of formative and summative assessment for a dance or cardiovascular fitness unit. Improvement of both score and difficulty level would indicate that a student has improved. The learner's dance ability is not formally assessed through the final score given by the game. Teacher or peer assessment through the use of a rubric or checklist could be useful in assessing individual dance ability. This could be done by assessing specific characteristic of dance (e.g. rhythm, flow, movement, and body awareness). Another form of assessment could involve children creating their own dance combinations by utilizing movements that they learned by participating in the *Zumba* activity. This summative assessment could be completed as a group or individually, and would connect the dance movement that were practiced through a virtual means back to reality. Rubrics could be used to help assessment dance combination and allow students to better understand the requirements of the activity.

Cost

The cost of the *Zumba* game itself varies by system and release date of the game. Older versions of the game cost less both in new or used condition. *Zumba Kids*, which is intended for elementary students, costs $9.99. The Wii and PlayStation Move versions of the game includes a hands free belt that allows the dancer to perform movements without keeping ahold of a game controller. This could be a useful tool for children with difficulty or simply allowing them to move more freely. Purchasing additional belts costs $9.99 per belt. An app version of *Zumba* is available for the Apple iOS, Android, and Windows phone. There is a "lite" version of the app, *Zumba Dance*, which is available for $1.99. A full version of the *Zumba Dance* app costs $24.99, which unlocks additional songs and includes full three classes. The app version of *Zumba* requires a smart device, such a tablet or phone, to initiate game play.

Conclusion

Educators need to be patient as they are finding themselves becoming more comfortable with the technology and implementing it into the classroom. It is important to note that it will take time to get acclimated to creating an effective learning environment for optimal exergame implementation. Classroom routines and specific exergaming procedures are extremely important. For example, when students enter the classroom or gymnasium, they are not permitted to use the equipment unless instructed to do so at the beginning of the unit. Then, as the unit progresses, children can immediately begin using the equipment when they enter the area to increase physical activity time. In lieu of being in a classroom at recess, students can participate in exergames in the gymnasium.

Technology is a part of daily life. The new generation of children have been raised, and surround by this ever advancing technology. It is now common place for these technologies to be integrated into educational instruction to engage all learners. The same strategies can apply into the physical education classroom setting. Exergaming systems can be used as a tool to help address academic content standards. These systems can be utilized by all students, regardless of age, size, ability, or fitness level. This is very important when the student population comes from a large variety of backgrounds (socioeconomic, multi-cultural, religious, and different household dynamics). Exergames also appeal to different learning styles by displaying interactive challenges in the form of a projected image. The very visual, technology-based instruction has the potential to change a lot of learner's views and attitudes about being physically active.

As technology continues to evolve, education needs to reform to meet the needs of the learners. The current exergames motivate learners while increasing physical activity in their classroom. By following the recommendations outlined in this chapter, educators can create positive classroom environments where students can enjoy being physically active.

References

Adkins, M., Brown, G. A., Heelan, K., Ansorge, C., Shaw, B. S., & Shaw, I. (2013). Can dance exergaming contribute to improving physical activity levels in elementary school children? *African Journal for Physical, Health Education, Recreation & Dance, 19*(3), 576–585.

American Academy of Pediatrics. (2013, November). *Children, adolescents, and the media, 132*(5). Retrieved from http://pediatrics.aappublications.org/content/132/5/958

American Academy of Pediatrics. (2015). *Media and children*. Retrieved from https://www.aap.org/en-us/advocacy-and-policy/aap-healthinitiatives/pages/media-and-children.aspx

Centers for Disease Control and Prevention. (2012). *TV watching and computer use in the U.S. youth ages 12–15*. Retrieved from http://www.cdc.gov/nchs/data/databriefs/db157.pdf

Common Sense Media. (2013). *Zero to eight: Children's media use in America*. Retrieved from https://www.commonsensemedia.org/file/zerotoeightfinal2011pdf-0/download

Gao, Z. (2013). The impact of an exergaming intervention on urban school children's physical activity levels and academic outcomes. *Asian Journal of Exercise & Sports Science, 10*(2), 1–10.
Gao, Z., Huang, C., Liu, T., & Xiong, W. (2012). Impact of interactive dance games on urban children's physical activity correlates and behavior. *Journal of Exercise Science & Fitness, 10*(2), 107–115.
Gao, Z., Chen, S., & Stodden, D. F. (2015). A comparison of children's physical activity levels in physical education, recess, and exergaming. *Journal of Physical Activity & Health, 12*(3), 349–354.
Gao, Z., Zhang, P., & Podlog, L. W. (2014). Examining elementary school children's level of enjoyment of traditional tag games vs. interactive dance games. *Psychology, Health & Medicine*, 19(5), 605–613.
George, A. M., Rohr, L. E., & Byrne, J. (2016). Impact of Nintendo Wii games on physical literacy in children: Motor skills, physical fitness activity behaviors, and knowledge. *Sports, 4*(3), 2–10.
Graf, D., Pratt, L., Hester, C., & Short, K. (2009). Playing active video games increases energy expenditure in children. *Pediatrics, 124*(2), 534–540.
Hong, J., Tsai, C., Ho, Y., Hwang, M. T., & Wu, C. (2013). A comparative study of the learning effectiveness of a blended and embodied interactive video game for kindergarten students. *Interactive Learning Environments, 21*(1), 39–53.
Li, B. J., Lwin, M. O., & Jung, Y. (2014). Wii, myself, and size: The influence of proteus effect and stereotype threat on overweight children's exercise motivation and behavior in exergames': Correction. *Games for Health, 3*(3), 192.
Maloney, A., Bethea, T., Kelsey, K., Marks, J., Paez, S., Rosenberg, A., … Sikich, L. (2008). A pilot of a video game (DDR) to promote physical activity and decrease sedentary screen time. *Obesity, 16*(9), 2074–2080.
Martin, N. J., Ameluxen-Coleman, E. J., & Heinrichs, D. M. (2015). Innovative ways to use modern technology to enhance, rather than hinder, physical activity among youth. *The Journal of Physical Education, Recreation & Dance, 86*(4), 46–53.
National Heart, Lung, and Blood Institute. (2012). *Expert panel on integrated guidelines for cardiovascular health risk reduction in children and adolescents*. Retrieved from https://www.nhlbi.nih.gov/files/docs/peds_guidelines_sum.pdf
Nintendo. (2015). *Wii fit plus*. Retrieved from http://wiifit.com/
O'Donovan, C., Roche, E. F., & Hussey, J. (2014). The energy cost of playing active video games in children with obesity and children of a healthy weight. *Pediatric Obesity, 9*(4), 310–317.
Perron, R. M., Graham, C. A., Feldman, J. R., Moffett, R. A., & Hall, E. E. (2011). Do exergames allow children to achieve physical activity intensity commensurate with national guidelines? *International Journal of Exercise Science, 4*(4), 257–264.
Rudella, J. L., & Butz, J. V. (2015). Exergames: Increasing physical activity through effective instruction. *The Journal of Physical Education, Recreation & Dance, 86*(6), 8–15.
Sheehan, D. P., & Katz, L. (2012). The impact of a six week exergaming curriculum on balance with grade three school children using the Wii FIT. *International Journal of Computer Science in Sport, 11*(3), 5–23.
Sun, H. (2012). Exergaming impact on physical activity and interest in elementary school children. *Research Quarterly for Exercise Science and Sport, 83*(2), 212–220.
Sun, H. (2013). Impact of exergames on physical activity and motivation in elementary students: A follow-up study. *Journal of Sport and Health Science, 2*(3), 138–145.
Toscano, L., Ladda, S., & Bednarz, L. (2014). Moving to the beat: From Zumba to hip-hop hoedown. *Strategies: A Journal for Physical and Sport Educators, 27*(2), 31–36.
Ubisoft Entertainment. (2015a). *Just Dance Games*. Retrieved from http://just-dance.ubi.com/en-US/games/index.aspx
Ubisoft Entertainment. (2015b). *Just Dance Now*. Retrieved from www.justdancenow.com
Ubisoft Entertainment. (2015c). *Wii Fit U for Wii U*. Retrieved from http://wiifitu.nintendo.com/

US Games. (2016). *Wireless idance gaming system*. Retrieved from http://www.usgames.com/wireless-idance-gaming-system

Vernadakis, N., Papastergiou, M., Zetou, E., & Antoniou, P. (2015). The impact of an exergame-based intervention on children's fundamental motor skills. *Computers & Education, 83*, 90–102.

World Health Organization. (2016). *Global strategy on diet, physical activity and health*. Retrieved from http://www.who.int/dietphysicalactivity/factsheet_young_people/en/

YouTube. (2015). *Just dance for kids search*. Retrieved from https://www.youtube.com/results?search_query=just+dance+for+kids

Dr. Jennifer L. Rudella is currently an Assistant Professor at Lock Haven University of Pennsylvania in the Department of Health Science and has been teaching in higher education for over three years. Her teaching career began in public education where she taught elementary physical education, adapted physical education, high school health education, high school physical education, and lifetime fitness for five years. Research interests include exergames, fitness testing, integrating technology in health and physical education curricula, skills-based health education, and student motivation. Her Pennsylvania licensures include an Instructional II teaching certification in health and physical education and a supervisory certification in curriculum and instruction. She is also a Certified Health Education Specialist from the National Commission for Health Education Credentialing, Incorporated. Dr. Rudella completed her undergraduate degree at Lock Haven University of Pennsylvania in the Health and Physical Education program. Her master's degree in Exercise Science and Health Promotion was acquired from California University of Pennsylvania. Her doctoral degree in Curriculum and Instruction was completed at Indiana University of Pennsylvania.

Ms. Jennifer V. Butz is a health and physical education teacher at Northern Lehigh School district. Research interests include exergames, lifetime fitness, increasing physical activity in children, academic achievement and physical activity, and innovative technology practices in health and physical education. She is certified in health and physical education and currently holds an Instructional II permanent teaching certification from Pennsylvania. She has been teaching elementary health and physical education in the public school setting since 2007. Ms. Butz completed her undergraduate degree at Lock Haven University in the Health and Physical Education program. Her master's degree in Classroom Technology was completed at Wilkes University and she is currently an all but disseration (ABD) doctoral candidate in Curriculum and Instruction at Indiana University of Pennsylvania.

Chapter 7
Understanding the Relationship Between Dog Ownership and Children's Physical Activity and Sedentary Behavior

Hayley Christian, Carri Westgarth, and Danny Della Vedova

Children and dogs are as necessary to the welfare of the country as Wall Street and the railroads.

– Harry S Truman, President of the United States, 1945–1953

Introduction

Dogs have played a significant role in human lives for thousands of years. In modern society, pet dogs are present in 24% of UK (Pet Food Manufacturers Association, 2014), 39% of Australian (Animal Health Alliance, 2013), and 44% of USA (American Pet Products Association, 2015) households. Living closely with animals can significantly influence human life, but it is only more recently that the impact of pet dogs on human health has become an area of scientific interest. There is a growing body of evidence suggesting that pet ownership is associated with a number of physical, mental and emotional health benefits (Allen, 1997; Herzog, 2011; McNicholas et al., 2005). Suggested benefits of pet ownership include lower systolic blood pressure, plasma cholesterol and triglyceride levels (Anderson, Reid, & Jennings, 1992), lower rates of mortality after a heart attack (Friedmann, Katcher, Lynch, & Thomas, 1980; Friedmann, Thomas, Stein, & Kleiger, 2003), less feelings of loneliness, stress and depression (Garrity, Stallones, Marx, & Johnson, 1989; Katcher, 1982; Stallones, Marx, Garrity, & Johnson, 1991) and fewer annual visits to the doctor (Headey & Grabka, 2007).

H. Christian (✉) · D. Della Vedova
The University of Western Australia, Crawley, Australia
e-mail: hayley.christian@uwa.edu.au

C. Westgarth
University of Liverpool, Liverpool, UK
e-mail: carri.westgarth@liverpool.ac.uk

H. Brewer, M. R. Jalongo (eds.), *Physical Activity and Health Promotion in the Early Years*, Educating the Young Child 14,
https://doi.org/10.1007/978-3-319-76006-3_7

The most significant research evidence in terms of quality and size surrounds the association between dog ownership and physical activity. A review of 29 studies published between 1990 and 2010 provides evidence that in adults dog ownership is associated with increased physical activity and that this is due to the increased physical activity facilitated from walking a dog (Christian et al., 2013). Across studies, dog owners reported more minutes per week of physical activity (median = 329 min/week) than non-dog owners (median = 277 min/week), and specifically more walking (Dog owners: 129 min/week; Non-owners: 111 min/week) (Christian et al., 2013). Dog owners are also more likely than non-owners to meet the recommended level of physical activity for health benefit (150 min/week of moderate to vigorous physical activity) (Christian et al., 2013; Coleman et al., 2008; Cutt, Giles-Corti, Knuiman, Timperio, & Bull, 2008). Moreover, a 2013 American Heart Association Scientific Statement on 'Pet Ownership and Cardiovascular Risk' recommended that there is robust data for a relationship between dog ownership and cardiovascular disease risk reduction (Levine et al., 2013).

While there is mounting evidence of a positive relationship between dog ownership and physical activity, the data also indicates that not all people who own a dog walk with it; the review found that across studies approximately 40% of dog owners do not walk with their dog. Of those dog owners who do walk with their dog (60%) they walk a median duration and frequency of 160 min per week and 4 walks per week, respectively. Thus, while about half of all dog owners walk their dog regularly the other half do not, highlighting the potential population-level physical activity benefits if this group of non-dog walkers could be encouraged to commence dog walking. Interventions to increase community levels of dog walking require a clear understanding of the barriers and motivators for dog walking.

A number of individual, social environment and physical environment factors influence physical activity behaviours (Stokols, 1996) including dog walking. A 2014 review paper applied the socio-ecological theory to dog walking, and summarised the available evidence on the correlates of dog walking (Westgarth, Christley, & Christian, 2014). The review found that there is good evidence that physical environmental and neighbourhood factors can influence dog walking behaviour, as dog walking is associated with accessibility to aesthetically pleasing walking environments (e.g., high quality local parks). The review also found that dog owners have specific needs and that a dog-friendly environment is important, in particular the ability to let the dog off leash. However, the most striking finding was a consistent strong association and large effect size between dog walking and the nature of the dog-owner relationship; described in a variety of ways including attachment, and feelings of support, motivation and obligation provided by the dog for walking (Brown & Rhodes, 2006; Christian nee Cutt, Giles-Corti, & Knuiman, 2010; Hoerster et al., 2011). There is some evidence suggesting that children are also more likely to report walking their dog if they have a high attachment to it (Westgarth et al., 2013). It appears there is something special about the bond between people and their dogs that motivates them to walk regularly with them. The joyful experience of dog walking and the translation of this into a sense of fulfilling a dogs needs is likely a significant motivator for walking.

While a significant proportion of studies investigating the physical activity and health benefits of dog ownership in adults, there is mounting evidence of a positive relationship between dog ownership and physical activity in children. The following sections provide an overview of the relationships between dog ownership and children's health, specifically physical activity, sedentary behaviour and overweight and obesity.

Dog Ownership and Child Health

A number of studies provide evidence of the psychological and physical health benefits of pet ownership for children. Pet ownership is associated with a stronger immune system, social-emotional development, increased feelings of safety, self-confidence, family cohesion and increased physical fitness (Smith, 2012). One of the main mechanisms through which pets, in particular dogs, may facilitate improved health outcomes in children may be through increased physical activity associated with owning, walking and playing with a family dog. A high proportion of households with children own a dog. It is estimated that between 50 and 70% of US and Australian households with children have dog (Australian Bureau of Statistics, 1995; Mathers, Canterford, Olds, Waters, & Wake, 2010; Salmon, Timperio, Chu, & Veitch, 2010). Dog ownership levels are higher in families with school aged children (Albert & Bulcroft, 1988; Melson, 1998; Paul & Serpell, 1992; Westgarth et al., 2007, 2010) and this may relate to parental beliefs that pets help children learn responsibility, develop a sense of identity and independence, are sources of unconditional love and loyalty and are a stimuli for certain kinds of cognitive learning (Soares, 1985).

Given the high levels of physical inactivity, sedentary behaviour and overweight and obesity in children (Active Healthy Kids Australia, 2014; Commonwealth of Australia, 2014; U.S. Department of Health and Human Services, 2015), effective child-friendly strategies to combat these high levels of unhealthy behaviours in the community are required. One such potential strategy may be the physical activity facilitated by owning a family dog. While much of the evidence to date suggests that dog ownership is associated with increased levels of physical activity in children (Christian, Trapp, Lauritsen, Wright, & Giles-Corti, 2012; Martin, Wood, Christian, & Trapp, 2015; Owen et al., 2010; Salmon et al., 2010) it also highlights that a large proportion of children are not engaged in any dog-facilitated physical activities, in particular dog walking (Westgarth et al., 2013). Dog-facilitated physical activity in children can also be encouraged through a number of other ways. For example, dogs may facilitate active play in children through active games such as fetch and chase. However, the primary source of dog-facilitated physical activity in children is dog walking done with family members or independently either with friends, siblings or on their own.

Given the emerging evidence that dog ownership is associated with increased levels of physical activity in children it is plausible that dog ownership may also be helpful for reducing levels of sedentary time as well as overweight and obesity in children. Evidence of the relationship between dog ownership and physical activity, sedentary behaviour and overweight/obesity in children is presented below. Differences in the nature of these relationships for boys and girls and different age groups of children (early years, middle childhood, and adolescence) are also described.

Dog Ownership and Children's Physical Activity

To date, thirteen studies have investigated the relationship between dog ownership and physical activity in children. Overall, the findings suggest that dog ownership is associated with increased physical activity levels in children however, the relationship varies according to the age and gender of children and the type of physical activity measured.

The majority of studies examining the relationship between dog ownership and children's physical activity have focused on school age children or adolescents. For example, an Australian study of 1218 10–12 year olds found that dog ownership was associated with an average of 29 more minutes of walking, and 142 more minutes of physical activity per week (Christian et al., 2012). Children with a dog were also 49% more likely to achieve the recommended level of weekly physical activity (420 min) and 32% more likely to have walked in their neighborhood in the last week, compared with non-dog owners (Christian et al., 2012). In support of these findings more than one-third of primary school aged children and one quarter of secondary school students reported that they walked with their dog at least once in the past week, with dog walking being amongst the most common play activities, particularly for girls (Martin et al., 2015). In addition, secondary school students who reported walking the dog or playing with pets were 80% more likely to meet national physical activity recommendations of 60 min of moderate-vigorous physical activity per day compared with secondary school students who did not report any pet-related activity (Martin et al., 2015).

Studies using objective measures of children's physical activity levels have yielded similar results. An English study using accelerometers to measure children's physical activity levels found that children with a dog spent significantly more time per day in light, moderate to vigorous, and vigorous physical activity and recorded more overall activity counts and steps per day compared with non–dog owners (Owen et al., 2010). For example, compared with non-owners dog owners spent 5 more min/day in light intensity physical activity, 3 more min/day in moderate-vigorous physical activity and did an additional 357 steps/day (Owen et al., 2010). A US study of adolescents (mean age 15 years) found that dog ownership was associated with higher levels of accelerometer measured physical activity (mean daily accelerometer counts/min), even after adjusting for age, puberty, gender, race, number of household members, and socio-economic status (Sirard, Patnode, Hearst, & Laska, 2011).

A few studies have stratified their results by gender and reported significant gender differences in the relationship between dog ownership and physical activity. For example, in school aged children, boy, but not girl, dog owners walked significantly more min/week and were more likely to walk in their neighborhood than non-dog owners (Christian et al., 2012). Furthermore, girl, but not boy, dog owners were more likely to achieve recommended levels of physical activity and did more minutes of physical activity than non-dog owners (Christian et al., 2012). It is possible that differences in the relationship and interaction boys and girls have with their dog explains this variation. For example, boys are generally more independently mobile than girls are and thus may be allowed to walk with their dog on their own; this would contribute more to their overall walking levels. In contrast, girls may engage in active play with their dog and this contributes more to their overall physical activity levels. Research is required to further investigate gender differences in how boys and girls interact with the family dog, the types of dog-facilitated physical activity undertaken and the effect this has on children's overall physical activity levels.

Only three studies to date have examined the relationship between dog ownership and physical activity in young children. One American study reported no significant difference in parent-report physical activity of dog owning vs. non-dog owning children (4–10 years) visiting a pediatric clinic, however it is not clear how physical activity was measured (Gadomski et al., 2015). Two Australian studies analyzed the same data set of 294 5–6 year olds (Salmon et al., 2010; Timperio, Salmon, Chu, & Andrianopoulos, 2008) and found that approximately 77% never walked a dog, 11% walked a dog 1–2 times/week, 12% walked a dog three times/week and 24% reported walking a dog as a family at least once per week, regardless of dog ownership (Timperio et al., 2008). When physical activity was measured objectively using accelerometers, dog ownership was associated with an additional 29 min per day of physical activity among 5–6 year old girls but not boys (Salmon et al., 2010). Importantly, families that reported regular family dog walking spent more time per week physically active, compared with dog owners who reported never or rarely walking the dog as a family (Salmon et al., 2010). Similarly, in a qualitative study of mother's perceptions of children's barriers and facilitators for physical activity, dog ownership was found to encourage increased walking, particularly via children prompting parents to take the dog for a walk (Veitch, Hume, Salmon, Crawford, & Ball, 2013). While these studies highlight that family dog walking is an important source of physical activity for some dog-owning households, they also indicate that a large proportion of children are not physically active with their family dog. This is supported by findings from a UK study showing that 15.4% of children reported walking with any dog (their own or belonging to a friend or family member) once daily or more, 14.1% several times a week, 27.6% once a week or less, and 42.8% never (Westgarth et al., 2013). Promoting family dog walking may be an effective way for both parents and children to increase their overall levels of physical activity. Moreover, family dog walking may provide opportunity to develop the bond between children and their dog which may facilitate children's interest in dog walking. Family dog walking may also assist in teaching young children the health benefits of dog walking (both for dogs and humans) and thus assist with establishing good physical activity habits early in life.

A potential source of dog-facilitated physical activity in older children is the physical activity derived from children being independently mobile and being able to walk their dog on their own, with siblings or with friends. Children's independent mobility (i.e., a child's ability to walk or cycle without adult supervision) has been found to be associated with children's dog walking behavior (Christian et al., 2014). In a sample of children from dog owning families, those who reported walking their dog were more independently mobile than children who had a dog but did not walk it. Moreover, significantly more dog walkers than non-dog walkers reported having walked in the neighborhood, played in the street, and played in yard in the last week (Christian et al., 2014). These findings highlight that active outdoor play near home is an important source of dog-facilitated physical activity. They also suggest that independent walking with a dog may provide opportunities for children to become more aware and knowledgeable about the neighborhood they live in and interact with other children and adults in their neighbourhood (Underwood, 2011). Independent walking with a dog also aids increased physical activity. Furthermore, travelling with a dog may provide benefits in terms of safety (Cutt, Giles-Corti, Knuiman, & Burke, 2007; Cutt, Giles-Corti, Wood, Knuiman, & Burke, 2008) and companionship (Christian nee Cutt et al., 2010; Cutt et al., 2007; Cutt, Giles-Corti, & Knuiman, 2008; Cutt, Giles-Corti, Wood et al., 2008) for children. This may positively influence parent and child perceptions of how safe it is to engage in walking without adult supervision, which in turn facilitates the likelihood of being independently mobile and physically activity (Christian et al., 2014). Further research is needed to examine strategies for encouraging more children to be independently mobile with their dog.

Considering a large proportion of western households with children have a dog but up to 60–75% of children do not participate in physical activity with their dog (Christian et al., 2014; Mathers, Canterford, Olds, Waters, & Wake, 2010; Salmon et al., 2010), there is a need to find effective intervention strategies for encouraging increased dog-facilitated physical activity in children. A recent review of intervention studies (mostly in adults) found that the promotion of dog walking among dog owners who do not routinely walk their dogs may be an effective strategy for encouraging more physical activity (Christian et al., 2016). The review found that some of the most effective strategies were those that emphasize the value of dog walking for both dogs and people, enhance the social-interaction benefits, encourage family dog walking, and ensure dog walking-friendly public space is available.

Despite an emerging evidence base showing that dog ownership is associated with higher levels of physical activity in children, our search located only two small pilot intervention studies conducted to date. A small 2013 German cross over case study involving twelve obese children aged between 8 and 12 years old found that the presence of a therapy dog for two 10-min sessions during a 19-min exercise program increased the amount of accelerometer measured physical activity, compared to only having a human trainer present (Wohlfarth, Mutschler, Beetz, Kreuser,

& Korsten-Reck, 2013). Despite the small sample size, and temporary use of a therapy dog rather than actual pet dog, the findings suggest that dogs may enhance motivation for physical activity in obese children. Although the limited sample may not be representative of the wider population, incorporating dogs into obesity intervention programs may help to motivate children to undertake physical activity and improve the weight status.

Another intervention pilot study conducted is an exploratory assessor blinded random control trial involving twenty eight Scottish families (Morrison et al., 2013). Families were allocated to either a 10week dog-based physical activity intervention or a control group. The dog-based physical activity intervention included three home visits, two phone calls, and two text messages targeting parents, children and the dog to be active together, including playing games. The study found no significant difference in child accelerometer measured moderate-vigorous physical activity/week or parent-report weekly minutes of dog walking between groups. The impact of the intervention may have been underestimated as outcomes were measured in the period immediately after the intervention rather than during the final week, however participants reported the study was successful in providing sufficient information for safe dog walking and motivation to increase dog walking (Morrison et al., 2013). Despite this being a pilot intervention study and thus limited by its small sample size, the feasibility and acceptability of the intervention and outcome measures was high for participating families suggesting that future intervention studies should focus on using dogs as an agent of lifestyle change in physical activity interventions targeting children and their parents.

Given the large proportion of children who do not engage in physical activity with their dog, and the high level of pet ownership in many Western countries, the promotion of dog walking and pet play to support children's physical activity is warranted. Furthermore, there is a need for prospective studies in order to determine the longitudinal effects and further clarify the relationship between dog ownership and physical activity in children.

Dog Ownership and Children's Sedentary Behavior

Four studies to date have investigated the association between dog ownership and children's sedentary behavior. In an Australian study of 10–12 year olds, dog ownership status and parent report screen use were not significantly associated, even after adjustment for parent and child socio-demographic factors (Christian et al., 2012). Similarly, a US study reported no significant difference in parent-report screen time of ≤ 2 h/day among dog owning and non-dog owning children 4–10 years (Gadomski et al., 2015). Furthermore, a study using accelerometers found no significant association between dog ownership and accelerometer measured sedentary time in 9–10 year olds from the UK (Owen et al., 2010). A family based dog walking pilot intervention study also observed no significant difference in objectively measured sedentary behavior between control and intervention groups at follow-up

(Morrison et al., 2013). Although there is a growing evidence base suggesting that dogs may be an important facilitator of children's physical activity, the impact dog ownership has on reducing childhood sedentary behaviors is likely to be negligible. The findings to date are consistent with research indicating that the determinants of physical activity are different from those for sedentary behavior (Owen, Leslie, Salmon, & Fotheringham, 2000). However, further studies using pet dogs as agents for health-enhancing lifestyle changes in children are warranted. These studies should include self-report and objective measures in order to clarify the value of promoting the switch from sedentary behaviors (e.g., screen use) to active play with the family dog.

Dog Ownership and Children's Overweight and Obesity

It is possible that the increased physical activity facilitated by dogs contributes to an increase in energy expenditure and thus positively influences child overweight and obesity levels. To date, only a handful of studies have investigated the relationship between dog ownership and overweight and obesity in children with mixed findings. For example, an Australian study found that dog ownership amongst a random sample of 10–12 year olds was not associated with childhood overweight/obesity (23.3% in both dog-owner and non-owner groups), even after adjustment for sociodemographic and environmental factors (Christian et al., 2012). Another Australian study, also of 10–12 year olds observed no significant association between weight status and dog ownership or frequency of dog walking per week (Timperio et al., 2008). Similarly, a US study reported no significant difference in objectively measured BMI or weight status for dog owning compared with non-dog owning 4–10 year olds (Gadomski et al., 2015). A separate study in the UK (n = 7,759) analysing both cross-sectional (7 year olds) and longitudinal data (between 7 and 9 years) from the Avon Longitudinal Study of Parents and Children (ALSPAC) study also found no association between dog ownership and body mass index (BMI), even after adjustment for a number of factors (e.g., parental obesity, maternal smoking during pregnancy, child gender, birth weight, TV watching, sleep) (Westgarth et al., 2012).

However, there is some evidence that dog ownership is associated with reduced odds of overweight/obesity in younger children. In a sample of 281 Australian children aged 5–6 years, children who had a family dog had a 50% reduced likelihood of being overweight or obese (Odds Ratio = 0.5, 95% Confidence Interval = 0.3–0.8), yet no significant association was observed with frequency of dog walking or family dog walking (Timperio et al., 2008). Thus, pet interactions (such as informal play with the family dog) could help younger children to maintain a healthy weight status. It is possible that the relationship between dog ownership and weight status may be mediated by physical activity in younger (but not older children) (Salmon et al., 2010). It is important to consider that obesity is a complex outcome, influenced by both energy intake and expenditure. Future research should investigate if physical activity mediates the relationship between dog ownership and weight status in children and if this differs by age, gender and dietary intake.

Studies conducted with adolescents also highlight how interaction with pets may assist with children maintaining a healthy weight status. A study involving 928 adolescents found that 5.5% of pet owners were obese compared with 10.5% of non-pet owners (Mathers et al., 2010). In contrast, 20.4% of adolescent pet owners were overweight compared with 17.1% of non-pet owners. However, the association between weight status (non-overweight, overweight, obese) and pet ownership was non-significant for any pets as well as dog, cat and horse ownership. Despite this study reporting that 89% of adolescents owned a pet (72% owned a dog), 75% reported no interaction with their pets (Mathers et al., 2010). In contrast, Martin et al found 44% of secondary school students interacted with their pets in pet play although the correlation between playing with pets and obesity was not examined (Martin et al., 2015).

Again, these findings highlight the need for further studies to understand the relationship between dog-facilitated physical activity and the effect on levels of overweight and obesity in children. These studies should focus on the mechanisms or pathways (e.g., via active play with dog, family dog walking) through which pets, in particular dogs, assist in reducing children's level of overweight/obesity. Furthermore, more research is needed to understand the relationship between dog ownership and dog-facilitated physical activity and overweight/obesity for different age groups of children (early years, middle childhood, adolescence) and the effect of children's dietary intake on these relationships. Finally, there is an urgent need for studies with a stronger design (i.e., longitudinal and intervention studies) to better understand how dog-facilitated physical activity can help curb the obesity epidemic in children.

Discussion

Overall, there is evidence that dog ownership is associated with increased physical activity in children and this relationship is mostly consistent across different ages and gender. However, there is less convincing evidence that dog ownership further translates to reduced levels of overweight and obesity in children especially in older children with some limited evidence in younger children. Finally, it appears from the few studies conducted that there is no evidence that dog ownership is associated with sedentary behaviour in children.

Overall, future studies of the relationship between dog ownership, dog-facilitated physical activity, and health behaviours require stronger study designs (i.e., longitudinal and intervention), and more rigorous research methodology (i.e., random sampling, adjustment for confounders known to be associated with physical activity or weight status, such as diet, and the use of objective and context-specific measures). Observation research may provide a greater understanding of the context in which dog-facilitated physical activity in children occurs and the factors

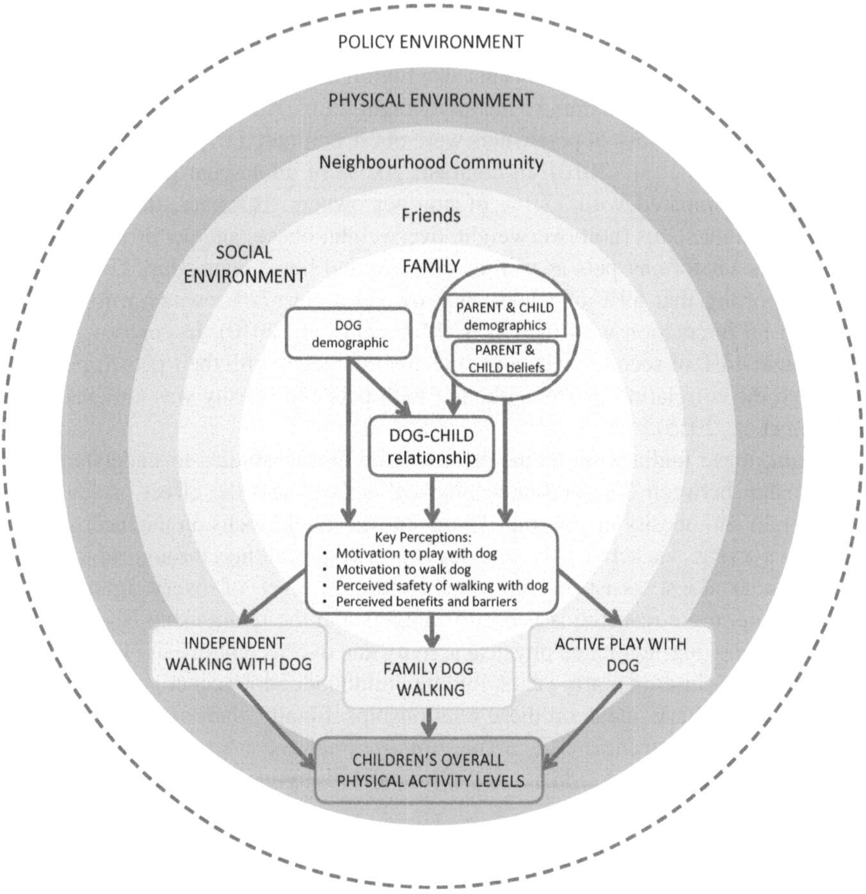

Fig. 7.1 Social-ecological model of the factors influencing dog-facilitated physical activity in children. (Adapted from Westgarth et al. 2014)

that may affect this. The social-ecological framework provides a useful theoretical framework for understanding the factors associated with dog-facilitated physical activity in children. These factors are represented in Fig. 7.1.

A number of evidence gaps exist that should be the focus of future enquiry. These include:

- Investigation of the contribution of:
  - Family dog walking and independent dog walking, to children's structured physical activity,
  - Active play with a dog to children's unstructured physical activity; and
  - How these relationships differ by gender and across different child ages (early years, middle childhood and adolescence).

- Further research into the role of parent (and educator) perceptions as facilitators or barriers for dog-facilitated physical activity.
- Investigation of the correlates of dog-facilitated physical activity in children – are they the same or different to the correlates of dog walking in adults?
- What dog-specific factors (e.g., dog size, breed, age, temperament, health status; attachment to dog; interaction with dog and other family members and friends; sense of responsibility to care for and walk dog; access to local parks supportive of dog walking) specifically influence children's dog-facilitated physical activity.
- Examination of dog-facilitated physical activity across different behaviour settings; the home (indoors, outdoor yards), local parks and streets, family and friends houses.
- Intervention research to identify strategies for increasing children's physical activity levels through dog-facilitated physical activity (e.g., developing a child's self-efficacy to walk the dog by actively involving them in the process through holding the lead with and then without parent assistance).
- Use of objective measures of physical activity (e.g., accelerometers) to determine the contribution of different types of dog-facilitated physical activity to children's overall physical activity levels (duration, frequency and intensity of physical activity).
- Context-specific (and objective) measures of children's dog-facilitated physical activity and play behaviors (e.g., active play with dog outdoors and indoors, independent walking with dog, family dog walking).

Despite the benefits of dog-facilitated physical activity in children being an emerging area of research, there are a number of practice-relevant implications that need consideration. Considering a large proportion of households with children already own a dog, physical activity focussed interventions should incorporate dog walking and active play with a dog as a strategy to increase children's physical activity levels. There are a number of practice-relevant issues to consider:

- It is important that future physical activity interventions and programs take a 'whole of family' approach to increasing children's physical activity levels via dog-facilitated physical activity. Since parents are the gatekeepers to their children's behaviour, parent perceptions of dog-facilitated physical activity can be either motivators or barriers to children being more physically active with their dog. For example, parents who perceive their dog as difficult to control when on lead may be less likely to allow their child to take the dog for a walk on their own, compared with parents who perceive their dog as well-behaved on lead.
- The social influence of significant others such as other family members, friends, local veterinarian and educators may also be key for encouraging dog-facilitated physical activity in children.
- Given the widespread attachment of children to their dogs, and the strong evidence in favour of the influence of the dog-owner bond on owner walking behaviour, programs that promote how much dogs love going 'walkies' and the benefits of exercise for dogs, may encourage children and their families to begin walking

for the sake of their dog. In older children, encouragement of walking the dog on their own, with siblings or friends may facilitate children's independent mobility and positively contribute to physical activity levels.
- Active play with the family dog is a potentially effective strategy that can be facilitated by encouraging parents to switch screen time for outdoor or even indoor play with the dog. A list of active games children and pets can play together (in and out of home) that were developed as part of the Children and Pets Exercising Together intervention (Morrison et al., 2013) are outlined in Table 7.1.

Dog walking and active play with a dog is an easy, affordable, and readily accessible activity for children to partake in which provides a number of physical activity and health benefits. However, it is important to acknowledge a number of ethical issues associated with the promotion of dog-facilitated physical activity. Dog ownership (adoption, rescue or purchase) should not be done for the primary purpose of increasing children's physical activity levels (Levine et al., 2013). Individuals acquire a dog for a variety of reasons and although one may be as a motivator for exercise, there are many other aspects to factor in (Voith, 2009). Responsible dog ownership requires meeting a number of obligations including the provision of shelter, food, veterinary care and exercise appropriate to that individual dog. If dogs are to facilitate our wellbeing, consideration of their welfare is paramount.

There are a number of health and safety issues to consider when promoting the benefits of dog-facilitated physical activity in children. The issues of dog attacks and bites, and the fear from dogs being seen as 'out of control' whilst in public are a significant risk to individuals and contribute to community concern about dogs in public places (Toohey & Rock, 2015; Voith, 2009). Dogs should be well socialized from birth so that they are friendly to 'unknown' dogs and people, as well as being sufficiently trained in manners and impulse control (wait, walking on a loose leash, recall to a sit) so that they are amenable to instruction and are pleasurable to walk (Fox & Stelzner, 1967; Seksel, 2015). A reward-based dog trainer should be sought for advice on teaching these skills using non-aversive methods. Any risks specific to children walking and playing with dogs should also be avoided, through comprehensive training, age-appropriate supervision and the appropriate use of dog-related equipment. For example, the use of harnesses and head collars to assist with training to prevent pulling on the leash, and age-appropriate decisions as to who holds the lead, which games can be played, and the level of parental supervision required. It is recommended that no child should ever be left alone with a dog or be held responsible to supervise a dog. Careful consideration of the ability of adolescents to meet the responsibilities of walking a dog should be made depending on the individual child and their dog.

Finally, it is important that the local policy and physical environment is supportive of both adults and children walking with their dog. Key factors include access to high quality of public open space, community education programs, a consistent regulatory and educational approach across local government, and balancing the

Table 7.1 Indoor and outdoor games children can play with their dogs[a]

Name of game	Instructions
Find It	Whilst your dog waits and watches, have your child hide a treat and then tell your dog to find it. Give your dog lots of praise when they are successful, and after several attempts, hide the object in less visible locations so that they work harder to find it. Ensure that your child is being active throughout the entire process.
Hansel and Gretel Food Trials	Whilst keeping your dog near, give your child a small bowl of treats and get them to make a trail for your dog to follow. Ask your child to return once the path is complete and then let your dog and child follow along celebrating at each successful find.
Commando Crawl	Ask your child to lay a trail of treats by crawling under furniture (e.g., dining table, line of plastic patio chairs) from one end of the room to the other. Teach your dog to belly crawl across the floor to get the treats. Ask your child to follow along the trail behind your dog celebrating at each successful find.
Hide & Seek	Whilst holding your dog, get your child to hold your dog's favorite treat or toy and hide somewhere outside or in another room. As soon as your child is hidden let your dog go. Encourage your child to help your dog find them by calling your dog's name. Celebrate when your child is found, offering your dog lots of petting, praise, as well as the toy/treat. Alternatively, involve your child in the seeking by hiding the toy/treat from them both.
Dog Bowling	Arrange empty 2L plastic bottles in a bowling triangle outside or in the hallway, then, holding your dog at the opposite end, have your child stand behind the bottles with a treat and call your dog's name. The aim is for your dog to score a 'strike' before the game is finished.
Fetch	Your dog will first need to know how to fetch. Then have your child throw an item while telling your dog to 'fetch'. Whilst your dog is fetching your child should be jumping, dancing, or skipping on the spot. When your dog returns, tell your child to give them the 'drop it' command, and then give your dog lots of praise when they drop the item. If you are absolutely sure that your dog is not possessive of objects, advance the previous game by having a race between your dog and child to reach the toy. Make sure your child and dog are still when you throw the item. You may have to give your child a head start by positioning them closer to the toy.
Clean Up Your Toys	Get a bucket and scatter a number of toys in a small area nearby, and get your dog to pick them up one at a time and place them in your hand. Give your dog a treat for each item they pick up, before placing it in the bucket. If your dog is confident at this behavior, you can make it increasingly difficult for your dog to put the item in your hand, while maintaining the fun of the game. As your dog is cleaning up the toys, your child should be doing star jumps, or bunny hops on the spot and counting how many they can complete before all items are returned.
Football	Have your child gently kick the ball so it rolls on the ground toward your dog. When your dog uses his nose to push the ball around ensure your child gives them lots of praise. Your dog and child can then kick and push the ball between them whilst running around.

(continued)

Table 7.1 (continued)

Name of game	Instructions
Circuit Training	Locate four obstacles in the yard or park, and decide on a circuit and a number of laps to be completed. Your child should have your dog on a lead and then run with it around the circuit. At the end of a full circuit give your dog a treat. Advance the circuit training by asking your child and dog to jump over small obstacles, or to crawl under an object
Recall	While holding your dog by the collar, ask your child to run a few paces away, stop and turn around, and then let your dog go when the child calls their name. Reward your dog with a treat once they sit down next to your child. Advance the previous game by asking your child to run to a further distance and stop. Once your dog arrives at the child, go to them, take hold of your dog again, and ask your child to run off in a different direction.
Rounders	Set up four markers in a square then, holding your dog, throw a ball towards your child. Your child hits the ball and runs around the four markers, whilst your dog is released to go and fetch the ball and return it. Try to hit the last marker with the ball before your child completes the circuit.

[a]Adapted with permission from the Children, Parents and Pets Exercising Together (CPET) study (Morrison et al., 2013). Ensure that your dog is friendly around food items and toys before undertaking these games

benefits of increased dog walking with community concerns about dogs in public places (Christian et al., 2016; Cutt et al., 2007; Cutt, Giles-Corti, Wood et al., 2008; Westgarth et al., 2014). For example, provisions should be made so that all dog faeces are appropriately disposed of to minimise the risks to public health of zoonotic disease and to protect the aesthetics of the environment. The provision of dog-related infrastructure (dog litter bags and bins, dog drinking water facilities, dog-related signage) in parks supports more dog walking in adults and is likely to be important for children and families who walk (and play) with their dog at local parks.

Summary

Considering the high levels of physical inactivity in children coupled with the high levels of dog ownership in many households, dog facilitated physical activity is a potentially viable strategy for increasing physical activity levels and improving child health and well-being. Since up to 70% of households with children have a dog, dog owning families are an important target group for physical activity interventions. Understanding the factors that encourage children to walk with their dog and engage in active play with their dog will help to develop population health strategies aimed at increasing the overall amount of physical activity children undertake on a regular basis.

References

Active Healthy Kids Australia. (2014). *Is sport enough? 2014 report card on physical activity for children & young people*. Adelaide, South Australia: Active Healthy Kids Australia.

Albert, A., & Bulcroft, K. (1988). Pets, families, and the life course. *Journal of Marriage and the Family, 50*(2), 543–552.

Allen, D. T. (1997). Effects of dogs on human health. *American Veterinary Medical Association, 210*, 1136–1139.

American Pet Products Association. (2015). *APPA National Pet Owners Survey 2015–2016*. Greenwich, CT: American Pet Products Association.

Anderson, W. P., Reid, C. M., & Jennings, G. L. (1992). Pet ownership and risk factors for cardiovascular disease. *Medical Journal of Australia, 157*, 298–301.

Animal Health Alliance. (2013). *Pet ownership in Australia summary 2013*. Canberra, Australia: Animal Health Alliance.

Australian Bureau of Statistics. (1995). *Australian Social Trends, 1995 (ABS Cat. no. 4102.0)*. Canberra, Australian Capital Territory.

Brown, S. G., & Rhodes, R. E. (2006). Relationship among dog ownership and leisure-time walking in western Canadian adults. *American Journal of Preventive Medicine, 30*(2), 131–136.

Christian, H., Bauman, A., Epping, J., Levine, G. N., McCormack, G., Rhodes, R. E., ... Westgarth, C. (2016). Encouraging dog walking for health promotion and disease prevention. *American Journal of Lifestyle Medicine*. doi:10.1177/1559827616643686.

Christian, H., Trapp, G., Lauritsen, C., Wright, K., & Giles-Corti, B. (2012). Understanding the relationship between dog ownership and children's physical activity and sedentary behaviour. *Pediatric Obesity, 8*(5), 392–403.

Christian, H., Trapp, G., Villanueva, K., Zubrick, S. R., Koekemoer, R., & Giles-Corti, B. (2014). Dog walking is associated with more outdoor play and independent mobility for children. *Preventive Medicine, 67*, 259–263.

Christian, H., Westgarth, C., Bauman, A., Richards, E., Rhodes, R., Evenson, K., ... Thorpe, R. (2013). Dog ownership and physical activity: A review of the evidence. *Journal of Physical Activity and Health, 10*(5), 750–759.

Christian nee Cutt, H., Giles-Corti, B., & Knuiman, M. (2010). "I'm just a-walking the dog" correlates of regular dog walking. *Family & Community Health, 33*(1), 44–52.

Coleman, K. J., Rosenberg, D. E., Conway, T. L., Sallis, J. F., Saelens, B. E., Frank, L. D., & Cain, K. (2008). Physical activity, weight status, and neighborhood characteristics of dog walkers. *Preventive Medicine, 47*(3), 309–312.

Commonwealth of Australia. (2014). *More than half of all Australian adults are not active enough*. Canberra, Australia: Department of Health, Australian Government.

Cutt, H., Giles-Corti, B., & Knuiman, M. (2008). Encouraging physical activity through dog walking: Why don't some owners walk with their dog? *Preventive Medicine, 46*, 120–126.

Cutt, H., Giles-Corti, B., Knuiman, M., & Burke, V. (2007). Dog ownership, health and physical activity: A critical review of the literature. *Health & Place, 13*, 261–272.

Cutt, H., Giles-Corti, B., Knuiman, M., Timperio, A., & Bull, F. (2008). Understanding dog owners' increased levels of physical activity: Results from reside. *American Journal of Public Health, 98*(1), 66–69.

Cutt, H. E., Giles-Corti, B., Wood, L. J., Knuiman, M. W., & Burke, V. (2008). Barriers and motivators for owners walking their dog: Results from qualitative research. *Health Promotion Journal of Australia, 19*, 118–124.

Fox, M., & Stelzner, D. (1967). The effects of early experience on the development of inter and intraspecies social relationships in the dog. *Animal Behaviour, 15*(2–3), 377–386.

Friedmann, E., Katcher, A., Lynch, J., & Thomas, S. (1980). Animal companions and one-year survival of patients after discharge from a coronary care unit. *Public Health Reports, 95*(4), 307–312.

Friedmann, E., Thomas, S. A., Stein, P. K., & Kleiger, R. E. (2003). Relation between pet ownership and heart rate variability in patients with healed myocardial infarcts. *The American Journal of Cardiology, 91*, 718–721.

Gadomski, A., Scribani, M., Krupa, N., Jenkins, P., Nagykaldi, Z., & Olson, A. L. (2015). Pet dogs and children's health: Opportunities for chronic disease prevention? *Preventing Chronic Disease, 12*(205), 1–10.

Garrity, T. F., Stallones, L., Marx, M. B., & Johnson, T. P. (1989). Pet ownership and attachment as supportive factors in the health of the elderly. *Anthrozoös, 3*(1), 35–44.

Headey, B., & Grabka, M. M. (2007). Pets and human health in Germany and Australia: National longitudinal results. *Social Indicators Research, 80*(2), 297–311.

Herzog, H. (2011). The impact of pets on human health and psychological well-being: Facto, fiction, or hypothesis? *Current Directions in Psychological Science, 20*(4), 236–239.

Hoerster, K. D., Mayer, J. A., Sallis, J. F., Pizzi, N., Talley, S., Pichon, L. C., & Butler, D. A. (2011). Dog walking: Its association with physical activity guideline adherence and its correlates. *Prevention Medicine, 52*(1), 33–38.

Katcher, A. H. (1982). Are companion animals good for your health? *Aging, 331–332*, 2–8.

Levine, G. N., Allen, K., Braun, L. T., Christian, H. E., Friedmann, E., Taubert, K. A., ... Lange, R. A. (2013). Pet ownership and cardiovascular risk: A scientific statement from the American heart association. *Circulation, 127*(23), 2353–2363.

Martin, K., Wood, L., Christian, H., & Trapp, G. (2015). Not just "A Walking the dog": Dog walking and pet play and their association with recommended physical activity among adolescents. *American Journal of Health Promotion, 29*(6), 353–356.

Mathers, M., Canterford, L., Olds, T., Waters, E., & Wake, M. (2010). Pet ownership and adolescent health: Cross-sectional population study. *Journal of Paediatrics and Child Health, 46*(12), 729–735.

McNicholas, J., Gilbey, A., Rennie, A., Ahmedzai, S., Dono, J., & Ormerod, E. (2005). Pet ownership and human health: A brief review of evidence and issues. *British Medical Journal, 331*(7527), 1252–1254.

Melson, G. F. (1998). The role of companion animals in human development. In C. C. Wilson & D. C. Turner (Eds.), *Companion animals in human health* (pp. 219–236). Thousand Oaks, CA: Sage Publications.

Morrison, R., Reilly, J. J., Penpraze, V., Westgarth, C., Ward, D. S., Mutrie, N., ... Yam, P. S. (2013). Children, parents and pets exercising together (CPET): Exploratory randomised controlled trial. *BMC Public Health, 13*(1096), 1–12.

Owen, C., Nightingale, C., Rudnicka, A., Ekelund, U., McMinn, A., van Sluijs, E., ... Whincup, P. (2010). Family dog ownership and levels of physical activity in childhood: Findings from the child heart and health study in England. *American Journal of Public Health, 100*(9), 1669–1671.

Owen, N., Leslie, E., Salmon, J., & Fotheringham, M. (2000). Environmental determinants of physical activity and sedentary behavior. *Exercise and Sport Science Reviews, 28*(4), 153–158.

Paul, E. S., & Serpell, J. (1992). Why children keep pets: The influence of child and family characteristics. *Anthrozoös, 5*(4), 231–244.

Pet Food Manufacturers Association. (2014). *Pet population 2014 Report* (Vol. 2013). London, UK.

Salmon, J., Timperio, A., Chu, B., & Veitch, J. (2010). Dog ownership, dog walking, and children's and parent's physical activity. *Research Quarterly for Exercise and Sport, 81*(3), 264–271.

Seksel, K. (2015). Puppy socialization classes. *Veterinary Clinics of North America: Small Animal Practice, 27*(3), 465–477.

Sirard, J. R., Patnode, C. D., Hearst, M. O., & Laska, M. N. (2011). Dog ownership and adolescent physical activity. *American Journal of Preventive Medicine, 40*(3), 334–337.

Smith, B. (2012). The 'pet effect' health related aspects of companion animal ownership. *Australian Family Physician, 41*(6), 439–442.
Soares, C. J. (1985). The companion animal in the context of the family system. *Marriage and Family Review, 8*(3/4), 49–62.
Stallones, L., Marx, M. B., Garrity, T. F., & Johnson, T. P. (1991). Pet ownership and attachment in relation to the health of U.S. adults, 21 to 64 years of age. *Anthrozoös, 4*(2), 100–112.
Stokols, D. (1996). Translating social ecological theory into guidelines for community health promotion. *American Journal of Health Promotion, 10*(4), 282–298.
Timperio, A., Salmon, J., Chu, B., & Andrianopoulos, N. (2008). Is dog ownership or dog walking associated with weight status in children and their parents? *Health Promotion Journal of Australia, 19*(1), 60.
Toohey, A., & Rock, M. (2015). Newspaper portrayals, local policies, and dog-supportive public space: Who's wagging whom? *Anthrozoös, 28*(4), 549–567.
U.S. Department of Health and Human Services. (2015). *Step It Up! The surgeon general's Call to action to promote walking and walkable communities.* Retrieved from http://www.surgeongeneral.gov/library/calls/walking-and-walkable-communities/
Underwood, C. (2011). *The influence of walking a pet dog has on children's independent mobility and physical activity.* Paper presented at the 2011 Annual Meeting of the International Society for Behavioral Nutrition and Physical Activity, Melbourne, Australia.
Veitch, J., Hume, C., Salmon, J., Crawford, D., & Ball, K. (2013). What helps children to be more active and less sedentary? Perceptions of mothers living in disadvantaged neighbourhoods. *Child: Care, Health and Development, 39*(1), 94–102.
Voith, V. (2009). The impact of companion animal problems on society and the role of veterinarians. *Veterinary Clinics of North America: Small Animal Practice, 39*(2), 327–345.
Westgarth, C., Boddy, L., Stratton, G., German, A., Gaskell, R., Coyne, K., ... Dawson, S. (2013). A cross-sectional study of frequency and factors associated with dog walking in 9-10 year old children in Liverpool, UK. *BMC Public Health, 13*(822), 1–10.
Westgarth, C., Christley, R. M., & Christian, H. E. (2014). How might we increase physical activity through dog walking? A comprehensive review of dog walking correlates. *International Journal of Behavioral Nutrition and Physical Activity, 11*, 83.
Westgarth, C., Heron, J., Ness, A. R., Bundred, P., Gaskell, R. M., Coyne, K., ... Dawson, S. (2012). Is childhood obesity influenced by dog ownership? No cross-sectional or longitudinal evidence. *Obesity, 5*(6), 833–834.
Westgarth, C., Heron, J., Ness, A. R., Bundred, P., Gaskell, R. M., Coyne, K. P., ... Dawson, S. (2010). Pet ownership during childhood: Findings from a UK birth cohort and implications for public health research. *International Journal of Environmental Research and Public Health, 7*, 3704–3729.
Westgarth, C., Pinchbeck, G. L., Bradshaw, J. W. S., Dawson, S., Gaskell, R. M., & Christley, R. M. (2007). Factors associated with dog ownership and contact with dogs in a UK community. *BMC Veterinary Research, 3*, 1–9.
Wohlfarth, R., Mutschler, B., Beetz, A., Kreuser, F., & Korsten-Reck, U. (2013). Dogs motivate obese children for physical activity: Key elements of motivational theory of animal-assisted interventions. *Frontiers in Psychology, 4*(796), 1–7.

Dr. Hayley Christian leads a research program on the development, evaluation and translation of strategies for improving children's physical activity levels, health and well-being through multilevel interventions focussed on the child, family, social and built environment. A focus of this work is on improving children's physical activity levels through identifying and testing intervention strategies to increase active play and walking with the family dog. Hayley is a Senior Research Fellow and holds an Australian National Heart Foundation Future Leader Fellowship.

Dr. Carri Westgarth is a Research Fellow and holds a UK Medical Research Council Fellowship in 'Understanding dog ownership and walking for better human health'. With a background in animal behaviour, veterinary epidemiology and human public health, she leads a portfolio of projects related to the role pets in enhancing human wellbeing and the role of owners in enhancing pet welfare. In particular her work focuses on physical activity, obesity and dog bites.

Danny Della Vedova graduated from The University of Western Australia with majors in Population Health and Conservation Biology. He has interned as a research assistant within the Centre for the Built Environment and Health under the guidance of Dr. Hayley Christian. This led him to develop a research-informed dog walking intervention as part of a Masters level health promotion unit. He is currently volunteering in Madagascar as a project development intern for an NGO, helping to implement their health and environmental projects.

Chapter 8
Integrating Pedometers in Early Childhood Settings to Promote the Development of Positive Health Trajectories

Leah E. Robinson, E. Kipling Webster, Kara K. Palmer, and Catherine Persad

Integrating Pedometers in Early Childhood Settings to Promote the Development of Positive Health Trajectories

Promoting and sustaining physical activity in children is a global quest and aids in supporting a positive health trajectory (Robinson et al., 2015). Obesity and physical activity rates of American children remain a concern (Ogden, Carroll, Kit, & Flegal, 2012). The United States recommends children between the ages of 2–5 years acquire 120 min of daily physical activity, with approximately half of this time being of moderate to vigorous intensity (Institute of Medicine, 2011; National Association for Sport and Physical Education, 2009). Recommendations for older children (ages 6–17 years), state they should engage in at least 60 min of physical activity each day (Physical Activity Guidelines for Americans, 2008). Evidence clearly indicates that children accumulate approximately half of their daily physical activity recommendations (i.e., 60 min) in childcare settings (Pate, Pfeiffer, Trost, Ziegler, & Dowda, 2004) and schools (Siedentop, 2009). Therefore, it is imperative that preschools and schools are providing children with an environment conducive for physical activity.

Children's need to accumulate physical activity throughout the school day supports the development of policies and practices to encourage movement and physical activity within preschools and schools. The Health and Medicine Division of the National Academies of Sciences formerly the Institute of Medicine (IOM, 2011) and

L. E. Robinson (✉) · K. K. Palmer · C. Persad
University of Michigan, Ann Arbor, MI, USA
e-mail: lerobin@umich.edu; palmerka@umich.edu; ccpersad@umich.edu

E. Kipling Webster
School of Kinesiology, Louisiana State University, Baton Rouge, LA, USA
e-mail: kipwebster@lsu.edu

H. Brewer, M. R. Jalongo (eds.), *Physical Activity and Health Promotion in the Early Years*, Educating the Young Child 14,
https://doi.org/10.1007/978-3-319-76006-3_8

Early Childhood Obesity Prevention Policies recommend that preschools provide children opportunities to engage in at least 15 min of physical activity per hour, endorse specific modifications to the preschool environment to support the attainment of the physical activity goal, adopt teaching/learning activities that promote physical activity, and provide indoor and outdoor environments that are conducive to physical activity. For school-age populations, Educating the Student Body Taking Physical Activity and Physical Education to School recommends creating a whole-of-school approach toward physical activity that fosters at least 60 min per day of vigorous or moderate-intensity physical activity through various contexts in the school (IOM, 2013). A whole-of-school approach is a multi-component school initiative where all aspects of the school community work collectively together to positively influence the health and well-being of children (e.g., active transport, recess, physical education, classroom integration, curriculum, policy, and environmental strategies).

Impact of Physical Activity on Academic Performance

The health benefits of physical activity during a child's developmental years are unquestionable (Janssen & LeBlanc, 2010; Logan Webster, Getchell, Pfeiffer, & Robinson, 2015; Robinson et al., 2015). Physical activity also has an essential association with school success and academic performance. Palmer, Miller, and Robinson (2013) found that, compared to engagement in a sedentary task, a 30-min movement and physical activity session resulted in preschoolers demonstrating better sustained attention. Similarly, Webster, Wadsworth, and Robinson (2015) found that a 10-min physical activity break in the classroom led to more time on-task engagement during classroom activities. These findings align with other reviews that support the beneficial effect of physical activity on academic performance (CDC, 2010; Hillman, Erickson, & Kramer, 2008). A recent review of 50 studies found a positive relationship between participation in physical activity and academic performance in over half the studies (50.5%) as well as non-detrimental effects in 48% of the remaining studies (Rasberry et al., 2011). High levels of physical fitness and physical activity have been associated with higher levels of academic performance (Hillman, Castelli, & Buck, 2005; Hillman et al., 2009).

Despite movement and physical activity's contribution to health trajectories in children (Robinson et al., 2015), data support that young children spend 80% of their day in sedentary behaviors even when given the opportunity to engage in outdoor and indoor physical activities (Brown et al., 2006). The established relationship between physical activity and cognition as well as the established low-levels of classroom physical activity clearly demonstrate the need for modification or better inclusion techniques to bring more physical activity in the classroom. Children's physical activity could be improved through various instructional and organizational practices or by incorporating recommendations set forth by the IOM reports (IOM, 2011, 2013). We hope that this chapter will provide early childhood educators with a better understanding of the importance of incorporating physical activity into the classroom as well as practical examples of how to effectively accomplish this goal.

Pedometers and Evidence to Support Integration in Classroom Settings

Pedometers are the most commonly used objective physical activity measurement tool in clinical settings (Trost & O'Neil, 2014). They are lightweight devices that do not interfere with normal daily activities. Pedometers are a low-cost device ($10–$20) that effectively calculate an individual's step-count. These devices can be easily integrated into any classroom to help monitor children's physical activity (Robinson & Wadsworth, 2010). Pedometers provide simplistic feedback as it relates to the number of steps acquired which allows children to actively use and understand this feedback from an informative and motivational standpoint, but it is also meaningful information (i.e., step count) to teachers and/or parents who can use this information to reinforce and encourage a healthy model for physical activity. Pedometers could get preschoolers excited about being physically active and moving. There has not been studies to examine the motivational effects of pedometers in preschoolers. But step-count feedback from pedometers were a motivating factor in increasing physical activity (i.e., number of steps) in school-age children (Butcher, Fairclough, Stratton, & Richardson, 2007; Gardner & Campagna, 2011). Although a step count recommendation for preschool-age children is not established, acquiring 12,000 and 15,000 steps per day is recommended for girls and boys between 6 and 12 years, respectively (Tudor-Locke et al., 2011). It is possible for a preschool teacher to establish daily step count goals for students (e.g., 5000–7000 steps during school hours) or obtain a baseline measure of step counts for a class over a 3 or 4-day period. This step count baseline could be used to establish a goal for your classroom to meet and eventually surpass. The remainder of the chapter will focus on practical approaches that early childhood educators could use within their classroom to promote their student's physical activity and movement.

Effective Strategies for Implementing Pedometers into the Classroom

This section provides effective strategies and approaches for implementing pedometer usage in your classroom as well as discusses different strategies to meet cross-curriculum goals of integrating both physical activity and learning opportunities. Opportunities to reinforce learning concepts with movement provide new ways for children to apply information and create novel approaches for reinforcing classroom concepts. The following examples are just a few highlighted strategies that have been shown to be effective approaches for integrating pedometers into the classroom.

Converting Steps to Mileage

Step counts from pedometers provide an easy representation of the most popular physical activity, ambulatory movements (i.e., walking). Converting step counts to a distance covered is an easy and effective way for a child to visualize their physical activity engagement. Although physical activity behaviors vary from person to person, most researchers use the estimation that 2000 steps are equivalent to one mile of walking (Shape Up America! 2015). From this estimation, you can use step counts to determine how many miles students' walk in 1 day, 1 week, or one school year. You may also combine the entire class's step counts to calculate class totals and see how many miles your classroom can walk in a specified period of time. This step count equivalent can also be integrated in academic lessons as you might see if the class can "walk" to a different city, country, or – over extended periods of time even to a different planet! A paper from Robinson and Wadsworth entitled "Stepping toward Physical Activity Requirements: Integrating Pedometers into Early Childhood Settings" provides some additional teaching activities like – Seeing the World (2010). Integrating academics with physical activity behaviors can be an invaluable and easy way to get children excited about accumulating steps and reinforce academic concepts, such as geography, social studies, earth science, or even math. Classrooms can also compete against each other to accumulate the most steps over a period of time. The last section of the chapter provides an array of activities that teachers use to integrate pedometers with teaching and learning along with additional resources to provide support.

Setting SMART Activity Goals

Using pedometers in the classroom provides children with a unique opportunity to learn about goal setting (i.e., enhancing problem solving skills). The instant availability of feedback allows children to make attainable short-term and/or long-term goals. For instance, children may set goals toward meeting the United States physical activity recommendations/guidelines giving them a chance to learn about physical activity recommendations and what if feels like to meet these recommendations.

When using pedometers in the classroom, teachers may begin with a baseline measurement of activity. Teachers will have children wear pedometers for a few days or a week to determine what their regular physical activity behaviors resemble. From here, teachers and their students can work together and evaluate how much

S	**Specific** • Clearly defines the goal you are hoping to achieve, and providing ample detail on each component of your goal.
M	**Measurable** • A goal needs to have the ability to be measured so that you can determine if you are achieving what you set out to do
A	**Attainable** • Realistic goals will help students realize what they are able to achieve and build self-confidence and self-efficacy
R	**Relevant** • A goal should be pertinent and related to what you set out to accomplish
T	**Timely** • Creating a well-defined timeline will help to track progress towards your goal

Fig. 8.1 SMART goal

physical activity they are acquiring and then set goals for how much they want to increase their physical activity. This collaborative effort could be an excellent math integration scenario reinforce addition, multiplication, or percentages. Students could establish a goal to walk 100 more steps per day, they might want to walk twice as much, or they might want to increase weekly step counts by 10%. With pedometers, students have the opportunity for immediate feedback to see if they are achieving their goals. If students are not on track to meet their goal, they can create a plan on how to modify their behavior to accomplish the desired goal.

Using SMART (**S**pecific, **M**easurable, **A**ttainable, **R**elevant, and **T**imely; Fig. 8.1) Goals are a simple and easy approach to help your students with goal setting. Goal setting is a tool that we will use across our lifespan, so establishing effective goal setting strategies early might prove to be fruitful later in life. In particular, setting and accomplishing physical activity goals in early childhood may establish the confidence and self-efficacy to be physically active long after pedometer usage is complete. SMART Goals include a **S**pecific desired behavioral outcome (100 more steps/day) that is a **M**easurable (quantifiable), **A**ttainable (realistic), **R**elevant (working towards daily step count), and **T**imely (include specific timeline). An example of a SMART goal for pedometer usage could be as follows: to increase step count from 9000 to 10,000 steps per day by walking to school for the next 5-days. This specific goal involves an increase of 1000 steps per day (measurable) by walking to school (attainable/relevant) over the course of the week (timely). This kind of goal setting highlights how pedometers may also be important in teaching children self-management skills as children learn how to set and accomplish goals. The example provided is a short-term goal (1-week), but the SMART technique can be used to set short and long-term goals alike.

Pedometers in the Classroom

Pedometers are a cost-effective, practical tool that can be integrated into the classroom setting to support physical activity. Teachers can include pedometers in their lesson plans or use them to create effective opportunities for increasing daily physical activity within their classroom. Using pedometers are relatively simple and should not overwhelm teachers with learning a new technology. In this section, we discuss practical approaches and ideas for how teachers can use pedometers to reinforce academic content and create physical activity opportunities in the classroom.

Reinforcing Academic Content

Pedometers can be used in the classroom to create opportunities for students to work cooperatively towards a group goal. This activity requires teamwork, communication, and encouragement that may foster social cohesiveness and group responsibility. As there are many curricular implications for the usage of step counts, classrooms may offer incentives toward reaching certain step count goals as a group. A classroom may set a SMART goal to accumulate the numbers of steps equivalent to the distance between the classroom and the zoo within 1 month. When students accomplish this goal, the teacher may prepare a special lesson plan or classroom activity based on zoo animals. Depending on your class content, there are multiple integration possibilities that could reinforce academics while promoting a group goal or activity.

Math The possibilities of using pedometers in math lessons are limitless. Pedometers measure a physical step, something most young children have personal experience with, giving concrete meaning to a numerical value. Teachers can use this to their advantage by using the pedometer as a tool for mathematical concepts. In preschools, pedometers can be used to help teach basic mathematical principles such as greater than or less than. Teachers may have children wear pedometers during work time or on the playground. When work time or outdoor playtime is over, teachers can look at children's pedometers and report on who took the most steps or the fewest steps. This simple activity introduces children to the idea that some mathematical values are higher or lower than others.

Teachers of older children can use pedometers in more concrete mathematical lessons such as addition or subtraction. To use pedometers in an addition lesson, have children walk around the classroom for 5-min. After the 5-min, record how many steps each child took. Have the children use these values and calculate different measures from the class such as: how many steps did the whole class take? or did the boys or the girls in the class take more steps? Figure 8.2 shows a sample worksheet where pedometers were used to teach addition. Once children start answering these types of questions, they may start to develop questions of their

Name: ______________________

How many steps did you take on…
Monday? _________
Tuesday? _________
Wednesday? _________
Thursday? _________
Friday? _________

TOTAL_______________

Now ask a friend.

How many steps did your friend take:

Monday? _________
Tuesday? _________
Wednesday? _________
Thursday? _________
Friday? _________

TOTAL_______________

Who took the most amount of steps during the week?
You or your friend? How do you know?

Fig. 8.2 Example of Pedometer Math worksheet

own. Encourage children to think about addition or subtraction questions that can be answered using the pedometers. Have the children write these questions down and try to solve the math themselves.

Science Teachers can implement several outdoor and indoor science activities that will integrate movement and physical activity with learning. Taking your class outside during science lessons is a great way to introduce children to a plethora of science concepts from botany to meteorology. These lessons can be easily modified for teaching a variety of science concepts across different ages. Though not the central focus of the lesson, pedometers may facilitate children's engagement during science outdoor adventures.

Nature Walks (Outdoor Activity) Nature walks can give children a hands-on experience for learning a range of science concepts including life science, geography and even meteorology. Life science nature walks can accommodate a spectrum of learning objectives such as identifying plants or insects and may be easily modified for children's developmental level (preschool to second grade). Preschoolers may want to find three differently colored leaves whereas second graders may want to find leaves from two different conifers or deciduous trees. Teachers can ask children to use their pedometers and count how many steps they took from the school to each tree and together the class can determine which tree is the farthest or closest to the classroom door. Children can use this information and make a map to the trees on the same display where they present their leaves. Simple modifications can be made to highlight different content areas such as insects, clouds, or different animal habitats that may fit into your particular lesson plan.

Similarly, teachers can use nature walks to teach geography. Students could walk through several different terrains: level ground, hills, and forested areas. Teachers can ask students to make observations about how weather affects the flora and fauna in a given area. Teachers can also prompt children to read their pedometers after each walk. Did children take more steps on the flat ground or in the hills? Why might this be?

Physiology (Indoor Activity) Pedometers also provide opportunities to learn about the body and how movement and physical activity impact our biological system. For example, have the children take 10 steps in 1-min. What happens to their body? Does their heart rate increase? Do they start to sweat? What happens when they take 100 steps in a 1-minute? Does their body have the same response as it did with only 10 steps? Use this small experiment to launch into conversations about the importance of exercise, especially for heart and musculoskeletal health.

Reading Reading periods pose an especially difficult challenge for young children. Sitting still and listening to a story for an extended period of time may or may not be feasible for a child in preschool or early elementary school. A simple fix to this dilemma is to make a story active. Have the children re-enact the story. If the main character is walking to school, have the children walk around the classroom; if the main character is skiing in the mountains have the children pretend to ski around the classroom. Teachers can also work with their class to write their own "Book of Activities". This book can focus on specific words the class is learning while incorporating some of the classrooms' favorite movements.

Physical Activity Breaks In just as little as 10 min teachers can incorporate physical activity into their classroom by implementing physical activity breaks. The possibilities for how to structure a physical activity break are fluid and can be built around your classroom schedule and students' abilities. Breaks can range from a dance session, to a short physical activity game, or even to a structured workout routine. We recommend making a list of possible break activities to have on hand. Authors of a recent study made physical activity cards and during each break teachers selected a set number of physical activity cards to do with their class (Webster et al., 2015). This approach is simple and practical for teachers and offers a variety of activities for the children. Think about it, if you had 10 different activity cards and only use 4 cards during each break, you have over 5000 possible ways to structure your break!

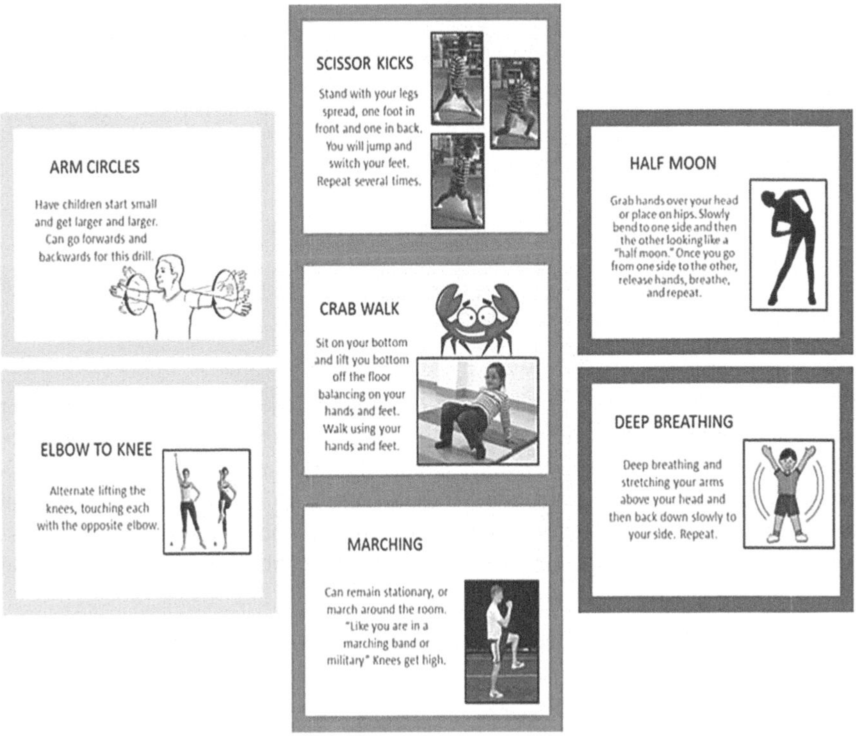
SCISSOR KICKS
Stand with your legs spread, one foot in front and one in back. You will jump and switch your feet. Repeat several times.
ARM CIRCLES
Have children start small and get larger and larger. Can go forwards and backwards for this drill.
HALF MOON
Grab hands over your head or place on hips. Slowly bend to one side and then the other looking like a "half moon." Once you go from one side to the other, release hands, breathe, and repeat.
CRAB WALK
Sit on your bottom and lift you bottom off the floor balancing on your hands and feet. Walk using your hands and feet.
ELBOW TO KNEE
Alternate lifting the knees, touching each with the opposite elbow.
DEEP BREATHING
Deep breathing and stretching your arms above your head and then back down slowly to your side. Repeat.
MARCHING
Can remain stationary, or march around the room. "Like you are in a marching band or military" Knees get high.

Fig. 8.3 Example of physical activity break cards. Yellow cards are warm-up, green are intense activities, and blue are cool-down

Cards can also be created and grouped by intensity or purpose of the exercise. You may create a card for arm circles. Arm circles promote flexibility and muscular endurance in young children but are not a very intense exercise so they might be categorized as a warm-up or cool-down activity. Marching in place or jumping jacks are more intense physical activities, so these may be utilized in the middle of the break to increase students' heart rate and cardiorespiratory endurance (after the warm up but before the cool down) and may be labeled as an intense or vigorous activity. An example of a 10-min break using a predetermined warm up, intense exercises, and cool down cards is provided in Fig. 8.3.

Classroom-based activity breaks are becoming more popular in preschool and elementary classrooms. A project by Mahar et al. (2006) found that by implementing a short, 10-min break in the classroom children increased their in-school physical activity by an average of 780 steps compared to classes that did not conduct breaks! These results plus the extremely flexibility in break structures make physical activity breaks a simple and sustainable way of increasing children's daily physical activity.

Exercise Bingo

Jumping Jacks	Frog Jumps	Balance on 1-foot	Push Ups
March in Place	Lunges	Side to side jumps	Trunk Twists
Scissor Kicks	Shoulder Rolls	Toe Touches	Squats
Run in Place	Arm Circles	Bicycles	Crab Walk

Fig. 8.4 Example of Exercise Bingo

Physical Activity Games Physical activity games are a good substitute for outdoor recess and a clever way to have students get rid of excess energy in-between structured lesson plans. Physical activity games are particularly useful when recess is canceled due to poor weather conditions. Contrary to common belief, physical activity games do not all require large spaces and can be played safely in a classroom. Below are several examples and ideas of simple, physical activity games that can be implemented in your classroom.

Four corners is a crowd favorite among any age group of students and is easy to do in a typical classroom space. The game requires very little setup and can be modified to relate back to school subjects. If you are teaching about the early presidents of the United States, write down the name of the first four presidents on a piece of paper or an index card and place each index card in one of the four corners of the classroom. The teacher stands in the middle of the classroom and counts to ten while the students silently walk (hop, skip, leap...get creative!) to one of the corners of the room. After the 10 seconds, the teacher will call out the name of a president and the students in that corner with that president's card have to get 25 steps on their pedometer (or any other fun, physical activity) before the next round can begin. Fun and simple, this game can be easily changed to encompass a broad variety of school subjects as well as modified for different ages.

Students can also take part in designing physical activity games in the classroom. Students and teachers can work together to create a game of "Exercise Bingo" (Fig. 8.4). In lieu of numbers, fill each BINGO space with a different activity. Each time the teacher calls out a space on your board, you must get up and complete the activity before you mark it off. Make one large game board for the class or multiple game boards for each student! Have the children use their pedometers and keep track of how many steps they can accumulate throughout a single game. A teacher can use these steps to transition into a math or science lesson.

Physical activity games can be structured like Four Corners or Bingo, but can also be as simple and unstructured as an impromptu dance party! The important part about these games is that your students see that playing these games and having fun can also increase their step counts. Children are more likely to do something that they enjoy with the added benefit of being physically active.

Conclusion

With children spending most of the waking hours in schools there is a need for school policies and practices to ensure that school environments provide opportunities for children to move and be physically active during school hours. The early childhood years are a critical period of human development. Although we understand the importance of physical activity to our health, often we do not understand the pivotal role movement and physical activity has toward the total well-being of children. Ultimately, movement and physical activity support positive developmental trajectories of health that contribute to healthy growth and development (Robinson et al., 2015). Regular participation in physical activity helps to build strong bones and muscles, controls weight, and may play a role in improving blood pressure and cholesterol (Bouchard, Blair, & Haskell, 2012; Janssen & LaBlanc, 2010; Janz et al., 2010). All before of the systems of the body are positively affected by physical activity participation.

Many factors affect physical activity participation in children. Children's engagement in physical activity can be influenced by external factors: where they live, whether they are a girl or a boy, race/ethnicity, age, socioeconomic status – as well as internal factors: motivation, enjoyment of physical education or recess, and motor skill competency. Motor skills or movement behaviors that help individuals manipulate objects and to a navigate themselves through space are essential for lifelong physical activity participation (Robinson et al., 2015; Logan et al., 2015). Motor skills do not naturally develop, they must be taught, practiced, and reinforced for children to adequately acquire the knowledge and skill set needed to participate in physical activities later in life (Robinson, 2011; Robinson & Goodway, 2009). Since movement behaviors are crucial to the healthy development of children there is a need for evidence-based interventions that promote motor skills and physical activity in early childhood settings (Logan, Robinson, Webster, & Barber, 2013; Robinson, Webster, Logan, James, & Barber, 2012; Robinson, 2011; Robinson & Goodway, 2009).

In terms of socio-emotional development, movement and physical activity provide an opportunity for children to socially interact and engage with peers and helps to reduce stress, improve self-esteem, and facilitate emotional well-being (Sallis, Prochaska, & Taylor, 2000; Strong et al., 2005; Van Sluijs, McMinn, & Griffin, 2007). From a public health standpoint, there has been an increased focus on walking, for example the U.S. Surgeon General's Call to Action (Step it up!). The goal of the call is to get Americans of all ages and abilities to walking to improve their health (USHHS, 2008). By getting Americans walking and more physically active, this will significantly reduce the risk of chronic disease and premature death while supporting positive mental health (USHHS, 2008). By providing movement and physical activity opportunities during the early childhood years, young children are moving forward toward meeting the physical activity recommendations. Evidence also strongly supports that cognitive development and physical activity have a reciprocal relationship (Singh, Uijtdewilligen, Twisk, Van Mechelen, & Chinapaw, 2012; Tomporowski, Davis, Miller, & Naglieri, 2008). Existing and emerging evidence clearly supports that early childhood programs need to find ways to adopt approaches that integrate movement and physical activity in teaching and learning (i.e., using a movement-based approach). These practices and policies are also supported by the Health and Medicine Division of the National Academics of Sciences formerly the Institute of Medicine (IOM, 2011, 2013).

In closing, when using pedometers to incorporate movement and physical activity into your classroom children have the opportunity to learn through movement. This integration may reinforce classroom and academic goals, and allows for easy incorporation of pedometer steps into curriculum items to reinforce academic subjects. With ample opportunity to bolster children's awareness and participation for movement and physical activity more cognitive benefits and academic behaviors may coincide with increased incidence or physical activity and bolster healthy development in young children.

References

Bouchard, C., Blair, S. N., & Haskell, W. (2012). *Physical activity and health*. Champaign, IL: Human Kinetics.

Brown, W. H., Pfeiffer, K. A., McIver, K. L., Dowda, M., Almeida, M. J. C. A., & Pate, R. R. (2006). Assessing preschool children's physical activity: The observational systems for recording physical activity in children preschool version. *Research Quarterly for Exercise and Sport, 77*, 167–176.

Butcher, Z., Fairclough, S., Stratton, G., & Richardson, D. (2007). The effect of feedback and information on children's pedometer step counts at school. *Pediatric Exercise Science, 19*(1), 29–38.

Centers for Disease Control and Prevention (CDC). (2010). *The association between school based physical activity, including physical education, and academic performance* (Vol. 500, pp. 5–32). Atlanta, GA: Department of Health and Human Services.

Gardner, P. J., & Campagna, P. D. (2011). Pedometers as measurement tools and motivational devices: New insights for researchers and practitioners. *Health Promotion Practice, 12*(1), 55–62.

Hillman, C. H., Castelli, D. M., & Buck, S. M. (2005). Aerobic fitness and neurocognitive function in healthy preadolescent children. *Medicine & Science in Sports & Exercise, 37*(11), 1867–1974.

Hillman, C. H., Erickson, K. I., & Kramer, A. F. (2008). Be smart, exercise your heart: Exercise effects on brain and cognition. *Nature Reviews Neuroscience, 9*(1), 58–65.

Hillman, C. H., Pontifex, M. B., Raine, L. B., Castelli, D. M., Hall, E. E., & Kramer, A. F. (2009). The effect of acute treadmill walking on cognitive control and academic achievement in preadolescent children. *Neuroscience, 159*, 1044–1054.

Institute of Medicine (IOM). (2011). *Early childhood obesity prevention policies*. Washington, DC: The National Academies Press.

Institute of Medicine (IOM). (2013). *Educating the student body: Taking physical activity and physical education to school*. Washington, DC: The National Academies Press.

Janssen, I., & LeBlanc, A. G. (2010). Systematic review of the health benefits of physical activity and fitness in school-aged children and youth. *International Journal of Behavioral Nutrition and Physical Activity, 7*(40), 1–16.

Janz, K. F., Letuchy, E. M., Gilmore, J. M. E., Burns, T. L., Torner, J. C., Willing, M. C., & Levy, S. M. (2010). Early physical activity provides sustained bone health benefits later in childhood. *Medicine & Science in Sports & Exercise, 42*(6), 1072.

Logan, S. W., Robinson, L. E., Webster, E. K., & Barber, L. T. (2013). Exploring preschoolers' engagement and perceived physical competence in an autonomy-based object control skill intervention: A preliminary study. *European Physical Education Review, 19*, 302–314.

Logan, S. W., Webster, E. K., Getchell, N., Pfeiffer, K., & Robinson, L. E. (2015). Relationship between fundamental motor skill competence and physical activity during childhood and adolescence: A systematic review. *Kinesiology Review, 4*, 416–426.

Mahar, M. T., Murphy, S. K., Rowe, D. A., Golden, J., Shields, A. T., & Raedeke, T. D. (2006). Effects of a classroom-based program on physical activity and on-task behavior. *Medicine & Science in Sports & Exercise, 38*(12), 2086–2094.

National Association for Sport and Physical Education (2009). Active start: A statement of physical activity guidelines for children from birth to age 5 (2nd Edition). Reston, VA: SHAPE America - Society of Health and Physical Educators.

Ogden, C. L., Carroll, M. D., Kit, B. K., & Flegal, K. M. (2012). Prevalence of obesity and trends in body mass index among US children and adolescents, 1999–2010. *Journal of the American Medical Association, 307*(5), 483–490.

Palmer, K. K., Miller, M. W., & Robinson, L. E. (2013). Acute exercise enhances preschoolers' ability to sustain attention. *Journal of Sport and Exercise Psychology, 35*(4), 433–437.

Pate, R. R., Pfeiffer, K. A., Trost, S. G., Ziegler, P., & Dowda, M. (2004). Physical activity among children attending preschools. *Pediatrics, 114*(5), 1258–1263.

Physical Activity Guidelines Advisory Committee. (2008). *Physical activity guidelines for Americans* (pp. 15–34). Washington, DC: US Department of Health and Human Services.

Rasberry, C. N., Lee, S. M., Robin, L., Laris, B. A., Russell, L. A., Coyle, K. K., & Nihiser, A. J. (2011). The association between school-based physical activity, including physical education, and academic performance: A systematic review of the literature. *Preventive Medicine, 52*, S10–S20.

Robinson, L. E. (2011). Effect of a mastery climate motor program on object control skills and perceived physical competence in preschoolers. *Research Quarterly for Exercise and Sport, 82*, 355–359.

Robinson, L. E., & Goodway, J. D. (2009). Instructional climates in preschool children who are at-risk. Part I: Object control skill development. *Research Quarterly for Exercise and Sport, 80*, 533–542.

Robinson, L. E., Stodden, D. F., Barnett, L. M., Lopes, V. P., Logan, S. W., Rodrigues, L. P., & D'Hondt, E. (2015). Motor competence and its effect on positive developmental trajectories of health. *Sports Medicine, 45*(9), 1273–1284.

Robinson, L. E., & Wadsworth, D. D. (2010). Stepping toward physical activity requirements: Integrating pedometers into early childhood settings. *Early Childhood Education Journal, 38*(2), 95–102.

Robinson, L. E., Webster, E. K., Logan, S. W., James, W. A., & Barber, L. T. (2012). Teaching practices that promote motor skills in early childhood settings. *Early Childhood Education Journal, 40*, 79–86.

Sallis, J. F., Prochaska, J. J., & Taylor, W. C. (2000). A review of correlates of physical activity of children and adolescents. *Medicine & Science in Sports & Exercise, 32*(5), 963–975.

Shape Up America! (2015). *10,000 Steps*. Retrieved from: www.shapeup.org

Siedentop, D. L. (2009). National plan for physical activity: Education sector. *Journal of Physical Activity & Health, 6*(2), S168.

Singh, A., Uijtdewilligen, L., Twisk, J. W., Van Mechelen, W., & Chinapaw, M. J. (2012). Physical activity and performance at school: A systematic review of the literature including a methodological quality assessment. *Archives of Pediatrics & Adolescent Medicine, 166*(1), 49–55.

Strong, W. B., Malina, R. M., Blimkie, C. J., Daniels, S. R., Dishman, R. K., Gutin, B., … Rowland, T. (2005). Evidence based physical activity for school-age youth. *The Journal of Pediatrics, 146*(6), 732–737.

Tomporowski, P. D., Davis, C. L., Miller, P. H., & Naglieri, J. A. (2008). Exercise and children's intelligence, cognition, and academic achievement. *Educational Psychology Review, 20*(2), 111–131.

Trost, S. G., & O'Neil, M. (2014). Clinical use of objective measures of physical activity. *British Journal of Sports Medicine, 48*(3), 178–181.

Tudor-Locke, C., Craig, C. L., Beets, M. W., Belton, S., Cardon, G. M., Duncan, S., … Rowe, D. A. (2011). How many steps/day are enough? For children and adolescents. *International Journal of Behavioral Nutrition and Physical Activity, 8*(1), 78–92.

USHHS. (2008). *Physical activity guidelines for Americans*. Washington, DC: U.S. Department of Health and Human Services.

Van Sluijs, E. M., McMinn, A. M., & Griffin, S. J. (2007). Effectiveness of interventions to promote physical activity in children and adolescents: Systematic review of controlled trials. *British Medical Journal, 335*(7622), 703.

Webster, E. K., Wadsworth, D. D., & Robinson, L. E. (2015). Preschoolers' time on-task and physical activity during a classroom activity break. *Pediatric Exercise Science, 27*(1), 160–167.

Leah E. Robinson is an Associate Professor and Chair of Movement Scienceat the University of Michigan, and directs the Child Motor, Activity, & Developmental Health Laboratory. Her research takes a developmental perspective to motor skill acquisition, physical activity, and developmental health. She examines how to promote motor skills and physical activity in pediatric populations through the design and implementation of an evidence-based intervention – CHAMP (the Children's Health Activity Motor Program). She has published 4 book chapters and has over 70 peer-reviewed publications. Her research has been funded by the National Institutes of Health and the Robert Wood Johnson Foundation. In recognition of scholarly achievement, she has received several national and international honors.

E. Kipling Webster is an Assistant Professor at Louisiana State University and completed post-doctoral research training in the School of Kinesiology at the University of Michigan. Her research interests focus on physical activity behaviors and motor skill competency in pediatric populations. She examines school-based programs that target positive health-related outcomes, such as reducing childhood obesity and increasing physical activity, fitness, motor skill competency, and psychological variables related to health. Her research has been published in peer-review journals and presented at international and national conferences.

Kara K. Palmer is a PhD Candidate in the School of Kinesiology at the University of Michigan and is a Graduate Research Assistant in the Child Motor, Activity, & Developmental Health Laboratory. She received her Masters of Education from Auburn University in 2013. Kara's research focuses on pediatric motor development and physical activity. Her research has been published in peer-reviewed journals and presented at both national and international conferences.

Catherine Persad is a Sophomore and participant in the Undergraduate Research Opportunity Program at the University of Michigan. She serves as an Undergraduate Research Assistant in the Child Motor, Activity, & Developmental Health Laboratory.

Chapter 9
Preschoolers with Developmental Delays, Adapted Physical Education, Related Services, Physical Activity, and Collaborative Teaching

Nathan M. Murata

"*It takes a village to raise a child*" is metaphoric for describing how a team of individuals may be needed to facilitate how preschoolers learn, interact with others, and engage with the environment. Educating preschoolers requires a synergistic approach whereby classroom teachers, parents, and others work collaboratively to enhance the child's developmental growth, learning, social skills, and life activities. With numerous educational mandates and priorities, suggesting that an individual albeit classroom teacher and teacher aide can singlehandedly enhance the educational experiences for preschoolers alone is a daunting requirement. Recognizing those priorities, the *village* (e.g., classroom) embarks on a quest to deliver the most salient, productive, and efficient methods to address these priorities. One such venue to assert is the notion of physical activity (i.e., motor domain) serving as the catalyst for promoting and engaging preschoolers in their educational, physical, social, and emotional growth. Notwithstanding are preschoolers with developmental delays who require more "*villagers*" (i.e., adapted physical education, related services professionals) to support and enhance the learning experience within the *village*.

This chapter is organized into four sections. It begins with a rationale for physical activity for preschoolers with and without developmental delays. Next, it discusses the research on the notion of play and physical activity on obesity and overweightness for all preschoolers. Then, it describes how related service (e.g., occupational therapy, physical therapy, speech-language pathology) personnel "*other villagers*" augment a preschoolers' educational milieu. The article concludes by advocating for collaborative teaching and service delivery to more effectively deliver instruction and guidance to preschoolers and their families.

N. M. Murata (✉)
College of Education, University of Hawai'i at Mānoa, Honolulu, HI, USA
e-mail: nmurata@hawaii.edu

H. Brewer, M. R. Jalongo (eds.), *Physical Activity and Health Promotion in the Early Years*, Educating the Young Child 14,
https://doi.org/10.1007/978-3-319-76006-3_9

There are physical, social, psychological, and educational benefits associated with physical activity (motor domain) for young children, often established during early childhood (Cliff, Okely, Smith, & McKeen, 2009; Li, Kwan, King-Dowling, & Cairney, 2015) and with the potential for collateral benefits for forming the bedrock for physical activities and healthy lifestyles (Tucker, 2008). In this connection, physical activity is a key element to maximizing growth and development for preschool children, a major component of a preschool program including special education (Murata & Maeda, 2002; Van Cauwenberghe, Labarque, Gubbels, De Bourdeaudhuij, & Cardon, 2012). Physical activity is also vital in addressing the increase prevalence of overweightness and obesity (Pate, Pfeiffer, Trost, Ziegler, & Dowda, 2004) and an integral part of a preschooler's developmental process (United States Department of Health and Human Services, 2015). While physical activity can bolster increased attention, memory and learning, there are still many preschoolers who do not receive the necessary amount of physical activity (National Association for Sport and Physical Education [NASPE], 2002), which can lead to higher obesity rates and overweightness in preschoolers.

Obesity rates continued to climb for preschool children in recent years (Bellows, Davies, Anderson, & Kennedy, 2013; Pathare, Piche, Nicosia, & Haskvitz, 2016). The prevalence of obesity and higher Body Mass Index (BMI) in preschoolers with developmental delays has been clearly documented (Dwyer, Higgs, Hardy, & Baur, 2008; Hwang, Wu, Chen, Cheng, & Chen, 2014; Pate et a., 2004). One effective way to address obesity and overweightness in preschoolers is to promote more quality physical activity (Beets, Bornstein, Dowda, & Pate, 2011; Bellows et al., 2013; NASPE, 2002) and proper nutritional intake and dietary habits (Derscheid, Umoren, Kim, Beverly, & Zittel, 2010). National Association for Sport and Physical Education position statement on physical activity indicate that preschoolers ages 3–5 years old engage in at least 60-min of daily physical activity that promotes health-related fitness and movement skills (NASPE, 2002).

Gallahue and Cleland-Donnelly (2003) noted that fundamental motor skills provide the infrastructure for learning more important games, sports and activities for daily living. Furthermore, Gallahue and Cleland-Donnelly posited that a child who does not develop adequate fundamental movements exhibits a lower self-concept and social development. This lack of developmentally appropriate motor skills can also negatively correlate with a preschooler's ability to learn the rudiments of games, sports, activities for daily living (Kirk & Rhodes, 2011) and may even contribute to the rise in obesity (Bellows et al., 2013). Consequently, Tucker (2008) posited that despite clear evidence on the benefits of physical activity, nearly 23% of American children do not engage in any free-time physical activity. Relatedly, Pate et al. (2004) found that preschoolers engage in only 7.7 minutes of moderate to vigorous physical activity during school hours when National guidelines suggest nearly eight times that amount of exercise, at least 60 minutes. Physical inactivity becomes more magnified when considering preschoolers with developmental delays (Pierce-Jordan & Lifter, 2005).

Preschoolers with Developmental Delays

Preschoolers with developmental delays are described as having challenges in one or more of the following areas: cognitive skills, communication skills, social/emotional functioning, behavior, fine and gross motor skills. These preschoolers may be eligible for special education services once parents agree to screening, formal assessment and Individualized Family Service Plan (IFSP) or Individualized Education Program (IEP) development. Public Law 108-446, Individuals with Disabilities Education Improvement Act of 2004, Part C, [para] states the need to provide "specially designed instruction to meet the unique needs of young children with disabilities, including infants and toddlers, receiving special education services." As a primary service, *physical education is specifically mentioned in the definition of special education* for pupils with Individualized Education Program (IEP) or IFSP (infants and toddlers;) (IDEA, 2004). Furthermore, IDEA (2004) stipulates that physical education means instruction in (a) physical and motor fitness; (b) fundamental motor skills and patterns; and (c) skills in aquatics, dance, and individual and group games and sports including intramural and lifetime sports. The promotion of physical education applies to preschoolers with developmental delays (Dummer, Connor-Kuntz, & Goodway, 1995). Preschoolers with developmental delays are entitled to a quality physical activity program that attunes with other related domains to prepare for school readiness, transition into kindergarten, and improved physical well-being and motor development.

Preschoolers with developmental delays need as much (and perhaps) more motor skills acquisition and competence in order to interact with their environment and learn skills. Whether this environment is the classroom, outside, during recess (Nicaise, Kahan, Reuben, & Sallis, 2012), or even at home, physical activity should be provided to preschoolers to increase higher levels of physical activity and to reduce the potential for being overweight or obese (Verbestel et al., 2011). Despite the environmental influences, there is a misconception that all children are "naturally" active and do not require any form of encouragement or support to be active. In some cases, preschoolers with developmental delays may need to be taught "how to play." Adapted physical education is taught to preschoolers primarily focusing on basic motor skills, balance, movement, coordination activities, fundamental gross motor skills, object control skills, and spatial/body awareness. Even the notion of "play" has significant positive developmental outcomes in preschoolers' with and without developmental delays.

Play

Play is defined as an activity that offers physical, social and emotional stimulation. Play fosters creativity, and provides educational and functional growth for preschoolers. Play has been used as a way for preschoolers to engage in their learning, enhance communication channels between adults, and improve social-emotional and motor skill development (Recchia, 2016). Play allows for perseverance, steadfast ability to overcome, gumption to be successful and inevitably how to even compromise with other children (Recchia, 2016). Some consider play as the "work" of children and toys are the "tools" for carrying out children's important work (Lifter, Mason, & Barton, 2011; Jansma, 1999). Early childhood education theorists (e.g., Vygotsky, Bruner, Piaget, and others) postulate that play is one of the most important ways in which young children learn (National Association for the Education of Young Children [NAEYC], 2012; Reifel, 2014). Play is so fundamentally important to a child's life that without enough time engaged in play, young children may develop a play deficit disorder. Acknowledging the possibility of having a "play deficit" requires our attention (Kretchmar, 2012). That is, play disabilities can be witnessed for some children who do not exhibit appropriate social behaviors. The extent of this chapter does not lend support to a detailed and thorough discourse on play; however, play is important to mention as a vital factor in learning and physical activity for preschoolers with and without developmental delays.

Conceivably, play can be in the form of either structured or unstructured play (Gunner, Atkinson, Nichols, & Eissa, 2005; Murata & Maeda, 2002). Structured play offers specific goals to be carried out and typically led by the teacher or adult. For instance, a classroom teacher may organize the playground with specific obstacles to have preschoolers work on various motor skills. Unstructured play is synonymous to "free play" where the children opt to initiate, pretend, and create activities and interactions. Yet many preschool teachers opt for a more play-like environment in order to compensate for the motor domain (Murata & Maeda, 2002). Consequently, promoting a play-like environment only with limited to no instruction does not correlate with an increase in motor competence and development for preschoolers with developmental delays. Despite efforts to promote a quality program, many preschool teachers have little knowledge, training and skills about motor development, yet, are left responsible for directing the motor skills program. Conversely, Alhassan et al. (2012) conducted a pilot study that demonstrated a teacher directed locomotor motor skills program can possibly improve along with a reduction in sedentary lifestyles for minority preschoolers. Jones et al. (2011) reported that physical activity programs with structured lessons can be implemented by a preschool staff that can increase the physical activity levels for preschoolers. However researchers do not specifically describe who belongs or qualifications as preschool staff. Researchers continue to show the benefits of a gross motor instructional skill programs for all preschoolers (Goodway, Crow, & Ward, 2003), including preschoolers from disadvantaged backgrounds (Goodway & Branta, 2003; Goodway, Robinson, & Crow, 2010), and preschoolers with development coordination disorder (Hodge, Leiberman, & Murata, 2012; Slater, Hillier, & Civetta, 2010). Most of these researchers mention that the preschool teacher provides the necessary instruction. Nonetheless, I would argue that a qualified individual be available to provide motor skill instruction (Woodson-Smith & Holden, 2015). Therefore, preschool teachers have multiple physical activity and gross/fine motor curricula at their disposal to implement a sound motor activity program. Curricular concepts such as basic movement forms, basic games, creative and rhythmic patterns, body management/movements, cooperative games, and fitness concepts all form the basis for a quality preschool movement and physical activity program.

To inherently address quality movement curricula, some notable programs (but not limited to) *SMART START Preschool Movement Curriculum* (Wessel & Zittel, 1995), SPARK, (www.sparkpe.org), Coordinated Approach to Child Health (CATCH); (www.catglobalfoundation.org), *Moving with a Purpose* (McCall & Craft, 2000) and Food Friends: *Get Movin with Mighty Moves* (The Food Friends Foundation, http://www.foodfriends.org/food-friends-programs/get-movin-mighty-moves/ have been in widespread use and mentioned throughout the early childhood and adapted physical activity literature. For example, preschool programs have *Get Movin with Mighty Moves* to be helpful in developing gross, fine motor competencies, and nutrition as well as addressing the obesity problem faced by preschoolers with and without developmental delays. The CATCH program includes three main components: (a) it's fun to be healthy; (b) structured physical activities; and (c) family education. While Hengstman (2001) promotes the *Movement ABC* guide by infusing and stimulating language development into a physical activity program. For example, this infusion of language into a physical activity program enhances both content areas by reinforcing skills and concepts that may have been previously taught. Given this myriad of quality physical activity programs available to preschool teachers, implementing a sound program can be accomplished. Unfortunately delivering a quality program to preschoolers with developmental delays requires the efforts of qualified and certificated personnel, including related services providers, working collaboratively as team to reach IFSP and motor development goals.

Related Services

Special education is a primary service that is specifically designed instruction to fulfill the instructional needs of infants, toddlers and young children with disabilities. Coupled with the implementation of special education instruction, many preschoolers with developmental delays require related services to benefit from special education instruction. Related services are:

> The Public Law 108-117 (Individuals with Disabilities Education Improvement Act) defined "Related Services" as transportation and such developmental, corrective, and other supportive services as are required to assist a child with a disability to benefit from special education, and includes speech-language pathology and audiology services, interpreting services, psychological services, physical and occupational therapy, recreation, including therapeutic recreation, early identification and assessment of disabilities in children, counseling services, including rehabilitation counseling, orientation and mobility services, and medical services for diagnostic or evaluation purposes. Related services also include school health services and school nurse services, social work services in schools, and parent counseling and training. (IDEA, 2004, U.S.C. §140(a)(17))[para]

Unfortunately the discourse surrounding related services cannot be addressed totally within this chapter; instead the focus will be on the most commonly used related services provided to preschoolers with developmental delays: Occupational Therapy (OT), Physical Therapy (PT) and Speech-Language Pathology (SLP). The American Occupational Therapy Association (AOTA), American Speech–Language Hearing Association (ASHA) and the American Physical Therapy Association (APTA), offer policies and procedures for family centered approaches to learning as well as collaboration for early intervention services (Campbell, Chiarello, Wilcox, & Milbourne, 2009; Colyvas, Sawyer, & Campbell, 2010). Collectively, these related services are quite common for preschoolers with developmental delays and actually can form the motor team (Menear & Davis, 2015). This notion of collaboration as mandated by these organizations is critical to acknowledging the positive impact such efforts have on the classroom teacher and preschoolers. Silliman-French et al. (2007) and Menear and Davis (2015) refer to a cadre of professionals as the Gross Motor Team for children with disabilities. Menear and Davis stated "*collaboration across these disciplines and others regarding the selected IEP goals for a child can improve the child's overall educational experience*" (Menear & Davis, 2014, p. 19). These related services have supported collaborative efforts as an appropriate service delivery model for preschoolers with and without developmental delays.

Occupational Therapy The acquisition of fine motor skills for preschoolers and young children is an important part of developmental growth and serves as a conduit for augmenting motor skills, play, physical activity, activities for daily living, education and social/emotional growth (Marr, Cermack, Cohn, & Henderson, 2003). IDEA (2004) defined an occupational therapist as someone using various techniques to (1) improve, develop, and/ore restore function impaired or list through illness, injury, or deprivation; (2) improve ability to perform task for independent functioning; and (3) prevent through early intervention initial or further impairment or loss of function. Watkins et al. (2014) reported that occupational therapy intervention for preschoolers may improve selected preschool motor skills. The authors surmised that even low-birth weight children can benefit from some form of occupational therapy intervention. Case-Smith (2000) concluded that occupational therapy can improve the fine and visual motor skills during play therapy. She articulated the relationship between both fine and visual motor, by implementing play and peer instruction experiences. Her findings reinforced the importance of therapeutic play in intervention (Case-Smith, 2000). Hermes (2007) found that occupational therapists utilize more than one service delivery model ranging from direct service to collaborative consultation. Irrespective of which service delivery model used, either method appears to be equally effective in meeting objectives for preschoolers with mild motor impairments (Hermes, 2007).

Being that the motor domain serves as a fundamental infrastructure for preschoolers with developmental delays to learn, it seems logical that the preschool teacher, adapted physical educator (APE) along with an OT can promote the necessary prerequisite skills to facilitate appropriate motor gains. Rule and Stewart (2002) posited that classroom teachers can be taught to augment fine motor activities into their daily routines. Murata and Tan (2008), Murata and Maeda (2007) surmised that specific physical activities across occupational therapy skills can be infused in a physical activity curriculum for preschoolers with and without disabilities. Murata and Maeda (2007) articulate that fine motor type activities (e.g., movement sequencing, motor memory, spatial awareness) can be infused with the overall physical activity curriculum to reinforce specific fine motor skills taught by an occupational therapist. For example, the classroom teacher can place poly spots, tie jump ropes between chairs, and place high/low objects around the room. Using music, preschoolers can move around the room without touching one another, demonstrating spatial awareness from a high and low perspective, moving within one's own space, and ending with seating properly in their own space.

Physical Therapy Physical Therapy addresses issues related to rehabilitation, muscle strength, mobility, and posture as they relate to educational programming and activities for daily living. A licensed physical therapist performs ongoing assessment/evaluations, develops and modifies the education plan that includes objectives and benchmarks, and provides direct and indirect services (Neal, Bigby, & Nicholson, 2004). Downing (2004) and the American Physical Therapy Association (2015) reported that licensed PT provides the following services: (1) treatment to increase joint function, muscle strength, mobility and endurance; (2) address gross motor skills involved in physical movement and range of motion; (3) help improve a child's posture, gait, and body awareness; and (4) monitor function, fit and proper mobility aids and devices. Specific to preschoolers with developmental delays, PT would first conduct an assessment, provide intervention and strategies, evaluate movement and motor skills, establish movement goals, and include/teach the family about the intervention and strategies to assist the child within the natural environment (Downing, 2004; Shapiro & Sayers, 2003; Silliman-French et al., 2007). Shapiro and Sayers surmised that PT traditionally provided intervention and treatment through a "pull out" method whereby therapy was provided in isolation. With amendments to IDEA, shortages of PT personnel, PT are spending more time in the classroom, gymnasium, during the preschoolers' regular schedule to enhance and augment skill taught within the learning environment (Shapiro & Sayers, 2003).

The benefits of PT intervention on young children have been well documented (Elgsti, Chandler, Robinson, & Bodkin, 2010; Palisano, 2006). In fact, Nervik, Martin, Rundquist, and Cleland (2011) found that children aged three to five with high BMI may have difficulty with gross motor skills. Given limitations, they offer that PT can take part in efforts to address childhood obesity. Specific to the motor domain, PT has many similarities with adapted physical education. Both PT and APE address gross motor needs, assist with movement and learning within least restrictive environment, conduct physical and motor assessment, provide input into IFSP and IEP goals, and prepare the preschooler with transition to kindergarten and school readiness. For instance, a preschooler with limited mobility uses crutches for ambulation can participate in an adapted physical education program whereby the adapted physical educator, classroom teacher, and physical therapist focus on eye-foot coordination skills. Kicking a stationary ball into a modified goal is the intent of this adapted physical education lesson. While the adapted physical educator provides prompts and cues, the physical therapist can monitor leg and foot extension, while offering suggestions for leg strengthening activities. Hence, these activities can be facilitated by the classroom teacher on days where there is no adapted physical education or direct physical therapy services.

Speech-Language Pathology Speech-language pathology services comprise the following: (1) identification of children with speech or language impairments; (2) diagnosis and appraisal of specific speech or language impairments; (3) referral for medical or other professional attention necessary for the habilitation of speech or language impairments; (4) provision of speech and language services for the habilitation or prevention of communicative impairments; and (5) counseling and guidance of parents, children, and teachers regarding speech and language impairments (IDEA, 2004). Speech-language pathology plays an important role in a preschooler's educational development (ASHA, 2008). The majority of preschoolers with developmental delays receiving special education services as mandated by Part B of Public Law 108-446 have a speech-language deficit that requires intervention from a qualified speech-language pathologist and/or audiologist. These speech-language deficits are found in (but are not limited to) articulation, expressive and receptive language, and flow with a plausible relationship to deficits in motor coordination (ASHA, 2008). To this, Watson and Bellon-Harn (2013) articulated how collaboration between a speech-language pathologist and general educator can be implemented through the Response-to-Intervention technique offering step-by-step tiers. Consequently, Scarborough and Dobrich (1990) reported that children with articulation problems may also have significant motor delays, and a correlation existed between a child's linguistic ability and motor skills. Connor-Kuntz and Dummer (1996) postulated that preschoolers with speech impairments who participated in a language-enriched physical education environment improved in language development. More recently, Macdonald, Lord and Ulrich (2013) stated that there may be a plausible relationship between motor skills and social communicative skills for children with autism. While Macdonald et al. (2013) utilized students ages 6–15, their initial findings do hold possible implications for even young children with developmental delays. In this connection, Sunderland (2004) synthesized that speech-language pathologist be used as an instructional support as intervention becomes infused within class activities.

Kaczmarek (1985) suggested that integration of language communication objectives should be infused into the total preschool curriculum, including the motor domain. Ellis, Schlaudecker, and Regimbal (1995) found that collaboration between classroom teachers, physical educators, university professors and speech-language pathologists can help increase basic concepts for kindergartners. Results of their study indicated that kindergartners who received collaboration showed improvements in basic concepts when compared to those kindergartners who did not receive treatment. Solomon and Murata (2008) reported that a link exists between physical education and language arts which may contribute to a child's alertness and thinking. They offer suggestions on how the interdisciplinary teaching model can be used effectively to augment and reinforce language arts during physical education classes. For example the adapted physical educator can reinforce simple one word phrases (e.g., stop, go, move, turn, up, down, right, left) taught by the preschool teacher during the physical activity lesson. The promotion of language and speech concepts can be augmented into a physical activity lesson for children and students by reinforcing language strategies and tactics (Murata, 2000, 2003). Lastly, the need to seriously consider collaboration with speech-language pathology by both the preschool teacher and adapted physical educator magnifies when augmentative and alternative communication devices are integrated within the learning environment (Hammond & Warner, 1996; Hustad, Keppner, Schanz, & Berg, 2008). As another example, the adapted physical educator and classroom teacher can utilize "predictable activities" which become familiar and easily handled by preschoolers. Offering the same daily warm-ups or doing the same cardio exercise (i.e., jogging around the field) creates predictability for all (Murata, 2003).

Given that the motor domain is viewed as a vital component in a child's overall educational milieu and mentioned as a primary (direct) service in the definition of special education, adapted physical educators, in particular, are in a prime position to facilitate and assist in the development of such motor programs. Preschoolers with developmental delays require a robust educational experience utilizing a multi-prong teaching approach in collaboration with all primary and related service providers. During the IFSP meeting, would be a good start to the collaboration process. To this end, the notion of collaborative teaching across academic and related services can be an effective and efficient service delivery option for preschool teachers (Klein & Hollingshead, 2015; Silliman-French et al, 2007).

Collaborative Teaching and Service Delivery

Collaboration is defined as individuals sharing information, bringing their expertise into common understanding, communicating openly and freely without the fear of rejection or argument (Downing, 2004; Murata & Tan, 2008). In fact, "many societal problems are viewed as too complex to be resolved by a single specialization" (Tomporowski, P. D., McCullick, B. A., & Pesce, C. 2015, p. 132). Collaboration involves continuous two-way and open communication, flexibility, and mutual respect for others. Collaboration provides the ability to assess progress and brings a sense of shared responsibility between experts while lessening the burden toward direct services particularly when shortages exist (Lawson & Sailor, 2000; Maeda & Murata, 2004; Silliman-French et al., 2007). More specifically, Lawson and Sailor (2000) highlighted interpersonal collaboration or service integration as another entity for collaborative service delivery and suggested that a transdisciplinary approach is an effective conduit for service delivery among children with special needs. Children with special needs or preschoolers with developmental delays have multiple needs and the services provided are all inter-related. Interestingly, the literature is replete with information on collaboration and its potential benefit to professionals and preschoolers. However, limited information about the actual efficacy on collaboration and its implementation within the motor domain is available. There are various reasons as to why such a collaborative teaching and service delivery model is promoted (time for service delivery, shortages, caseloads); however, simply arguing for more personnel does not necessarily equate to efficient services, actual empirical evidence on the efficacy of such service delivery in special education is critical and mandatory.

Collaboration among professionals (preschool educators, adapted physical educators, physical therapists, occupational therapists and speech-language pathologists) and content areas can be successfully achieved in early intervention programs. For instance, the Adapted Physical Education National Standards (Kelly, 2006) call for APE to *"understand the team approach for providing educational programs, understand the nature of group dynamics, and situational leadership"* (Kelly, 2006, p. 135). In a similar vein, AOTA supports collaborating between individuals particularly in association with the IEP or IFSP process (Clark, Polichino, & Jackson, 2004). The APTA guiding principles include *collaboration* as part of its organizational vision (https://www.apta.org/Vision/). ASHA mentions "collaborating with other professionals (e.g., planning lessons with educators)" [para] as an important component of its clinical services (http://www.asha.org/policy/SP2007-00283/). Given the brevity of education and related services supporting and advocating for collaborative service delivery model, it makes sense that such a model for early intervention of preschoolers with developmental delays be used more frequently. The issue of collaboration between professionals needs to be addressed in light of appropriate service delivery for preschoolers with limited supply of trained and qualified personnel. Moreover, Radonovich and Houck (1990) reported on the inefficient use of support services (schedules quickly filled with direct one-to-one therapy). The authors proposed a "change process" in which primary and related services commit to collaborative teaming.

Inasmuch that professional jargon frequently has different interpretations and meanings, collaboration essentially employs the use of multiple professionals working together toward a common goal; hence a child's educational program. Another benefit with collaboration particularly with parents involve skills taught and learned within the classroom and school context, reinforcing concepts in different environment, and may be generalized into a more naturalistic setting with parents at home (Kirk & Rhodes, 2011). The child may need to generalize skills and concepts into other settings (e.g., regular classroom, home and community) in order to facilitate the transition process into general kindergarten classes. The generalization of skills cannot be obtained if taught in isolation. For example, one family activity is to bike on a nearby bike path. Instead of "packing the child", preschooler teachers can teach the child to pedal a tricycle in and around the school. Allowing for bike riding at school, can also positively influence inclusion into the family activity at home. By employing the collaborative teaching model, parents, classroom teachers, adapted physical educators and related personnel will be able to promote quality of service in order to best meet preschoolers' goal and objectives, IEP, or IFSP goals (Menear & Davis, 2015). More specifically, Howie et al. (2014) noted that collaborative partnership between preschooler teachers and research interventionists by adapting a flexible, adaptive intervention to add additional physical activity opportunities throughout the school day. Neal et al. (2004) and Downing (2004) purported that collaboration can exist effectively between classroom teachers, occupational therapy, physical therapy, speech language pathology and other related services. Without collaboration, there may be disconnect between the classroom teacher and adapted physical educators since many may not participate in the IEP or IFSP process (Klein & Hollingshead, 2015; Silliman-French et al., 2007). And finally, how collaboration is actually implemented within the context of the classroom and outside environment can be demonstrated by either direct service or consultation services which are acceptable IEP approaches. Monitoring services can also be implemented whereby only a written document may be submitted to the IEP team for information. The information may include specifically designed services to ensure appropriate programming and equipment in order to inform preschool teachers and adapted physical educators of safe and successful instructions within the least restrictive environment (Silliman et al., 2007).

Conclusion

Physical activity is an area primed for collaborative teaching, particularly in early childhood programs (Helms & Boos, 1996). When considering preschoolers with developmental delays the concomitant of disabilities or special needs can significantly impact their ability to learn and engage with the environment. Specialized direct instruction, instruction in physical education, and related services intervention should be provided to these preschoolers to enhance their learning, growth and overall development. Related services such as PT, OT and speech-language are quite common for preschoolers with developmental delays to supplement their instruction and learning. As such, it is imperative that preschool teachers understand the specific roles adapted physical education and related services play in improving children's motor skills and health. Early childhood educators should work collaboratively to foster professional relationships with these professionals. Physical activity and play are areas where preschoolers can learn and interact socially and emotionally. To accomplish such outcomes requires the preschool teachers to collaborate with other professionals to improve educational, increased student learning and life skills outcomes for preschoolers with developmental delays (Menear & Davis, 2015). The communication and coordination of the educational program for preschoolers with developmental delays is enhanced with a collaborative team approach.

References

Alhassan, S., Nwakkelemeh, O., Ghazarian, M., Roberts, J., Mendoza, A., & Shitole, S. (2012). Effects of locomotor skill program on minority preschoolers' physical activity levels. *Pediatric Exercise Science, 24*, 435–449.

American Physical Therapy Association. (2015). *Licensure*. Retrieved from: http://www.apta.org/Licensure/

American Speech-Language-Hearing Association. (2008). *Roles and responsibilities of speech-language pathologists in early intervention: Position statement*. Retrieved from www.asha.org/policy

Beets, M. W., Bornstein, D., Dowda, M., & Pate, R. R. (2011). Compliance with national guidelines for physical activity in U.S. preschoolers: Measurement and interpretation. *Pediatrics, 127*, 658–664. https://doi.org/10.1542/peds.2010-2021

Bellows, L. L., Davies, P. L., Anderson, J., & Kennedy, C. (2013). Effectiveness of a physical activity intervention for head start preschoolers: A randomized intervention study. *American Journal of Occupational Therapy, 67*, 28–36.

Campbell, P. H., Chiarello, L., Wilcox, M. J., & Milbourne, S. (2009). Preparing therapists as effective practitioners in early intervention. *Infants and Young Children, 22*, 21–31.

Case-Smith, J. (2000). Effects of occupational therapy services on fine motor and functional performance in preschool children. *American Journal of Occupational Therapy, 54*, 372–380.

Clark, G. F., Policchino, J., & Jackson, L. (2004). Occupational therapy services in early intervention and school-based programs. *The American Journal of Occupational Therapy, 58*(6), 681–685.

Cliff, D. P., Okely, A. D., Smith, L. M., & McKeen, K. (2009). Relationship between fundamental movement skills and objectively measured physical activity in preschool children. *Pediatric Exercise Science, 21*, 436–449.

Colyvas, J. L., Sawyer, L. B., & Campbell, P. H. (2010). Identifying strategies early intervention occupational therapist use to teach caregivers. *American Journal of Occupational Therapy, 64*, 776–785. https://doi.org/10.5014/ajot.2010.09044

Connor-Kuntz, F. J., & Dummer, G. M. (1996). Teaching across the curriculum: Language-enriched physical education for preschool children. *Adapted Physical Activity Quarterly, 13*, 302–315.

Derscheid, L. E., Umoren, J., Kim, S.-Y., Henry, B., & Zittel, L. (2010). Early childhood teachers' and staff members' perceptions of nutrition and physical activity practices for preschoolers. *Journal of Research in Childhood Education, 24*(3), 248–265.

Downing, J. A. (2004). Related services for students with disabilities. *Intervention in School and Clinic, 39*(4), 195–208.

Dummer, G. M., Connor-Kuntz, F. J., & Goodway, J. D. (1995). Physical education curriculum for all preschool students. *Teaching Exceptional Children, 27*, 28–34.

Dwyer, G. M., Higgs, J., Hardy, L. L., & Baur, L. A. (2008). What do parents and preschool staff tell us about young children's physical activity: A qualitative study. *International Journal of Behavioral Nutrition and Physical Activity*. Retrieved from http://www.ijbnpa.org/content/5/1/66 . doi:https://doi.org/10.1186/1479-5868-5-66

Elgsti, H. J., Chandler, L., Robinson, C., & Bodkin, A. W. (2010). A longitudinal study of outcome measures for children receiving early intervention services. *Pediatric Physical Therapy, 22*(3), 304–313.

Ellis, L., Schlaudecker, C., & Regimbal, C. (1995). Effectiveness of a collaborative consultation approach to basic concept instruction with kindergarten children. *Language, Speech, and Hearing Services, 26*, 69–74.

Gallahue, D. L., & Cleland-Donnelly, F. (2003). *Developmental physical education for all children* (4th ed.). Champaign, IL: Human Kinetics.

Goodway, J. D., & Branta, C. F. (2003). Influence of a motor skill intervention on fundamental motor skill development of disadvantaged preschool children. *Research Quarterly for Exercise and Sport, 74*(1), 36–46.

Goodway, J. D., Crowe, H., & Ward, P. (2003). Effects of motor skill instruction on fundamental motor skill development. *Adapted Physical Activity Quarterly, 20*, 298–314.

Goodway, J. D., Robinson, L. E., & Crowe, H. (2010). Gender differences in fundamental motor skill development in disadvantaged preschoolers from two geographical regions. *Research Quarterly for Exercise and Sport, 81*(1), 17–24.

Gunner, K. B., Atkinson, P. M., Nichols, J., & Eissa, M. A. (2005). Health promotion strategies to encourage physical activity in infants, toddlers, and preschoolers. *Journal of Pediatric Health Care, 19*, 253–258.

Hammond, A., & Warner, C. (1996). Physical educators and speech-language pathologists: A good match for collaborative consultation. *The Physical Educator, 53*, 181–189.

Helms, J. H., & Boos, S. (1996). Increasing the physical educator's impact: Consulting, collaborating and teacher training in early childhood programs. *Journal of Physical Education, Recreation, and Dance, 68*(6), 50–55.

Hengstman, J. G. (2001). *Movement abc: An inclusive guide to stimulating language development*. Champaign, IL: Human Kinetics.

Hermes, S. S. (2007). An approach for inclusion of preschoolers with developmental delays. *Developmental Disabilities Special Interest Section Quarterly, 30*(2), 1–4.

Hodge, S. R., Lieberman, L. J., & Murata, N. M. (2012). *Essentials of teaching adapted physical education: Diversity, culture and inclusion*. Scottsdale, AZ: Holcomb Hathaway Publishers.

Howie, E. K., Brewer, A., Brown, W. H., Pfeiffer, K. A., Saunders, R. P., & Pate, R. R. (2014). The 3-year evolution of a preschool physical activity intervention through a collaborative partnership between research interventionists and preschool teachers. *Health Education Research, 29*(3), 491–502. https://doi.org/10.1093/her/cyu014

Hustad, K. C., Keppner, K., Schanz, A., & Berg, A. (2008). Augmentative and alternative communication for preschool children: Intervention goals and use of technology. *Semin Speech Language, 29*(2), 83–91. https://doi.org/10.1055/s-2008-1080754

Hwang, A., Wu, I., Chen, C., Cheng, H. K., & Chen, C. (2014). The correlates of body mass index and risk factors for being overweight among preschoolers with motor delay. *Adapted Physical Activity Quarterly, 31*, 125–143.

Individuals with Disabilities Education Improvement Act (IDEIA) of 2004, P.L. 108-446, 118 Stat. 2647 (2004).

Jansma, P. (1999). *Psychomotor domain training and serious disabilities* (5th ed.). Landham, MD: University Press of America.

Jones, R. A., Riethmuller, A., Hesketh, K., Trezise, J., Batterham, M., & Okely, A. D. (2011). Promoting fundamental movement skill development and physical activity in early childhood settings: A cluster randomized controlled trial. *Pediatric Exercise Science, 23*, 600–615.

Kaczmarek, L. A. (1985). Integrating language/communication objectives into the total preschool curriculum. *Teaching Exceptional Children, 17*, 183–189.

Kelly, L. E. (2006). *Adapted physical education national standards* (2nd ed.). Champaign, IL: Human Kinetics.

Kirk, M. A., & Rhodes, R. E. (2011). Motor skill interventions to improve fundamental movement skills of preschoolers with developmental delay. *Adapted Physical Activity Quarterly, 28*(3), 210–232.

Klein, E., & Hollingshead, A. (2015). Collaboration between special and physical education: The benefits of a healthy lifestyle for all students. *Teaching Exceptional Children, 47*(3), 163–167.

Kretchmar, R. S. (2012). Play disabilities: A reason for physical educators to rethink the boundaries of special education. *QUEST, 64*, 79–86.

Lawson, H. A., & Sailor, W. (2000). Integrating services, collaborating, and developing connections with schools. *Focus on Exceptional Children, 33*(2), 22–29.

Li, Y.-C., Kwan, M. Y. W., King-Dowling, S., & Cairney, J. (2015). Determinants of physical activity during early childhood: A systematic review. *Advances in Physical Education, 5*, 116–127.

Lifter, K., Mason, E. J., & Barton, E. E. (2011). Children's play: Where we have been and where we could go. *Journal of Early Intervention, 33*(4), 281–297.

Macdonald, M., Lord, C., & Ulrich, D. A. (2013). The relationship of motor skills and social communicative skills in school-aged children with autism spectrum disorder. *Adapted Physical Activity Quarterly, 30*(3), 271–282.

Maeda, J. K., & Murata, N. M. (2004). Collaborating with classroom teachers to increase daily physical activity: The gear program. *Journal of Physical Education, Recreation and Dance, 75*(5), 42–46.

Marr, D., Cermack, S., Cohn, E. S., & Henderson, A. (2003). Fine motor activities in head start and kindergarten classrooms. *American Journal of Occupational Therapy, 57*, 550–557.

McCall, R. M., & Craft, D. H. (2000). *Moving with a purpose: Developing programs for preschoolers of all abilities*. Champaign, IL: Human Kinetics.

Menear, K. S., & Davis, T. D. (2015). Effective collaboration among the gross motor assessment team members. *Strategies, 28*, 18–21.

Murata, N. M., & Maeda, J. K. (2002). Structured play for preschoolers with developmental delays. *Early Childhood Education Journal, 29*(4), 237–240.

Murata, N. M. (2000). Speech-language strategies for physical educators. *Journal of Physical Education, Recreation and Dance, 71*(2), 36–38.

Murata, N. M. (2003). Language augmentation strategies in physical education. *Journal of Physical Education, Recreation and Dance, 74*(3), 29–32.

Murata, N. M., & Maeda, J. K. (2007). Using occupational therapy strategies by adapted physical educators and classroom teachers for preschoolers with developmental delays. *Palaestra, 23*(2), 20–25. 59.

Murata, N. M., & Tan, C. A. (2008). Collaborative teaching for preschoolers with developmental delays. *Early Childhood Education Journal, 36*(6), 483–489.

National Association for Sport and Physical Education (NASPE). (2002). *Active start: A statement of physical activity guidelines for children birth to five years*. Reston, VA: NASPE.

National Association for the Education of Young Children (NAEYC). (2012). Retrieved from: http://www.naeyc.org/files/naeyc/files/Play%20references%20in%20NAEYC%20position%20statements%2011-12.pdf

Neal, J., Bigby, L., & Nicholson, R. (2004). Occupational therapy, physical therapy, and orientation and mobility services in public schools. *Intervention in School and Clinic, 39*(4), 218–222.

Nervik, D., Martin, K., Rundquist, P., & Cleland, J. (2011). The relationship between body mass index and gross motor development in children aged 3 to 5 years. *Pediatric Physical Therapy, 23*(2), 144–148.

Nicaise, V., Kahan, D., Reuben, K., & Sallis, J. F. (2012). Evaluation of a redesigned outdoor space on preschool children's physical activity during recess. *Pediatric Exercise Science, 24*(4), 507–518.

Palisano, R. J. (2006). A collaborative model of service delivery for children with movement disorders: A framework for evidence-base decision making. *Physical Therapy, 86*, 1295–1305. https://doi.org/10.2522/ptj.20050348

Pate, R. R., Pfeiffer, K. A., Trost, S. G., Ziegler, P., & Dowda, M. (2004). Physical activity among children attending preschools. *Pediatrics, 114*, 1258–1263.

Pathare, N., Piche, K., Nicosia, A., & Haskvitz, E. (2016). Physical activity levels of non-overweight, overweight, and obese children during physical education. *Journal of Teaching Physical Education, 35*, 76–80.

Pierce-Jordan, S., & Lifter, K. (2005). Interaction of social and play behaviors in preschoolers with and without pervasive developmental disorder. *Topics in Early Childhood Special Education, 25*(1), 34–47.

Radonovich, S., & Houck, C. (1990). An integrated preschool developing a program for children with developmental handicaps. *Teaching Exceptional Children, 22*(4), 22–26.

Recchia, S. L. (2016). Preparing for teachers for infant education. In L. Couse & S. Recchia (Eds.), *Handbook of Early Childhood Teacher Education* (pp. 89–103). New York, NY: Routledge.

Reifel, S. (2014). The definition of play. In NAECY, *Defining and advocating for play*. Retrieved from: www.naeyc.org/yc/pastissues/2014/
Rule, A. C., & Stewart, R. A. (2002). Effects of practical life materials on kindergartners' fine motor skills. *Early Childhood Education Journal, 30*(1), 9–13.
Scarborough, H., & Dobrich, W. (1990). Development of children with early language delay. *Journal of Speech Hearing Research, 33*, 70–83.
Shapiro, D. R., & Sayers, L. K. (2003). Who does what on the interdisciplinary team regarding physical education for students with disabilities? *Teaching Exceptional Children, 35*(6), 32–38.
Silliman-French, L., Candler, C., French, R., & Hamilton, M. L. (2007). I have students with physical and motor problems: How can an APE, OT, or PT help? *Strategies, 21*, 15–20.
Slater, L. M., Hillier, S. L., & Civetta, L. R. (2010). The clinimetric properties of performance-based cross motor tests used for children with developmental coordination disorder: A systematic review. *Pediatric Physical Therapy, 22*(2), 170–179.
Solomon, J. R., & Murata, N. M. (2008). Physical education and language arts: An interdisciplinary teaching approach. *Strategies, 21*(6), 19–23.
Sunderland, L. C. (2004). Speech, language, and audiology services in public schools. *Intervention in School and Clinic, 39*(4), 209–217.
Tomporowski, P. D., McCullick, B. A., & Pesce, C. (2015). *Enhancing children's cognition with physical activity games*. Champaign, IL: Human Kinetics.
Tucker, P. (2008). The physical activity levels of preschool-aged children: A systematic review. *Early Childhood Research Quarterly, 23*, 547–558.
United States Department of Health and Human Services. (2015). *Policy statement on inclusion of children with disabilities in early childhood programs*. Retrieved from: http://www2.ed.gov/policy/speced/guid/earlylearning/joint-statement-full-text.pdf
Van Cauwenberghe, E., Labarque, V., Gubbels, J., De Bourdeaudhuij, I., & Cardon, G. (2012). Preschooler's physical activity levels and associations with lesson context, teacher's behavior, and environment during preschool physical education. *Early Childhood Research Quarterly, 27*, 221–230.
Verbestel, V., Van Cauwenberghe, E., De Coen, V., Maes, L., De Bourdeaudhuij, L., & Cardon, G. (2011). Within- and between-day variability of objectively measured physical activity in preschoolers. *Pediatric Exercise Science, 23*, 366–378.
Watkins, S., Jonsson-Funk, M., Brookhart, M. A., Rosenberg, S. A., O'Shea, T. M., & Daniels, J. (2014). Preschool motor skills following physical and occupational therapy services among non-disabled very low birth weight children. *Maternal, Child, Health Journal, 18*, 821–828.
Watson, G. D., & Bellon-Harn, M. L. (2013). Speech-language pathologist and general educator collaboration: A model for tier 2 service delivery. *Intervention in School and Clinic, 49*(4), 237–243.
Woodson-Smith, A., & Holden, G. (2015). The strengths and weaknesses of physical education programs in selected preschools in central North Carolina. *Journal of Research Initiatives, 1*(3). Retrieved from: http://digitalcommons.uncfsu.edu/jri/
Wessel, J. A., & Zittel, L. L. (1995). *Smart start: Preschool movement curriculum designed for children of all abilities*. Austin, TX: Pro-Ed.

Nathan M. Murata taught adapted physical education in the Honolulu District Schools, Honolulu Hawaii for several years. He went on to receive his Ph.D. at The Ohio State University. He is currently Dean for the College of Education, University of Hawai'i at Mānoa. He was a Principal Investigator of an Office of Special Education Personnel Preparation Grant.

Chapter 10
Exploring Daily Physical Activity and Nutrition Patterns in Early Learning Settings: Observational Snapshots of Young Children in Head Start, Primary, and After-School Settings

Dolores Ann Stegelin, Denise Anderson, Karen Kemper, Jennifer Young Woods, and Katharine Evans

Introduction

Childhood obesity is a global health issue that threatens the life trajectories of many individuals and has been recognized as one of the most serious health problems for children in the United States (Schwartz & Puhl, 2003). The overweight and obesity trend among adults can be traced to increasing rates of childhood obesity; obese toddlers frequently become obese adolescents and then enter adulthood with the same overweight issues. This chapter focuses on the daily physical activity and nutrition patterns in typical early learning settings in the U.S., in an effort to better understand how the increasing rates of obesity might be related to daily routines. In the U. S., families rely heavily on community-based early care and education programs to provide safe and stimulating environments for their young children, and many children spend 6–10 h each day during the week in these settings (NICHD, 2006).

D. A. Stegelin (✉) · D. Anderson · K. Kemper
Clemson University, Clemson, SC, USA
e-mail: dstegel@clemson.edu; dander2@clemson.edu; KKaren@clemson.edu

J. Y. Woods
Southern Wesleyan University, Central, SC, USA
e-mail: jwoods@swu.edu

K. Evans
Clemson University, Clemson, SC, USA

Department of Recreation Management and Therapeutic Recreation,
University of Wisconsin-La Crosse, La Crosse, WI, USA
e-mail: kevans@uwlax.edu

H. Brewer, M. R. Jalongo (eds.), *Physical Activity and Health Promotion in the Early Years*, Educating the Young Child 14,
https://doi.org/10.1007/978-3-319-76006-3_10

The age range of 4–7 years was chosen because young children are at an important point in the development of attitudes, preferences, and daily physical activity and play routines (Gelman, 2009). Furthermore, in the U. S. over 25% of 2–5 year-old children are at risk for overweight and obesity (Birch & Ventura, 2009). Obesity factors among children under the age of 6 have not been well researched, and there is a need to understand the most effective ways to prevent obesity within this population. In February 2011, The *White House Task Force on Childhood Obesity* submitted a report identifying settings, programs and policies that support the prevention of obesity for children during their first 5 years of life (F as in Fat, 2010, p. 68). During these early years, children transition from consuming formula or breast milk into eating modified adult diets. Young children are exposed to thousands of meals, commercials, and other marketing strategies that shape their perceptions of what is normal, what and how much to eat, and what they like and dislike (Birch & Ventura, 2009). In other words, the age range of 4–7 years seems to be a sensitive period for developing long lasting attitudes and habits related to food preferences and levels of physical activity. Children are born with a preference for sweet tastes and by 4 months of age they also begin to prefer salty tastes. These preferences can make it challenging to promote healthy eating patterns if young children are repeatedly exposed to modern processed foods that are high in sugar and salt. However, research has shown that children can learn to prefer healthy foods if appropriate feeding practices in supportive and positive social contexts are used (Birch & Ventura, 2009). During these first 5 years of life, important behavioral norms have been established in terms of food preferences, cultural eating styles, and food expectations (Birch & Ventura, 2009).

Review of the Literature

While there is an increasing number of studies that focus on observing children and their eating and activity patterns, there are few research studies that focus on the daily routines of young children related to their physical activity and nutrition routines in community-based early learning settings. Recent research efforts are described below.

In a recent report (Administration for Children and Families, 2010), an effort was made to assess children's daily physical activity and nutrition in Head Start centers in the U. S. In the spring of 2006, Head Start Region III provided 53 Head Start programs with a 2.5-day training-of-trainers (TOT) event for up to five staff members per program. During the training, participants gained hands-on experience with the use of music and songs through several activities that featured an animated character named "Choosy" (Choose **H**ealthy **O**ptions **O**ften and **S**tart **Y**oung). The Region III trainers and staff encouraged Head Start participants to tailor the enhancements to their own individual programs, and Choosy was introduced in participating programs as a potential mascot or role model that encourages children to engage in physical activity and to practice healthy food choices and eating habits. Thus the use of an animated character was a central aspect of this study of preschoolers in Head Start. While the majority of these programs reported that children enjoyed activities, eight of 26 Stage 2 programs encountered some difficulties getting children to eat new foods or try new activities. To address this, teachers reported encouraging children to try small "no thank you" or "thank the cook" bites of food when new (or traditionally avoided) foods were offered. Teachers also worked with children who were reluctant or embarrassed to dance by giving them Choosy cutouts to wave until they got used to doing the movements and felt more comfortable (Choosy is the animated character described above). This study provided helpful insight into the nuances of working directly with such young children and the need to accommodate their preferences and existing attitudes toward food. The use of Choosy seemed to facilitate the learning process for the young participants.

According to another study of longitudinal data from the Framingham Children's Study, there is a strong effect of low levels of physical activity on body fatness of young children (Moore, Nguyen, Rothman, Cupples, & Ellison, 1995). In this study, children were observed from the age of 3–5 years though enrollment into first grade and demonstrated the importance that early childhood behaviors have on obesity risk. Another study examined the relationship between obesity in preschool-aged children and exposure to 3 household routines: (1) regularly eating the evening meal as a family, (2) obtaining adequate sleep, and (2) limiting screen-viewing time (Anderson & Whitaker, 2010). Using data from the Early Childhood Longitudinal Study (ECLS), researchers found that the prevalence of obesity was 14.3% among children exposed to all 3 routines and 24.5% among those exposed to none of the routines. Preschool-aged children exposed to the 3 household routines of regularly eating the evening meal as a family, obtaining adequate nighttime sleep, and having limited screen-viewing time had a 40% lower prevalence of obesity than those exposed to none of these routines. This study utilized secondary data and allowed the researchers to examine a large number of child behaviors and routines.

In another study, Goodway and Robinson (2006) developed and assessed an early intervention with young children: SKIPing toward an Active Start Promoting Physical Activity in Preschoolers. In an assessment of Project SKIP, the authors found ways to infuse regular physical activity into early childhood classrooms; witnessed significant improvement of motor skills and perceived physical competence of children receiving the curriculum; observed remediation of motor delays; and developed strategies to educate teachers about the importance of physical activity and the means to promote an active start (Goodway & Branta, 2003). This study provides helpful insight into the benefits of kinesthetic teaching and learning and details strategies to use to increase levels of general physical activity in early care and education classrooms.

Other studies have been conducted that focus on young children's thoughts and perceptions related to body size and ways to modify body size (Worobey & Worobey, 2014), which would be helpful in planning and designing classroom interventions for overweight children. In general, there are limited research studies that target children younger than 8 years of age (Sypsa & Simons, 2008). Foundational studies have set the framework for more refined research on physical activity and young children in order to better understand factors that can influence children's physical activity levels. These include health-related factors such as body mass index (BMI) and other health indicators. Two recent studies focused on possible relationships between physical activity and body mass index. In one study, the association between objectively measured physical activity (PA) and body mass index (BMI) of 281 children (55.9% boys) aged 4–6 years was examined. Physical Activity (PA) was measured by accelerometers (Vale et al., 2010). In this study, children were categorized as non-overweight and overweight/obese. Results indicated that vigorous and moderate intensity levels of PA were not associated with BMI; however, a higher proportion of overweight/obese children were classified as low-vigorous PA compared to their non-overweight peers (43.9% versus 32.1%, respectively). Logistic regression showed that children with low-vigorous PA had higher odds ratios to be classified as overweight/obese compared to those with high-vigorous PA. These data suggest that vigorous PA may play a key role in the obesity development already at pre-school age and needs further investigation.

In another study, conducted by Dunton et al. (2012), largely Hispanic and non-Hispanic white children (N = 4550) with a mean (SD) age at study entry of 6.60 years were studied to determine whether participation in organized outdoor team sports and structured indoor non-school activity programs in kindergarten and first grade predicted a subsequent 4-year change in body mass index during the adiposity rebound period of childhood. After adjusting for confounders, BMI increased at a rate 0.05 unit/year slower for children who participated in outdoor organized team sports at least twice per week compared with children who did not. For participation in each additional indoors non-school structured activity class, lesson, and program, BMI increased at a rate 0.05 unit/year slower, and the attained BMI level at age 10 years was 0.48 unit lower. Results from this study suggested that engagement in organized sports and activity programs as early as kindergarten and the first grade may result in smaller increases in BMI during the adiposity rebound period of childhood. Again, this study contributed to our increasing understanding of the factors that are associated with childhood obesity.

Childhood Obesity and Population Indicators

The research literature reflects higher rates of childhood obesity among low-SES, Hispanic, and African-American children. Thus, in the study being described in this chapter, an emphasis was placed on 4–7 year olds from those populations who are served by diverse community-based centers and agencies: Head Start, public school, and community-based after school programs. In the selected county in the southeast part of the U.S., the majority of low-SES children, including Hispanic and African-American children, are served in the federally funded Head Start programs and the state-funded 4K programs. Primary classrooms selected for this research project were in the same neighborhoods and communities as the Head Start and 4K classrooms. Community recreation centers also serve a cross section of SES child and parent populations in this county. High-quality, early childhood programs are seen as a critical route by which societal problems of poor health, education shortfalls, and crime can be prevented (Mission: Readiness, 2009). In the southeastern state in which the study being reported was conducted, 50% of 4 year olds were in a state or federally funded pre-kindergarten program in 2008 (2009). Head Start is the nation's largest kindergarten program for at-risk children (2009). Head Start has developed a promising obesity prevention and health promotion curriculum called "Hip-Hop to Health" which is currently being evaluated by the University of Illinois for its impact on body mass index and obesity related behaviors (ClinicalTrials.gov). Unfortunately, Head Start only has funding to serve fewer than half of the eligible children in the U.S. (2009). Thus, there is a need to expand and refine the research on possible relationships between low-income status, ethnicity, gender, and nutrition status at home and in the early childhood program, and levels of physical activity of young children 4–7 years of age.

Research Question

The purpose of this exploratory community-based research project was to gain a greater understanding of the daily routines of 4–7 year old children related to daily nutrition and physical activity routines. The settings selected included Head Start 4K, primary, and after-school learning environments in a mid-sized city in the southeast. Specifically, this exploratory and observational study of a subset and representative sample of 4–7 year olds in community-based early learning settings focused on the following research question: *What are typical daily physical activity and nutrition patterns in community-based early learning settings for young children 4–7 years of age in the United States?*

Methodology

The researchers obtained approval for the study through the Institutional Review Board-IRB protocol # IRB2011-059, entitled "Early Childhood Obesity Prevention & Healthy Living Network Project". All names used in the reporting of the findings were pseudonyms in order to assure confidentiality of participants. Three types of data collection sites were utilized for stratified random sampling: Head Start, Kindergarten and primary classrooms in a public school, and County Recreation District (CRD) community after school recreation centers for a total of 4 community-based sites. The children selected for the extended direct observation reported in this study were a subset of an overall sample and included children in Head Start, after-school, and 4-year-old kindergarten (4K)-primary public school classrooms. Two of the researchers conducted both quantitative and qualitative observations of the students, with one researcher observing three of the students and the other researcher observing two. Complete observational data were obtained on four of the five children selected. An observational tool was developed that consisted of a running record of child behavior and a time-sampling checklist that was completed on each child every 30 min for the duration of the regularly scheduled program day. The measures used were adapted from an earlier study of preschoolers' nonsedentary physical activity of preschoolers (Brown et al., 2009). Students were observed in 30 min blocks-of-time, with the researcher recording anecdotal notes of the behaviors observed. At the conclusion of each 30-min block, the researcher recorded the behaviors observed on the quantitative time sampling measure in the appropriate category (outdoor context or indoor context). Observations began at the beginning of the program day in each of the community-based centers and ended when the child left to go home. Thus the entire daily routine was observed and recorded for each child participant.

Results

In this section, quantitative results of this observational study are presented first, followed by qualitative results.

Quantitative Findings

To determine the types of physical activity children participated in, a time sampling checklist was utilized that looked at both outdoor and indoor contexts for large motor physical activities (the actual activities and routines in which these activities occurred). A total of four students were observed ranging in ages from 5–8. One Latino student (Tony, male, age 5) was observed in a Head Start 4K program, two African American students (Luke, male, age 6 and Lisa, female, age 7) were observed in an after-school setting, while one Latino (Bobby, male, age 8) was observed in an elementary school setting. Observations for each child were comprised of 30-min blocks of time throughout the entire daily schedule for each setting and lasted approximately 6.5 h for each child in the Head Start 4K program and elementary school, while observations for each child in the after-school program lasted approximately 3 h. This research was conducted in a large county in the southeastern part of the country.

Outdoor Contexts for Large Motor Physical Activities

When looking at large motor physical activities that occurred in an outdoor context, it must be noted that the after-school program did not take the students outside during either observation. Data reported in this section will only outline observations

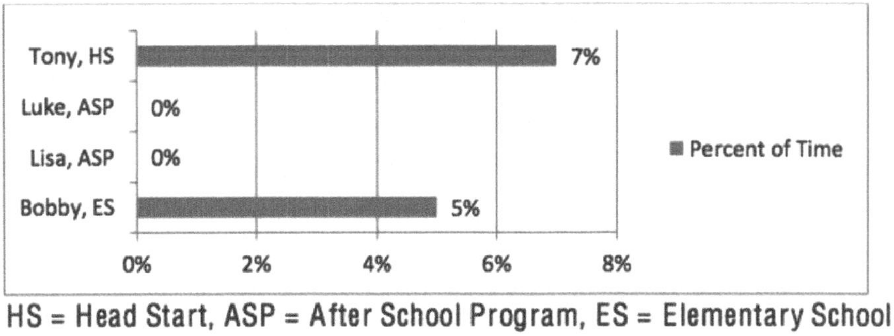

Fig. 10.1 Percent of time outdoors, direct physical activity

Table 10.1 Outdoor contexts for large motor physical activities

	Bobby, ES	Lisa, ASP	Luke, ASP	Tony, HS	Total
Fixed Equipment	1 CD			2 CD	3 CD
Game – Free or unstructured	1 CD			2 CD	3 CD
Open space				2 CD	3 CD

CD Child Directed. Each Activity was Chosen by the child to participate in not the teacher
ES Elementary School, *ASP* After School Program, *HS* Head Start

conducted in the Head Start, 4K and elementary school, which were both observed for approximately 6.5 h. Refer to Fig. 10.1 regarding the opportunity each child had for direct physical activity in an outdoor context.

Most of the activities the two children engaged in during outdoor contexts were initiated by the child, not teacher directed; outdoor environmental features associated with child-initiated physical activity included open spaces for running, swings and slides, and natural surfaces such as grass, sand, and dirt. Bobby played on fixed equipment and in an unstructured or game-free environment for a 20-min period. Specifically, Bobby played on the fixed equipment for half of his recess time, most of his time climbing up the stairs, then sliding down the sliding board. He then left the fixed equipment and started running, chasing, crawling, and hopping around the playground. Tony stayed outside for approximately 25 min and played on fixed equipment, in an unstructured or game-free environment, and in open space on the playground. On two separate occasions, Tony climbed on the jungle gym. When not playing on equipment, Tony was running, chasing friends, and pushing. Refer to Table 10.1 to see the number of times each child participated in different activities in an outdoor context.

Indoor Contexts for Physical Activities

Indoor activities observed included reading books, drawing, gross motor (i.e. shooting a basketball), working with manipulatives, singing/listening/dancing to music, sociodramatic play, and writing. Figure 10.2 illustrates the percentage of time each child participated in teacher directed physical activity in an indoor context (i.e. movement to music, exercise, and non-academic centers). Figure 10.3 illustrates the percentage of time each child participated in student directed physical activity in an indoor context (i.e. free-style basketball, running, kicking, and jumping). Only activities that involved direct physical activity were calculated. Reading, drawing, the use of manipulatives, watching videos, and writing were not included in the calculations of direct physical activity.

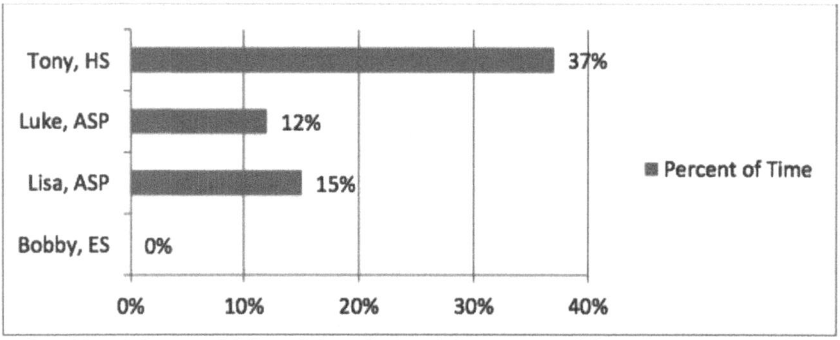

HS = Head Start, ASP = After School Program, ES = Elementary School

Fig. 10.2 Percent of time indoors, teacher initiated direct physical activity

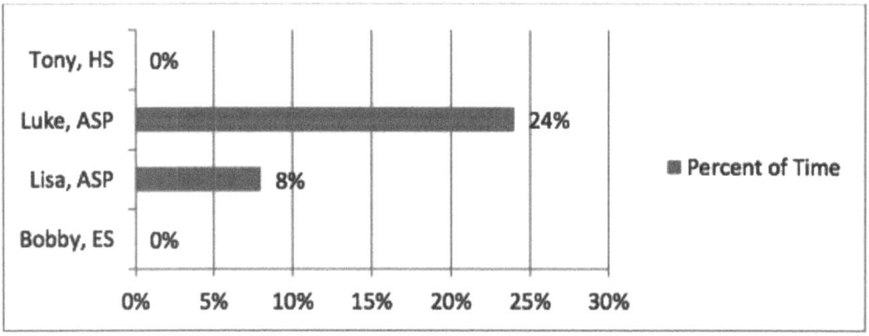

HS = Head Start, ASP = After School Program, ES = Elementary School

Fig. 10.3 Percent of time indoors, child initiated direct physical activity

Table 10.2 Indoor contexts for large motor physical activities

	Bobby, ES	Lisa, ASP	Luke, ASP	Tony, HS	Total
Books	2 TD	3 CD		1TD	3 CD, 3 TD
Drawing	1 TD		4 CD, 1 TD		4 CD, 2 TD
Gross Motor		1 TD	2 CD, 1 TD		2 CD, 2 TD
Manipulative	1 CD, 1 TD		3 CD, 1 TD	4 TD	4 CD, 6 TD
Music	1 CD, 5 TD	1 TD	1 TD	1 TD	1 CD, 8TD
Sociodramatic	1 TD			1 TD	2 TD
Videos/TV			1 CD		1 CD
Writing	1 CD, 5 TD	1 CD, 1 TD	4 CD		6 CD, 6 TD

CD Child Directed. Each activity was chosen by the child to participate in, not the teacher
TD Teacher Directed. Each activity was chosen by the teacher to participate in, not the child
HS Head Start, *ASP* After School Program, *ES* Elementary School

The only activity that all four students experienced was the inclusion of music. In all but one case, the teacher initiated the singing, listening, or dancing to the music. Bobby sang *Do Re Mi* to himself while completing his seatwork at one point during the observational period. Reading books was an activity that three out of four children participated in, with half the activity being teacher initiated and the other half being student initiated (if finished work early, would read or chose to go to the reading center over a different center). While Luke was observed drawing multiple times and was child initiated, Bobby only drew once and it was a teacher-initiated activity. Gross-motor activities were only observed at the after-school program: shooting basketball for both Lisa and Luke. This activity occurred after homework had been completed. The use of manipulatives was observed across all three settings. Lisa was the only student who did not utilize manipulatives; however, her homework was making sentences from her spelling words. More than half of the observations included the teacher initiating the use of manipulatives (i.e. tally marks), while the students initiated the use of manipulatives for the other portion of the observations (i.e. using fingers to add/subtract). Sociodramatic play was observed in the Head Start 4K program and at the elementary school. However, it was only observed one time for one student in each program. At the Head Start 4K program, it was observed when the teacher played music and the kids participated in the chicken dance and touched their heads, shoulders, knees, and toes. In the elementary school, sociodramatic play was observed during related arts (music class). Writing was observed at both the after-school program and elementary school. Six of the writing observations were child initiated, and the teacher initiated 6 of the writing observations. It is important to note that Bobby only initiated writing once out of the six different children initiated writing observations. Refer to Table 10.2 to see the number of times each child participated in different activities in an indoor context.

Indoor Routines

Indoor routines observed included centers, group time, nap (for Head Start 4K only), and self-care, seat work, snacks, and transitions. The teacher initiated both group time and naptime in all observed settings. Group time included sitting on the rug listening to the teacher read and whole group instruction. Naptime occurred for approximately an hour for the student observed at Head Start 4K. Centers were initiated eight times for both students observed at the Head Start 4K program and elementary school. The two students observed at the after-school program did not go to centers. Bobby went to centers during four different observation periods for individual or paired work. However, these centers were reading, writing, math, and computer. The teacher designated centers the students would rotate in and out of during the course of the day. Centers at the Head Start 4K program included sand box, kitchen, dress-up, and reading. Tony stayed in the same teacher initiated center for over 90 min (sand box). This center was included in Fig. 10.2 as it was not an academic center and teacher directed physical activity was observed. All students participated in self-care activities throughout each observation. Designated restroom breaks were observed in all three settings, with students initiating self-care activities at the Head Start 4K program and elementary school. At the Head Start 4K program, both students were observed participating in self-care routines on six different occasions. Half of these observations were teacher initiated and the other half were student initiated. It was observed that after playing in centers and outdoor recess, students automatically went to wash their hands. Self-care routines were not observed as frequently at the elementary school or after-school programs. Bobby participated in self-care routines three times, with one of these being child initiated. Lisa and Luke only used the restroom under the direction of the teacher. Seatwork was observed across all settings and was completed by three out of the four students observed. Tony at the Head Start 4K program did not complete seatwork, as it was not part of the routine that day. At the elementary school, all seatwork observed was initiated by the teacher. However, in the after school program, seatwork was initiated by both the teacher and the children being observed. Seatwork included writing, drawing, and coloring.

Nutrition

In all three settings, food being served (i.e. breakfast, lunch, snacks) was evident. All designated food routines were teacher directed, except for one where Lisa asked a friend if she could have his crackers. At the Head Start 4K program, students ate breakfast and lunch in a family-style manner in the classroom. Breakfast consisted of an apple and cereal. Tony ate all of his cereal, but only took one bite of the apple before throwing it away. He used approximately half of the milk from the carton in his cereal and did not drink the rest. Lunch consisted of green beans, French fries

Table 10.3 Indoor contexts for large motor physical routines

	Bobby, ES	Lisa, ASP	Luke, ASP	Tony, HS	TOTAL
Centers	4 TD			4 TD	8 TD
Group time	3 TD	3 TD	4 TD	4 TD	14 TD
Nap/Rest				2 TD	2 TD
Self care	1 CD, 2 TD	1 TD	2 TD	3 CD, 3 TD	4 CD, 8 TD
Seat work	3 TD	2 CD, 1 TD	3 CD, 2 TD		5 CD, 6 TD
Snacks	1 TD	1 TD	1 TD	1 CD, 1 TD	1 CD, 4 TD
Transition	10 TD	4 TD	1 CD, 5 TD	6 TD	1 CD, 25 TD

CD Child Directed. Each activity was chosen by the child to participate in, not the teacher

with ketchup, hot dog bun with chili (no weenie), and milk. Tony ate all of his French fries with ketchup. He scraped the chili off the hot dog bun and ate all of the bread. He did not eat the chili or the green beans. He did drink all of his white milk. At the elementary school, lunch consisted of fried chicken, macaroni and cheese, pinto beans, cornbread, and kiwi. Bobby ate almost his entire kiwi, ate some of his chicken leg and ¾ of his macaroni and cheese. He did not eat the cornbread or pinto beans. In the after-school program, students were offered a snack after they completed their homework and before unstructured play. Snacks included a piece of fruit and juice box for Luke during one observation and crackers and orange juice for Lisa during another observation. They both ate their entire snack and drank their entire beverage.

Transitions

Each of the four students observed were involved in transitions during various portions of the day. All but one of the transitions was teacher directed (i.e. moving from seatwork to recess, from group time to lunch, etc.). The one child initiated transition was when Luke stopped playing basketball during unstructured game time indoors to chase a girl. Refer to Table 10.3 to see the number of times each child participated in different routines in an indoor context.

Qualitative Findings

Following data collection, we independently analyzed the observational transcripts following two guiding questions: What are the behavior patterns of children in the various settings, and what impacts the behavior choices of the children? While we did view the data through the lens of these questions, we chose not to establish nor use *a priori* codes (Creswell, 2007, p. 152). Rather, each researcher organized the data into tentative codes based on the observational transcripts of each child. Each researcher then combined the codes into larger themes that were common across all of the children observed (2007). Following completion of the initial analysis, we compared the individual themes we identified independently for inter-rater reliability. We then sorted the tentative themes into common groupings creating two overarching themes.

Two overarching themes were identified through data analysis: restriction of activity and restriction of physical movement. Within the physical movement theme three subthemes were identified: unstructured play, structured play, and fidgeting. The first theme, restriction of activity, was very apparent within the settings Bobby, Tony, Lisa, and Luke were in. Each child was scheduled very strictly within his/her respective environment. Bobby, observed in an elementary school, experienced a traditional school day. His day was largely spent sitting: sitting at his desk, sitting on the floor in his classroom, and sitting on the floor in the music room. While there was movement between activities (from desk to floor, classroom to music room), physical activity was not built into the academic activities as each was completed sitting down. Tony also spent the majority of his time sitting during activities at the Head Start Center, although the restriction on Tony's time was also marked by extended periods of waiting during which he was unable to be physically active. Following breakfast, Tony waited 19 min from the time he was done cleaning up to the time the instruction began again. During this time, he was sitting on the floor, rather than being allowed to move about. Later in the morning when the class was transitioning to recess, Tony waited for 7 min standing quietly in line before the class was instructed to move outside. Lisa and Luke experienced similar types of restriction on their activity at the community center afterschool program. Again, their time was structured from beginning to end. For both, the first of their 2 h spent at the program was spent sitting down working on homework. For each of the four children, the main restriction to their physical activity was the schedule at their school, Head Start, or afterschool program. While this scheduling kept the children from participating in physical activity, some form of physical activity was built into each schedule for at least a short amount of time.

Each child did experience some form of physical activity during their time at their program. Bobby and Tony had the shortest amount of time for physical activity built into their schedules at the elementary school and the Head Start center. Bobby spent a total of 20 min at recess at his elementary school and Tony spent a total of 25 min at recess at the Head Start Center. For Lisa and Luke, the community center offered them the opportunity to participate in a more extended period of physical activity. The amount of time varied based on when the children were picked up, but amounted to 45 min for Lisa and almost 2 h for Luke. Within these scheduled physical activity allotments, the children chose to use this time in different ways. Bobby and Tony largely spent their time participating in free-form unstructured play. They were running, sliding, climbing on playground equipment, crawling, and hopping during their recess time. Neither Bobby nor Tony engaged with other children while playing, but rather chose to interact with their environment, using the playground equipment as the focus of their play. Luke also largely spent his time participating in unstructured play alone. He jumped on and off the bleachers in the gym, walked, hopped, and ran around the gym. Luke also mixed in sitting and lying down into his physical activity. He would, for instance, run from one corner of the gym to another and then lie down, then get up and repeat the process. Lisa was the only child that exhibited social participation in her physical activity as she played with at least one other child during her 45-min block of activity. Lisa also largely participated in structured play, the next subtheme within physical activity participation.

Lisa and Luke also chose to participate in some structured play. Lisa played basketball with friends for half of the time she spent participating in physical activity. Lisa and Luke were also given, and took advantage of, the opportunity to participate in structured play as games and exercises were lead for them by adult leaders at their afterschool program. These activities included adult-led exercises (jumping, hopping, running back and forth) and whole group games (tag games, basketball games). However, this scheduled time did not contain the only physical activity that was observed.

While the children's physical activity was most notable during the structured physical activity time built into their schedules, one other notable finding was that all of the children displayed a desire to move during the times allotted for academic endeavors. This subtheme was defined as fidgeting and was marked by movements made by the children while they were being asked to sit still for activities. Bobby was consistently squirming in his chair, rocking back and forth while sitting at his desk or on the floor, biting his fingernails, dancing while waiting in line to go back to his classroom after music class and while waiting for lunch, and running back and forth between his desk and cubby hole or his desk and the activity area he was working in. Tony also rocked back and forth while sitting, and standing up and sitting down repeatedly while working on an activity. Luke, during the first hour of the afterschool program while working on homework, was consistently fidgeting in his chair. He would stand up, sit down, shift the leg he was sitting on, and shift his weight in his chair. While waiting in the bleachers during snack time, Luke moved from step to step, jumped off the bleachers, sat back down, and repeated. Lisa, while still fidgeting, was subtler in her movements. During homework time, she did not focus well on her homework. Rather, she would move to find an adult to ask a question, go back to her back to get more paper, move to find an adult to ask another question, and moving in her chair to position herself to talk to other afterschool participants. For each child, within each setting, movement and fidgeting was a constant part of the time they were required to sit and work.

Limitations and Future Research

There are limitations when drawing conclusions from the data collected in this study. The sample size was small and the study was conducted in one specific county. Additionally, the students observed were not all the same age nor in the same grade. For example, the student in the elementary school was in 2nd grade and may not have been provided the same opportunities for direct physical activities due to his age/grade as other students in other settings (4 year old kindergarten and after-school). Future research needs to be conducted to look at a multitude of students, across early learning settings, of the same age. The data do suggest, however, that physical activity routines in all 3 community-based learning environments reflected restriction of activity and restriction of physical movement.

Discussion and Recommendations

In this section an overview of the quantitative and qualitative findings is presented. In addition, recommendations are provided based on the outcomes of this study within the context of current trends in school settings to encourage physical activity. Successful models are described that may facilitate enhanced policies and practices in community-based settings for 4–7 year old children.

Quantitative Discussion

These data suggest that the percentage of time students in the Head Start 4K and after-school program have to engage in teacher initiated direct physical activities is greater when compared to students in a typical elementary school setting. Data further suggest that the percentage of time students in an after-school program have to engage in child initiated direct physical activities is greater when compared to students in more structured settings, like Head Start 4K or elementary schools. However, when looking at the percentage of time to engage in direct physical activity, regardless of who initiates the activity, both the Head Start 4K and after-school programs provided similar amounts of time (see Fig. 10.4). Both the Head Start 4K

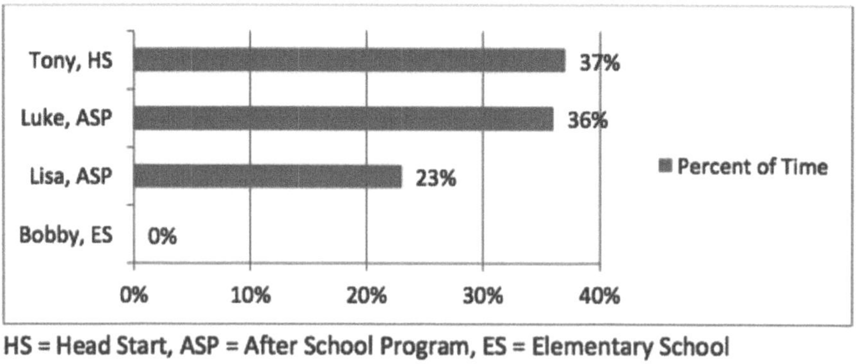

Fig. 10.4 Total percent of time indoors, direct physical activity

and after-school programs observed did allot time for the completion of academic work, but also ensured that students had both teacher initiated and child initiated direct physical activities in which to participate. Bobby, the student observed in a traditional elementary school, was not observed participating in any direct physical activity while indoors.

While there were many different activities for students in all three locations in which to participate, the majority of activities at the elementary school was academically focused and did not involve gross motor movement. For example, there were 10 different transitions for Bobby at the elementary school, while both Tony and Luke experienced 6 and Lisa experienced 4. The results from the quantitative data also suggest that children in school, afterschool and Head Start settings will take advantage of time allotted for physical activity whether or not that time is unstructured or instructor-led. While the settings varied in the amount of each type of physical activity (unstructured or instructor-led) in which children had the opportunity to participate, the willingness of the children to participate in the physical activity did not. The quantitative data also suggest that, overall, students in Head Start and afterschool programs had the smallest amount or proportion of time dedicated to physical activity, but the literature would suggest that this may have a detrimental effect on the academic success of students (Davis et al., 2011; Taras, 2005; Tomporowski, Davis, Miller, & Naglieri, 2008).

Nutrition Discussion

In all three settings in which students were observed, food was served primarily in a structured manner. The Head Start 4K classroom included several meal routines: breakfast, snack and lunch. These routines were characterized by a nurturing family-style setting in which children relaxed at tables of 8 with a teacher, and they seemed to enjoy their food over an extended period of time that encouraged conversation. While the quality and quantity of food in the Head Start 4K classroom were adequate, such foods as French fries and macaroni and cheese might be considered unhealthy from a caloric and fat content perspective. The snacks served at the after-school program were healthy and consisted of fruit, crackers, juice and water. The lunch served at the public school elementary school consisted of fried chicken, macaroni and cheese, pinto beans, cornbread, and kiwi.

When considering the nutrition routines within the context of the overall observed daily routines of physical activity and movement, we recommend that administrators and teachers in all three settings carefully review the nutrition routines (quantity/quality of food and manner of serving). Current practices suggest that food quantity and quality should be reconsidered within the context of a daily schedule that restricts physical activity and movement throughout the day. Limiting high calorie and fatty foods and increasing fresh fruits and vegetables along with increased physical activity and movement within the program's instructional routine are highly recommended.

Qualitative Discussion

The results from the observation data suggest that children in school, afterschool and Head Start settings want to be physically active and will do so when given the opportunity. While children may not require any type of structured play to be physically active, current activity guidelines in the United States require both structured and unstructured physical activity for optimal health in early childhood. In this study, all of the children observed chose to be physically active even when structured games or instructor-led physical activity was not provided. Further, our data suggest that children also take advantage of structured play when it is available. For instance, both Lisa and Luke played independently, but joined in when instructors at their afterschool program offered structured physical activities. As such, when building in or expanding physical activity offerings in school, afterschool or head start settings, administrators should bear in mind that children do not necessarily need structured, instructor-led physical activity options. Based on our observations, simply offering unstructured time during which children are allowed to be physically active will result in children taking advantage of the opportunity to move.

Next, our results suggest that two settings in which children may be in need of more opportunities for physical activity are in elementary school and Head Start programs. Unlike Lisa and Luke at the afterschool program, the amount of time allotted for physical activity was very limited in both the elementary school and Head Start settings. In addition, the only time available for any type of physical activity was a short recess. That is, physical activity was not built into the educational lessons or the classroom in any way. This presented a problem, as our data suggest that the children had a difficult time sitting still during lessons, which may have been detrimental to their focus and academic growth (all were observed fidgeting, squirming, rocking in their chairs, etc.). Recent literature supports the notion that physical activity is an important aspect in the cognitive function and academic achievement of children in school (Davis et al., 2011; Taras, 2005; Tomporowski et al., 2008). While administrators may be concerned that taking any time away from a strict academic focus may be detrimental to the success of their students, the literature suggests this may not be true. Taras (2005) noted that the "short-term cognitive benefits of physical activity during the school day adequately compensate for time spent away from other academic areas" (p. 218). As such, one solution may simply be to provide expanded opportunities for children to participate in physical activity during the school day. Another option in working to increase the amount of physical activity children participate in during the school day would be to work towards creating a generally more active school routine that engages children in kinesthetic and physically active learning across the curriculum.

A recent trend in increasing physical activity in schools is a model dubbed Action Schools (Naylor, Macdonald, Zebedee, Reed, & Mackay, 2006). This "active school" model is intended to encourage schools to create individualized plans for increasing the levels of physical activity in schools. The model directs schools to address six "Action Zones" within schools: the school environment, scheduled physical education, classroom action, family and community, extra-curricular, and school spirit (Naylor et al., 2006, p. 414). For instance, in the classroom action zone, teachers are tasked with providing a minimum of 15 additional minutes of physical activity for students per day. The Action School program has found success and empirical support of its efficacy and this, or a similar program, may be beneficial for schools to consider adopting (Naylor et al., 2006; Reed, Warburton, Macdonald, Naylor, & McKay, 2008).

In addition to a whole-school program for increasing physical activity during the school day such as the active school model, based on our observations, there are also smaller steps that schools may be able to implement more quickly (Castelli, Carson, & Kulinna, 2014). First, administrators can help guide teachers in building physical movement into lessons. For instance, in our study, Bobby participated in a music class while at school, but was required to remain seated on the floor during the music lesson. In this example, the students could have been allowed to dance, or move around the room while participating in music class. A final recommendation is for school and head start programs to examine the amount of downtime that, while potentially unscheduled, is present in their daily schedule. In our time at the Head Start program, Tony was observed spending over 25 min waiting for the next activity to begin. By identify the down time that is unintended, administrators or teachers can work towards eliminating wasted time. Doing so could potentially provide time for another 25-min recess or for physical activity breaks within the classroom. In short, anecdotal qualitative records written during each of the four observational sessions indicate that students seek opportunities for movement throughout their day. During transitional periods it was also discovered that students spent a lot of time waiting on adult- or school-initiated schedules.

Implications for Future Practice and Research

This exploratory study contributed to our understanding of typical routines of young children in representative community-based early care and educational settings. As described above, Head Start is a large federally funded early childhood program designed primarily for young children from lower-income homes and neighborhoods. Head Start serves a large percentage of young children in most communities and is moving towards serving an increasing number of very young children from infancy through preschool age. From our review of the literature and our own direct experience in Head Start classrooms, Head Start should be commended for providing meaningful and effective materials and learning strategies for both children and parents related to the issues of childhood overweight and obesity. We found the directors and classroom teachers to be very knowledgeable about childhood obesity, the need for nutrition education for the children and parents, and a commitment to try to new strategies to support young children's choices in food selection. In addition, Head Start parents demonstrated a high level of knowledge and awareness about childhood obesity, and many were at the point of transferring knowledge to personal practice in their own homes. We believe that Head Start is a good model of how childhood obesity can be addressed in a multi-faceted way: best practices in the classrooms, modeling by teachers and administrators, parent education and involvement, curriculum and instructional strategies for young children, and demonstration of an attitude of exploration and problem-solving by administrators.

This study also shed light on the typical routines of young children in public schools that have become increasingly sedentary. Our findings suggest that young children in 4K, 5K, and primary classrooms have some of the most restricted routines in early care and educational settings in the United States. This is a complex problem that is caused by such factors as an increased focus on seatwork and academics for very young children, classroom environments that are limited in space, school buildings that often do not have sufficient facilities for large motor activities, reduced and diminished recess policies and practices that lead to children not having access to outdoor play and activity either in time or quality, teachers and administrators who are not adequately prepared to deal with childhood obesity or believe that they do not have sufficient authority or power to make decisions that counter the district-level policies related to recess, active learning, and kinesthetic and integrated instructional approaches.

Perhaps least surprising in this study was the finding that community-based afterschool programs were the most physically active. Regardless of the limitations of these facilities, the after school agenda and schedule for all of the child participants reflected large chunks of very rigorous physical activity, variations in the schedule that included time for sedentary homework interspersed with time for free-choice play, team-based activities with rules and guidelines, and frequent study breaks that included healthy snacks and beverages. In addition, the afterschool directors and facilitators modeled high levels of physical activity and were skilled in connecting with all children and including them in team activities. In general, we found the after school settings to be most attuned to the need for increased levels of physical activity, consistency in healthy snack options, frequent breaks for water, and a variation in levels of physical activity for younger children.

Future research is needed that provides more in-depth understanding of the nuances of childhood obesity related to gender, race, socioeconomic status, and type of early care and educational setting. Furthermore, an examination of teacher preparation programs as well as administrator preparation is indicated. Those who make decisions on a regular basis related to young children's food choices and eating routines, daily schedules and planned activities, curriculum and instructional strategies, and the priorities of the classroom related to academics versus health-relate practices, are in need of a better understanding of the multiple factors that contribute to childhood overweight and obesity. More research is also indicated relative to the most effective ways to inform and engage parents of young children in the planning of at home activities, shared family events, and the importance of careful food selection and options. Parents are the most powerful role models for young children in the home and neighborhood settings while teachers and administrators are the most powerful role models for young children in early care and educational settings. In order to stem the tide of childhood obesity, an integrated and collaborative approach to holistic interventions in the home and schools is required. Foundational studies have prosvided essential information related to associations between food consumption and overweight, lack of physical activity and higher rates of overweight, early development of attitudes and preferences about food and physical activity, and the increased risks of children from lower SES homes to obesity and overweight. We are now ready for a more refined focus on the research that can impact the decision-making of parents, teachers, administrators, and the children themselves in order to address the complex health, social, and emotional issues related to childhood obesity.

References

Administration for Children and Families. (2010). *Efforts to meet children's physical activity and nutritional needs: Findings from the I am moving, I am learning implementation evaluation.* M. K. Fox, K. Hallgren, K. Boller, and A. Turner. Washington, DC: U.S. Department of Health and Human Services.

Anderson, S., & Whitaker, R. (2010). Household routines and obesity in US preschool-aged children. *Pediatrics, 125*(3), 420–428.

Birch, L. L., & Ventura, A. K. (2009). Preventing childhood obesity: What works? *International Journal of Obesity, 33*(1), 574–581.

Brown, W. H., Pfeiffer, K. A., McIver, K. L., Dowda, M., Addy, C. L., & Pate, R. R. (2009). Social and environmental factors associated with preschoolers' nonsedentary physical activity. *Child Development, 80*(1), 45–58.

Castelli, D. M., Carson, R. L., & Kulinna, P. H. (2014). Comprehensive School Physical Activity Programs. *Journal of Teaching in Physical Education, 33*(4), 435–439.

Creswell, J. W. (2007). *Qualitative inquiry & research design: Choosing among five approaches.* Thousand Oaks, CA: Sage.

Davis, C. L., Tomporowski, P. D., McDowell, J. E., Austin, B. P., Miller, P. H., Yanasak, N. E., ... Naglieri, J. A. (2011). Exercise improves executive function and achievement and altars brain activation in overweight children: A randomized, controlled trial. *Healthy Psychology, 30*(1), 91–98.

Dunton, G., McConnell, R., Jerrett, M., Wolch, J., Lam, C., Gilliland, M., & Berhane, K. (2012). Organized physical activity in young school children and subsequent 4-year change in body mass index. *Archives of Pediatric and Adolescent Medicine, 166*(8), 713–718.

F as in Fat. (2010). *How obesity threatens America's future. Issue report. Trust for America's health.* Robert Wood Johnson Foundation. Retrieved December 18, 2010, from www.healthy-americans.org

Gelman, S. A. (2009). Learning from others: Children's construction of concepts. *Annual Review of Psychology, 60*(1), 115–140.

Goodway, J. D., & Branta, C. F. (2003). Influence of a motor skill intervention on fundamental motor skill development of disadvantaged preschool children. *Research Quarterly for Exercise and Sport, 74*(1), 36–46.

Goodway, J. D., & Robinson, L. E. (2006). SKIPing toward an active start: Promoting physical activity in preschoolers. *Beyond the Journal: Young Children, 61*, 1–6.

Mission Readiness. (2009). *Ready, Willing and Unable to Serve*, Report by Mission: Readiness, Military Leaders for Kids. Retrieved December 18, 2010, from www.missionreadiness.org

Moore, L. L., Nguyen, U. S. D. T., Rothman, K. J., Cupples, L. A., & Ellison, R. C. (1995). Preschool physical-activity level and change in body fatness in young children – The Framingham Childrens Study. *American Journal of Epidemiology, 142*(9), 982–988.

National Institute of Child Health and Human Development, NIH, DHHS. (2006). *The NICHD Study of Early Child Care and Youth Development (SECCYD). Findings for children up to age 4 ½ years (05-4318).* Washington, DC: U.S. Government Printing Office.

Naylor, P. J., Macdonald, H. M., Zebedee, J. A., Reed, K. E., & McKay, H. A. (2006). Lessons learned from action schools! BC—An 'active school' model to promote physical activity in elementary schools. *Journal of Science and Medicine in Sport, 9*, 413–423.

Reed, K. E., Warburton, D. E. R., Macdonald, H. M., Naylor, P. J., & McKay, H. A. (2008). Action schools! BC: A school-based physical activity intervention designed to decrease cardiovascular disease risk factors in children. *Preventive Medicine, 46*(6), 525–531.

Schwartz, M. B., & Puhl, R. (2003). Childhood obesity: A societal problem to solve. *Obesity Reviews, 4*(1), 56–71.

Stegelin, D., Anderson, D., Kemper, K., Wagner, J., & Evans, K. (2014). Exploring daily physical activity and nutrition patterns in early learning settings: Snapshots of young children in head start, primary, and after-school settings. *Early Childhood Education Journal, 42*(2), 133–142.

Sypsa, C., & Simons, J. (2008). Questionnaires measuring the physical self children: A review. *European Psychomotricity Journal, 1*(2), 61–72.

Taras, H. (2005). Physical activity and student performance at school. *Journal of School Health, 75*(6), 214–218.

Tomporowski, P. D., Davis, C. L., Miller, P. H., & Naglieri, J. A. (2008). Exercise and children's intelligence, cognition, and academic achievement. *Educational Psychology Review, 20*(2), 111–131.

Vale, S., Santos, R., Soares-Miranda, L., Moreira, C, Ruiz, J., & Silva Mota, J. (2010). Objectively measured physical activity and body mass index in preschool children. *International Journal of Pediatrics, 2010,* Article ID 479439, 6 pages, 2010. https://doi.org/10.1155/2010/479439

Worobey, J., & Worobey, H. S. (2014). Body-size stigmatization by preschool girls: In a doll's world, it is good to be "Barbie". *Body Image, 11*, 171–174.

Dolores Ann Stegelin, Ph.D. is Professor Emerita at Clemson University where she provides university leadership in international study abroad and education, research in early childhood education, and support for innovative research in play. She serves on the advisory boards of the Emeritus College and the US Play Coalition at Clemson University.

Denise Anderson is a professor and currently serves as the Associate Dean of Undergraduate Studies in the newly organized College of Behavioral, Social and Health Sciences at Clemson University. She has conducted research, taught courses and published in peer-reviewed journals related to recreation and tourism for over a decade at Clemson University.

Karen Kemper is a professor in the Department of Public Health Sciences. While at Clemson, Dr. Kemper has served as the interim Director of the Joseph F. Sullivan Nursing Center, the Graduate Coordinator for the Public Health Sciences PhD program, and the Evaluator for the LiveWell Greenville Afterschool Initiative. Dr. Kemper has worked on numerous interdisciplinary research projects related to public health issues.

Jennifer Young Woods, Ph.D. is Assistant Professor of Special Education at Southern Wesleyan University, located in Central, South Carolina. She provides leadership for the special education department's programs and faculty development at SWU.

Katharine Evans, Ph.D. is Assistant Professor in the Department of Recreation Management and Therapeutic Recreation, University of Wisconsin-La Crosse, where she teaches and conducts research with undergraduate and graduate students.

Chapter 11
Using Physical Activity to Teach Academic Content: A Review of the Literature and Evidence-Based Recommendations

Stacie M. Kirk and Erik P. Kirk

Defining Early Literacy

A child's ability to read begins very early in a child's development providing a strong foundation for academic success (Gettinger & Stoiber, 2008; Kwak et al., 2009). The importance of early literacy as an essential content area in preschool curricula is widely recognized. Early literacy has been characterized as one of the new pre-K basics, along with language and numeracy skills (Christie & Roskos, 2006; Kibbe et al., 2011). In the past several decades, key literacy skills that develop during preschool are strongly correlated with the ability to read (Carlson et al., 2008; Miller & Votruba-Drzal, 2013; Reynolds, Temple, Robertson, & Mann, 2001). Many young children face significant challenges in learning to read because they lack essential early literacy skills (phonological awareness, letter knowledge, print awareness) when they begin school. In fact, children who are poor readers at the end of elementary school are most often those who failed to develop early literacy skills during preschool and kindergarten (Carlson et al., 2008; Castelli, Hillman, Buck, & Erwin, 2007; Rasberry et al., 2011). Furthermore, children growing up in poverty are at risk for lower-than-average levels of reading achievement through primary and secondary grades and are overrepresented in special education classrooms for students with learning disabilities (Gottlieb, Alter, Gottlieb, &

S. M. Kirk (✉)
Department of Teaching and Learning, Southern Illinois University, Edwardsville, IL, USA
e-mail: skirk@siue.edu

E. P. Kirk
Department of Applied Health, Southern Illinois University, Edwardsville, IL, USA
e-mail: ekirk@siue.edu

H. Brewer, M. R. Jalongo (eds.), *Physical Activity and Health Promotion in the Early Years*, Educating the Young Child 14,
https://doi.org/10.1007/978-3-319-76006-3_11

Wishner, 1994; Kozol, 1991; Miller & Votruba-Drzal, 2013; Schorr, 1988). Weaknesses in early literacy skills and subsequent reading failure are most common among low-income, non-White children and among children with limited proficiency in English (Miller & Votruba-Drzal, 2013). Compared to children from middle-income families, children from economically disadvantaged families experience significant difficulties learning to read and write because they enter school with less knowledge of letters and less familiarity with words (Basch, 2011; Efrat, 2011). The field of Early Childhood Education has placed an increased emphasis on program improvement and accountability based on children's outcomes. Several outcomes that are targeted includes development in the areas of literacy and language, which are critical to academic success later in life (Carlson et al., 2008; Coe, Pivarnik, Womack, Reeves, & Malina, 2006; Kwak et al., 2009; Miller & Votruba-Drzal, 2013). To this end, these findings emphasize the need for developing and establishing methods that can improve early literacy skills in preschoolers.

Lack of Physical Activity in Preschool Children

The National Association for Sport and Physical Education (2008) advises 120 min per day of physical activity (i.e., 60 min structured and 60 min unstructured) for young children. The National Association for the Education of Young Children (1998) recommends 60 min of outdoor activity per day. Currently, there is limited information about the physical activity levels of preschool children in community-based settings (Fulton & Shitabata, 1999; Pate, 2001). In particular, data regarding the contextual conditions associated with their activity is lacking (Sirard & Pate, 2001). Oliver, Schofield, and Kolt (2007) found that studies done with young children have shown levels of physical activity to be lower than expected. Sallis, Patterson, McKenzie, and Nader (1988) found that preschool children spent 60% of their outside playtime in sedentary activities and only 11% in moderate to vigorous activity.

Teachers and parents have assumed that preschool children are very active and engage in sufficient physical activity (Benham-Deal, 1993; Sallis et al., 1988). A systematic review by Tucker (Tucker, 2008) examined a total of 39 studies (published between 1986–2007) from seven countries (United States, Scotland, Finland, Australia, Chile, Estonia, Belgium) to establish an accurate reflection of the physical activity levels of preschool children. Nearly half of the studies included in the review reported less than 60 min per day of physical activity; therefore these children were insufficiently active according to NASPE guidelines (Active Start: A Statement of Physical Activity Guidelines for Children Birth to Five Years, 2008; Tucker, 2008). With only 54% of preschool children in this review found meeting the physically active recommendation and rising obesity rates within this age group (Ogden, Carroll, Kit, & Flegal, 2012), additional efforts are necessary to promote healthy activities in the preschool setting.

Recent work (Brown et al., 2009) replicated earlier findings in that their direct observation results indicated that children spent most of their time in sedentary activities (56% sedentary, 27% light, 17% moderate to vigorous physical activity). The same study also found that teachers rarely used intentional methods or teacher-arranged activities to increase physical activity. This demonstrates the need to target teacher involvement to increase preschool children's activity levels. It was also noted, through anecdotal observations, that preschool teachers are relatively passive with respect to encouragement and participation in children's outdoor physical activities. Intentional and active teacher involvement (i.e., organizing, modeling, encouraging) should be an integral part of any successful program to enhance children's physical activity (Brown et al., 2009). Over 60% of 3–5 year olds were served in center-based preschool settings in the United States in 2008 (Mamedova & Redford, 2015). With such large numbers of children in preschool and child care centers, early childhood professionals are in the unique position to support and encourage an active lifestyle among young children (Eastman, 1997).

Potential of Regular Exercise on Improving Academic Achievement in Preschoolers

Evidence suggests the importance of developing physical activity habits early in life to have the most beneficial effect on early literacy (Rasberry et al., 2011). Physical activity has been shown to improve literacy skills in children ages 6–18 years. However, the effects of increases in physical activity on literacy skills in preschool children (age three to five), a critical time in literacy development are not known. The National Association for Sport and Physical Education (2008) advises 120 min per day of physical activity (i.e., 60 min structured and 60 min unstructured) for young children. The National Association for the Education of Young Children (1998) recommends 60 min of outdoor activity per day. Despite these recommendations most preschool children do not meet these recommendations (Bornstein, Beets, Byun, & McIver, 2011; Eveline, Valery, Jessica, Ilse, & Greet, 2012), indicating a need for innovative strategies to increase daily physical activity. Integrating physical activity into preschool classrooms' academic lessons offers an innovative approach to increasing physical activity during the school day without decreasing the time devoted to academics.

Potential Mediators of the Association Between Physical Activity and Academic Achievement

Cardiovascular fitness and cognitive function. Despite the apparent relationship between fitness and academic achievement, only nine studies using true-experimental designs have been published in the extant literature. A meta-analysis of these studies found a positive association between physical activity and cognitive function in children age 4–18 years, suggesting that physical activity may be related to cognition during development (Sibley & Etnier, 2003). Specifically, participation in physical activity was related to cognitive performance along eight measurement categories (i.e., perceptual skills, intelligent quotient, achievement, verbal tests, mathematics tests, memory, developmental level/academic readiness, and other), and results indicated a beneficial relationship of physical activity on all categories, with the exception of memory (Sibley & Etnier, 2003). Of interest, the effect size observed by Sibley and Etnier (2003) in their meta-analysis on the association between physical activity and cognition in children was 0.32, which is apparently larger than that observed in Etnier (1997) meta-analysis of physical activity effects on cognition (ES = 0.25) across the lifespan (6–90 years), suggesting that physical activity may be more beneficial to children than adults. However, it should be noted that Sibley and Etnier (2003) classified cognition broadly and their meta-analysis did not include studies that measured either fitness or cognitive control. A more recent line of research by Hillman has indicated that both cardiovascular fitness (Buck, Hillman, & Castelli, 2008; Hillman, Buck, Themanson, Pontifex, & Castelli, 2009; Hillman, Castelli, & Buck, 2005) and single, acute bouts of moderate aerobic exercise (Hillman et al., 2009) influence neurocognitive function in 8–10 year old children. Specifically, when children are challenged with attentional tasks that require larger amounts of cognitive control (i.e., a subset of goal directed, self-regulatory processes that include planning, organization, abstract problem solving, working memory, motor control, and inhibitory control) those who are more fit perform better (i.e., shorter reaction time, higher response accuracy). Accordingly, this line of research indicates that both higher amounts of cardiovascular fitness and participation in acute exercise may improve cognitive health and function during tasks requiring greater amounts of attentional control. Given the nature and attentional requirements of reading comprehension and mathematical problem solving, basic indices of attention and processing speed, which are influenced by both fitness and exercise behavior, may provide some evidence of fitness/activity related improvements in academic performance.

Attention-to-task and academic achievement. Evidence suggests that physical activity breaks improve classroom behavior such as promoting on-task behavior (Barros, Silver, & Stein, 2009; Gabbard & Barton, 1979; Jarrett et al., 1998), less fidgeting (Jarrett et al., 1998) and better concentration scores (McNaughten &

Gabbard, 1993). Attention-to-task has recently been shown to improve in response to intermittent physical activity in children (Mahar et al., 2006).

For example, instructional periods that were kept short that were followed by even brief physical activity breaks has been shown to improve attention to task and work on cognitive tasks (Pellegrini & Bohn, 2005). Hillman et al. (2009) observed that student success increased when students were more actively engaged in learning during class time. Mahar (2011) noted the positive effects of participating in PA in the classroom through short breaks have on the amount of time students were actively engaged in learning, specifically to attention-to-task which significantly improved on-task behaviors. Attention-to-task is fundamental to learning (Manly et al., 2001) and includes other components of the classroom management such as discipline. That is, if students are presenting discipline problems, they are not attending to-task. Considering that classroom-based PA is relatively easy for teachers to implement in the classroom, it is recommended that children participate in short bouts (10 min) of classroom-based PA throughout the school day to sustain their on-task behavior.

Role of the Teacher

Research of Brown et al. (2009) found that teachers rarely use intentional methods or teacher-arranged activities to increase physical activity in young children. SHAPE America Active Start guidelines for preschoolers (2009), specifically state that "Caregivers and parents in charge of preschoolers' health and well-being are responsible for understanding the importance of physical activity and for promoting movement skills by providing opportunities for structured and unstructured physical activity (Active Start: A Statement of Physical Activity Guidelines for Children From Birth to Age 5, 2009). This demonstrates the need to target teacher involvement to increase preschool children's activity levels.

With that said, teachers play a critical role on integrating and encouraging increased physical activity throughout the day in preschool classrooms. Teachers are expected to serve as models for appropriate communication and social skills, as well as for appropriate self-help and cognitive skills. To this end, they should also be expected to serve as models for active movement and appropriate physical activities within the classroom setting. Specifically, Eastman states that "early childhood educators are in a unique position to support and encourage an active lifestyle among very young children" (Eastman, 1997). These supports can take the form of educational programs for parents related to physical activity, or changes to their daily programming to encourage more appropriate levels of physical activity (Ogden et al., 2012). Therefore, early childhood teachers should focus on encouraging both gross motor activity during outdoor play and movement during indoor play and activities.

Table 11.1 Example of incorporating weekly physical activities into the daily lesson plan

Time of day	Monday	Tuesday	Wednesday	Thursday	Friday
AM	Time: 10–10:15 am	Time: 10–10:15 am	Time: 10–10:15 am	Time: 10–10:15 am	Time: 10–10:15 am
	Moving with numbers	Dance party	Run/marching in place or around the room with rhymes	Animal action fun	Freeze dance
PM	Time: 3–3:15 pm	Time: 3–3:15 pm	Time: 3–3:15 pm	Time: 3–3:15 pm	Time: 3–3:15 pm
	"Simon says" movement game	Follow the leader	Music and movement CD	Same sound game	Hokey pokey

Academic Lessons Taught Using Physical Activity: Practical Examples and Strategies

A variety of literacy lessons may be used in the areas of picture naming (a measure of expressive language development), rhyming and alliteration (measures of phonological awareness). For example, the goal of a rhyming lesson is for children to find the rhymes within a particular poem or short story. The activity is designed to help children understand and identify rhyming words. During the lesson children will march in place while the teacher repeats several lines of a poem and the children identify the words that rhyme. Depending on the words that rhymed, the children could either act out the words or perform a certain number of jumping jacks (or other movement) before moving on to the next two lines of the poem and repeating the sequence throughout the poem. A detailed example of an activity lesson is found below. While these literacy concepts can be taught solely in large group time, reading, or other classroom activities, they can and should be integrated as lessons into a physical activity. Table 11.1 shows an example of how physical activities can be incorporated into the weekly lesson plan across both morning and afternoon activities.

Example: Physical Activity and Rhyming Awareness Lesson

Goal: In this lesson children are to find the rhymes. This activity helps children understand and identify rhyming words, while incorporating physical activities, like jumping jacks and touching toes.

Materials needed: Select a rhyming poem from the packet of poems. (E.g. Ten Little Bluebirds).

Instruction: When reading or reciting rhymes and rhyming stories, pause to identify words that rhyme. Use the word *rhyme* to describe the common ending sounds.

Activity Lesson: Children should march in place throughout the lesson. Begin by reciting the poem "Ten Little Bluebirds" two sentences at a time. After the first two sentences, identify the rhyming words "pine" and "nine" by saying "Do you know what? Pine and nine sound alike. They both end with the sound -ine. Pine and nine rhyme!" The children should then perform "nine" jumping jacks while counting out loud. Once completed with the nine jumping jacks the children should resume marching in place. Repeat for the remaining poem but use other activities such as touching toes, move arms up and down, jogging around the circle carpet. Repeat a second time so the children become familiar with the poem.

Advanced Lesson: In future lessons as the children become familiar with the poems ask the children to identify the rhymes as you read. For example, when reciting the poem "Ten Little Bluebirds," after the first two sentences, ask the children to identify the rhyming words. "I think there were two words that rhyme; can anyone tell me which words rhyme?" The children should indicate they know the answer by jumping up and down in place. Repeat for the remaining lines.

Below are examples of flip cards that can be printed and/or laminated to make a packet, so that teachers have a ready-made menu of physical activity-early literacy activities. The first page (Fig. 11.1) is a quick "Helpful Hints" guide to give teachers ideas of how to keep children engaged in the activity. Figures 11.2, 11.3, 11.4, 11.5, and 11.6 show examples of daily physical activity cards that would make up a 5 day

Physical Activity Routines

Helpful Hints:

- ❖ Think about different directions = up, down, low, high, sideways, forward, backward, right or left
- ❖ Key phrases to use: *How can you...?, See if you can..., How many ways can you...?*
- ❖ Options 1 and 2 are the morning/afternoon activities for the day.
- ❖ The Kids in Motion and the Miscellaneous CD are provided for use with some activities.

Fig. 11.1 Example of "Helpful Hints" guide for teachers for child engagement

Morning Activity Routine A

Option 1— Simon Says Movement Game (Teacher or aide is "Simon", encouraging students to do active movements, can be 1, 2 or 3 different movement commands for students to say and do)

Option 2— Hokey Pokey Game (put your right foot in, put your right foot out…..shake it all about!)

Cool Down— 2 minutes of sitting, relaxing

Afternoon Activity Routine A

Option 1— Animal Action Fun—teacher/student says name of an animal and the group has to move around the room like that animal (Kangaroo jumps, crocodile creep, bunny hops)

Option 2—Follow the Leader Marching Game—(have teachers and children take turns leading the group in marching, hopping, jumping, etc)

Cool Down— 2 minutes of sitting, lying still, etc

Fig. 11.2 Example of daily physical activity guide for Monday for teachers to use for integrating literacy and other pre-academic content into physical activities

Morning Activity Routine B

Option 1— Sleeping Giants/Waking Giants (Children pretend to be giants who like to jump, skip, hop, etc. Have children practice. Once children hear teacher say "Sleeping Giants", children stop and lie on floor. Teacher says "Waking Giants" and children get up and starting jumping, etc)

Option 2— Moving with Numbers (Take turns asking students to pick a number, then the rest of the group does the designated movement that number of times.) **Example— Jackie picks "4". The class jumps, slides, touches toes, etc. 4 times.**

Cool Down— 2 minutes of stretching, breathing, etc.

Afternoon Activity Routine B

Option 1— Same Sound Game (Teacher picks a letter of the alphabet and says the sound, then students jump, run in place, etc when they hear a word that starts with the same sound) (***example: C for cat, emphasize 'c' sound, then say cow, can, car, etc for students to listen for)***

Option 2—Jumping Beans Game (jumping up, down, forward, sideways, backward when a specific letter sound is heard)

Cool Down— 2 minutes of sitting, relaxing, etc.

Fig. 11.3 Example of daily physical activity guide for Tuesday for teachers to use for integrating literacy and other pre-academic content into physical activities

Morning Activity Routine C

Option 1 — Do What ....Does - (Pick one child to be leader. The child does a movement and the other children repeat the motion. Teachers emphasize the sound of the beginning letter of the motion. For example, emphasize the "j" sound if the motion is jumping.)

Option 2 — Music CD - (Play the CD and let the children dance to the songs.) Chicken Dance, YMCA, Cha Cha Slide, Wheels on the Bus, etc.

Cool Down — 2 minutes of stretching, breathing, etc.

Afternoon Activity Routine C

Option 1 — Hot Potato - One child has the "potato." Pass the potato around to each other. When the music stops, the children clap for the child with the potato so nobody is left out. The teacher asks the child to choose a word for the group to make a rhyme to. Restart the music and continue play.

Option 2 — Freeze Dance - Music from Kids in Motion or pick any kind of music. Have the kids dance to music and freeze when it stops. The teacher has the children count to a specific number before starting the music again.

Cool Down — 2 minutes of sitting, relaxing, etc.

Fig. 11.4 Example of daily physical activity guide for Wednesday for teachers to use for integrating literacy and other pre-academic content into physical activities

set of routines that teachers could choose from in the morning and afternoon. Each routine is meant to be implemented for 15 min, with one session in the morning and one session in the afternoon, for a total of 30 min of integrated learning through physical activity.

In each of the Figs. 11.2, 11.3, 11.4, 11.5, and 11.6, activities are listed for teachers to choose from for morning and afternoon activity routines that allow children to be physically active while also building their knowledge base in early literacy and pre academic content. To further illustrate the link between the physical activities

Morning Activity Routine D

Option 1 — Kids in Motion CD —(Free choice dance – the goal here is to have the children get moving and get their blood flowing. The teacher can incorporate letter sounds, counting, rhyming, etc into the motions of the children.)

Option 2 — Going on a Bear Hunt- (Follow the song on White CD—track #13. Children are working on auditory comprehension – following directions)

Cool Down — 2 minutes of stretching, breathing, etc.

Afternoon Activity Routine D

Option 1 — Musical Squares - (Have carpet squares for each child. Lay the carpet squares on the floor in a circle. The Children walk in a circle until the music stops. When the music stops, the children find a square. Then take a square away. Continue the process until there is one left. See how many children can fit on one square. This is a good activity for counting.)

Option 2 — Bean Bag Boogie - (Have a bean bag for each child. Can also use balls, scarves, or whatever you have in the room. They put the bean bag on the spot on their body where the music tells them. The teacher could have children sound out the name of the body part.)

Cool Down — 2 minutes of sitting, relaxing, etc.

Fig. 11.5 Example of daily physical activity guide for Thursday for teachers to use for integrating literacy and other pre-academic content into physical activities

and the content that teachers can incorporate, Table 11.2 lists the activities (in alphabetical order) and the corresponding content area that may be targeted through that activity. It should be noted that the content area possibilities included in Table 11.2 are in addition to auditory comprehension, which is an area that all activities can target and improve.

Morning Activity Routine E

Option 1 — Parachute (The children grab an end and shake it. The children each take turns throwing different sized ball on it or take turns running underneath it. The teacher could have children cross underneath when they hear a letter in their name, or when they are able to match a rhyming word to what the teacher says.)

Option 2 — Moving with Numbers (Take turns asking students to pick a number, then the rest of the group does the designated movement that number of times.) **Example— Jackie picks "4". The class jumps, slides, touches toes, etc. 4 times.**

Cool Down — 2 minutes of stretching, breathing, etc.

Afternoon Activity Routine E

Option 1 — Color Chants - (Teacher says a color and the child does a certain activity. Red-put hands on your head, Blue-put hands on your shoe, Green-Pretend to wash your face, pink- going to think, think, think (tap pointer finger against side of head as if thinking), Yellow-Wave to a friend, Purple-with both pointer fingers make circles in the air, Brown- turn yourself around and sit right down!)

Option 2 — Walk My Walk - (Challenge the students to walk like a particular person might. EX: tightrope walker, astronaut on the moon, ballerina, etc. This works on children's auditory comprehension.)

Cool Down — 2 minutes of sitting, relaxing, etc.

Fig. 11.6 Example of daily physical activity guide for Friday for teachers to use for integrating literacy and other pre-academic content into physical activities

Summary

Research is suggestive of an association between physical activity and academic achievement in children. There appears to be role of physical activity and academic achievement. Providing increased physical activity without decreasing academic instruction time is important in the current educational environment, where preschools are required to meet mandated school wellness policies. These policies require increased physical activity but are reluctant to decrease academic instruction

Table 11.2 Matching physical activities to early literacy and pre academic content area

Physical activity	Content area possibilities
1. Simon says movement game	Rhyming, counting
2. Hokey pokey game	Body parts, spatial relationships, motor coordination
3. Animal action fun	Animal identification, animal sounds, phonological awareness, motor coordination
4. Follow the leader marching game	Phonological awareness, counting, rhyming, body awareness, spatial relationships, motor coordination
5. Sleeping giants/ waking giants	Body awareness, spatial relationships, motor coordination, attention
6. Moving with numbers	Counting, motor coordination, attention
7. Same sound game	Phonological awareness, sound discrimination, sound identification
8. Jumping beans game	Phonological awareness, sound discrimination, motor coordination
9. Do what ….Does	Phonological awareness, sound discrimination, motor coordination
10. Music CD	Varies according to the song played, but may include motor coordination, spatial awareness, body awareness
11. Hot potato	Rhyming, counting, motor coordination
12. Freeze dance	Counting, body awareness, motor coordination
13. Kids in motion CD	Motor coordination, counting
14. Going on a bear hunt	Phonological awareness (sounds of the grass, mud, wind, etc.), body awareness
15. Musical squares	Counting, body awareness
16. Bean bag boogie	Motor coordination, body awareness, body parts
17. Parachute	Motor coordination, counting, rhyming, phonological awareness, sound identification, sound discrimination
18. Moving with numbers	Counting, number identification, motor coordination
19. Color chants	Color identification, motor coordination, body awareness
20. Walk my walk	Motor coordination, body awareness

time for fear of failing to meet mandated academic performance standards. Presented above are examples and practical strategies that have been incorporated into preschool classrooms, by teachers, to achieve this goal. In using these strategies, teachers can successfully work with preschool children to become more physically active during the day, while also retaining their focus on early literacy and other pre-academic skills.

References

Active Start: A Statement of Physical Activity Guidelines for Children Birth to Five Years. (2008) (pp. 5–11). Reston, VA: National Association for Sport and Physical Education (NASPE), an association of the American Alliance for Health, Physical Education, Recreation and Dance.

Active Start: A Statement of Physical Activity Guidelines for Children From Birth to Age 5. (2009). (2nd ed.).: Saddle Stitching.
Barros, R. M., Silver, E. J., & Stein, R. E. (2009). School recess and group classroom behavior. *Pediatrics, 123*(2), 431–436.
Basch, C. E. (2011). Physical activity and the achievement gap among urban minority youth. *Journal of School Health, 81*(10), 626–634.
Benham-Deal, T. (1993). Physical activity patterns of preschoolers during a developmental movement program. *Child Study Journal, 23*, 115–133.
Bornstein, D. B., Beets, M. W., Byun, W., & McIver, K. (2011). Accelerometer-derived physical activity levels of preschoolers: A meta-analysis. *Journal of Science and Medicine in Sport, 14*(6), 504–511.
Brown, W. H., Pfeiffer, K. A., McIver, K. L., Dowda, M., Addy, C. L., & Pate, R. R. (2009). Social and environmental factors associated with preschoolers' nonsedentary physical activity. *Child Development, 80*(1), 45–58.
Buck, S. M., Hillman, C. H., & Castelli, D. M. (2008). The relation of aerobic fitness to stroop task performance in preadolescent children. *Medicine and Science in Sports and Exercise, 40*(1), 166–172.
Carlson, S. A., Fulton, J. E., Lee, S. M., Maynard, L. M., Brown, D. R., Kohl, H. W., 3rd, & Dietz, W. H. (2008). Physical education and academic achievement in elementary school: Data from the early childhood longitudinal study. *American Journal of Public Health, 98*(4), 721–727.
Castelli, D. M., Hillman, C. H., Buck, S. M., & Erwin, H. E. (2007). Physical fitness and academic achievement in third- and fifth-grade students. *Journal of Sport and Exercise Psychology, 29*(2), 239–252.
Christie, J., & Roskos, K. (2006). Standards, science, and the role of play in early literacy education. In D. Singer, R. Golinkoff, & K. Hirsh-Pasek (Eds.), *Play = learning: How play motivates and enhances children's cognitive and social-emotional growth* (pp. 57–73). Oxford, UK: Oxford University Press.
Coe, D. P., Pivarnik, J. M., Womack, C. J., Reeves, M. J., & Malina, R. M. (2006). Effect of physical education and activity levels on academic achievement in children. *Medicine and Science in Sports and Exercise, 38*(8), 1515–1519.
Eastman, W. (1997). Active living: Physical activities for infants, toddlers, and preschoolers. *Early Childhood Education, 24*, 161–164.
Efrat, M. (2011). The relationship between low-income and minority children's physical activity and academic-related outcomes: A review of the literature. *Health Education & Behavior, 38*(5), 441–451.
Etnier, J. L. (1997). The influence of physical fitness and exercise upon cognitive functioning: A meta-analysis. *Journal of Sport and Exercise Psychology, 19*, 249–277.
Eveline, V. C., Valery, L., Jessica, G., Ilse, D. B., & Greet, C. (2012). Preschooler's physical activity levels and associations with lesson context, teacher's behavior, and environment during preschool physical education. *Early Childhood Research Quarterly, 27*(2), 221–230.
Fulton, J. E., & Shitabata, P. K. (1999). CO_2 laser physics and tissue interactions in skin. *Lasers in Surgery and Medicine, 24*(2), 113–121.
Gabbard, C., & Barton, J. (1979). Effects of physical activity on mathematical computation among young children. *Journal of Psychology, 103*, 287–288.
Gettinger, M., & Stoiber, K. (2008). Applying a response-to-intervention model for early literacy development in low-income children. *Topics in Early Childhood Special Education, 27*, 198–213.
Gottlieb, J., Alter, M., Gottlieb, B. W., & Wishner, J. (1994). Special education in urban America: It's not justifiable for many. *The Journal of Special Education, 2*(7), 453–465.
Hillman, C. H., Buck, S. M., Themanson, J. R., Pontifex, M. B., & Castelli, D. M. (2009). Aerobic fitness and cognitive development: Event-related brain potential and task performance indices of executive control in preadolescent children. *Developmental Psychology, 45*(1), 114–129.

Hillman, C. H., Castelli, D. M., & Buck, S. M. (2005). Aerobic fitness and neurocognitive function in healthy preadolescent children. *Medicine and Science in Sports and Exercise, 37*(11), 1967–1974.

Hillman, C. H., Pontifex, M. B., Raine, L. B., Castelli, D. M., Hall, E. E., & Kramer, A. F. (2009). The effect of acute treadmill walking on cognitive control and academic achievement in preadolescent children. *Neuroscience, 159*(3), 1044–1054.

Jarrett, O. S., Maxwell, D. M., Dickerson, C., Hoge, P., Davies, G., & Yetley, A. (1998). Impact of recess on classroom behavior: Group effects and individual differences. *Journal of Educational Research, 92*, 121–126.

Kibbe, D. L., Hackett, J., Hurley, M., McFarland, A., Schubert, K. G., Schultz, A., & Harris, S. (2011). Ten years of TAKE 10!((R)): Integrating physical activity with academic concepts in elementary school classrooms. *Preventive Medicine, 52*(Suppl 1), S43–S50.

Kozol, J. L. (1991). *Savage inequalities: Children in America's schools*. New York, NY: Crown.

Kwak, L., Kremers, S. P., Bergman, P., Ruiz, J. R., Rizzo, N. S., & Sjostrom, M. (2009). Associations between physical activity, fitness, and academic achievement. *Journal of Pediatrics, 155*(6), 914–918. e911.

Mahar, M. T. (2011). Impact of short bouts of physical activity on attention-to-task in elementary school children. [Review]. *Preventive Medicine, 52*(Suppl 1), S60–S64.

Mahar, M. T., Murphy, S. K., Rowe, D. A., Golden, J., Shields, A. T., & Raedeke, T. D. (2006). Effects of a classroom-based program on physical activity and on-task behavior. *Medicine and Science in Sports and Exercise, 38*(12), 2086–2094.

Mamedova, S., & Redford, J. (2015). *Early childhood program participation, from the National Household Education Surveys Program of 2012 (NCES 2013-029.REV)*. Washington, DC: National Center for Education Statistics, Institute of Education Sciences, U.S. Department of Education.

Manly, T., Anderson, V., Nimmo-Smith, I., Turner, A., Watson, P., & Robertson, I. H. (2001). The differential assessment of children's attention: The test of everyday attention for children (TEA-Ch), normative sample and ADHD performance. *Journal of Child Psychology and Psychiatry, 42*, 1065–1081.

McNaughten, D., & Gabbard, C. (1993). Physical exertion and immediate mental performance of 6th grade children. *Perceptual & Motor Skills, 77*, 1155–1159.

Miller, P., & Votruba-Drzal, E. (2013). Early academic skills and childhood experiences across the urban–rural continuum. *Early Childhood Research Quarterly, 28*(2), 234–248.

Ogden, C. L., Carroll, M. D., Kit, B. K., & Flegal, K. M. (2012). PRevalence of obesity and trends in body mass index among us children and adolescents, 1999–2010. *Journal of the American Medical Association, 307*(5), 483–490.

Oliver, M., Schofield, G. M., & Kolt, G. S. (2007). Physical activity in preschoolers: Understanding prevalence and measurement issues. *Sports Medicine, 37*(12), 1045–1070.

Pate, R. R. (2001). Assessment of physical activity and sedentary behavior in preschool children. *Pediatric Exercise Science, 13*, 129–130.

Pellegrini, A. D., & Bohn, C. M. (2005). The role of recess in children's cognitive performance and school adjustment. *Educational Researcher, 34*(1), 13–19.

Rasberry, C. N., Lee, S. M., Robin, L., Laris, B. A., Russell, L. A., Coyle, K. K., & Nihiser, A. J. (2011). The association between school-based physical activity, including physical education, and academic performance: A systematic review of the literature. *Preventive Medicine, 52*(Supplement (0)), S10–S20.

Reynolds, A. J., Temple, J. A., Robertson, D. L., & Mann, E. A. (2001). Long-term effects of an early childhood intervention on educational achievement and juvenile arrest: A 15-year follow-up of low-income children in public schools. *Journal of the American Medical Association, 285*(18), 2339–2346.

Sallis, J. F., Patterson, T. L., McKenzie, T. L., & Nader, P. R. (1988). Family variables and physical activity in preschool children. *Journal of Developmental and Behavior Pediatrics, 9*(2), 57–61.

Schorr, L. B. (1988). *Within our reach: Breaking the cycle of disadvantage*. New York, NY: Doubleday.

Sibley, B. A., & Etnier, J. L. (2003). The relationship between physical activity and cognition in children: A meta-analysis. *Pediatric Exercise Science, 15*, 243–256.

Sirard, J. R., & Pate, R. R. (2001). Physical activity assessment in children and adolescents. *Sports Medicine, 31*(6), 439–454.

Tucker, P. (2008). The physical activity levels of preschool-aged children: A systematic review. *Early Childhood Research Quarterly, 23*, 547–558.

Dr. Stacie M. Kirk teaches courses in Early Childhood Special Education and Early Intervention for Early Childhood Education and Special Education teacher candidates, as well as introductory special education and language development courses. Prior to joining SIUE, Dr. Kirk taught in both preschool and toddler-age early childhood classrooms, and has experience working with Early Head Start and Head Start programs. She has served as Principal Investigator, author and co-author for a number of grants, articles and presentations topics in the areas of Early Childhood Education, Early Childhood Special Education and Early Childhood Physical Activity and Health.

Dr. Erik P. Kirk teaches courses related the importance and effects of physical activity in children and adults. He has worked with both children and adults in weight management, nutrition education, and physical activity promotion. He has served as Principal Investigator, author and co-author for a number of grants, articles and presentations topics in the areas of Early Childhood Education, Early Childhood Special Education and Early Childhood Physical Activity and Health.

Chapter 12
Evaluating the Home for Promoting Motor Skill Development

Carl Gabbard and Priscila Caçola

Introduction

Contemporary theories and research on infant and early childhood development suggests quite convincingly that an optimal level of development occurs with a stimulating environment and strong contextual support (Bornstein & Bradley, 2012; Bronfenbrenner, 2005). Complementing this idea is the general contention that rich and enriched environments produce rich brains and optimal level of development occurs with strong contextual support (e.g., Bryck & Fisher, 2012; Davidson & McEwen, 2012). Increasing bodies of evidence underscore the idea that environmental stimulation plays a critical role in optimal human development during the early stages of life. Those early years mark powerful biological maturation and behavioral change, especially in motor behavior (Adolph & Berger, 2006; Piek, 2006). Of the various factors comprising the environment, few would disagree that the *home* is a primary agent for learning and developing the foundation for positive lifelong behaviors, especially during the early years (see review by Son & Morrison, 2010 and UNESCO (United Nations) report by Iltus, 2006).

This chapter begins with a discussion of the importance of the home environment in child development and the underlying theoretical notion that affordances in the home are critical to the developmental process, in this context, motor development.

C. Gabbard (✉)
Department of Health & Kinesiology (Motor Neuroscience), Texas A&M University, College Station, TX, USA
e-mail: c-gabbard@tamu.edu

P. Caçola
Department of Kinesiology, University of Texas at Arlington, Arlington, TX, USA

H. Brewer, M. R. Jalongo (eds.), *Physical Activity and Health Promotion in the Early Years*, Educating the Young Child 14,
https://doi.org/10.1007/978-3-319-76006-3_12

Next, is a brief description of contemporary assessment instruments and related research that have shown strong and promising potential for identifying affordances in the home. We complete the chapter with ideas for using this information in research, education, and clinical settings.

Role of the Home Environment and Affordances

Research findings strongly support the positive link between an adequate home environment and early developmental outcomes, including health, cognitive and motor development (Piek, Dawson, Leight, & Smith, 2008; Spencer et al., 2009; Treyvaud et al., 2012; Walker, 2010).

Of the home characteristics and of specific interest here, is the role of affordances. Affordances are characteristics of the environmental setting and opportunities that offer the individual potential for action, and consequently to learn and develop a skill or a part of the biological system. In addition to the more obvious set of affordances such as toys, materials, apparatus, and availability of space, stimulation and nurturing by parents (and others) provide the additional component of events. This view agrees with Stoffregen (2000) and Hirose (2002) in that events can be affordances—events offer the child opportunities for action. Hirose stated, "Affordances are opportunities for action that objects, events, or places in the environment provide for the animal" (p. 104). The idea that affordances in general can be conducive to stimulating child development was a part key element in Gibson's Ecological (*Affordance*) theory (Gibson, 1979, 2002). The home environment is a rich resource of opportunities that can be conducive to stimulating child development, especially at an early age.

Assessing the Home

This section describes selected instruments that have been used to assess various characteristics in the home environment that are associated with daily child activity and motor development.

The Home Observation for Measurement of the Environment (HOME) Inventory (Caldwell & Bradley, 1984)

The HOME inventory has been used in national longitudinal studies with the aim of identying factors provided by the family that influences a child's cognitive and emotional behavior. Whereas, the initial instrument and subsequent adaptations for different ages (infant to early adolescence) was not designed to assess 'motor affordances' specifically, the instruments do include a play (toy) component. Interestingly, and of specific interest here, one of the more intriguing findings from earlier large-scale national longiutudinal studies of the home and child development is the report that "availability of stimulating play materials" was a predictor of future mental behavior (Bradley et al., 1989; Mundfrom, Bradley, & Whiteside, 1993). What follows is a sample of work using the HOME inventory.

Poresky and Henderson (1982), using the *Bayley Scales* to assess motor development in 2-year-olds, reported that behavior was related to their home environment and socioeconomic status of the family. The researchers stated that Learning Materials and Involvement, HOME subscales, presented opportunities to learn through experience with the environment and affective support. In a similar study reported by La Veck and Hammond (1982), 3-year-olds from an advantaged environment scored higher on the Motor Scale of the McCarthy Scales than those from a less advantaged environment; the HOME Inventory was used to rate the general environment.

Parks and Bradley (1991) used the HOME instrument with 6-month-olds to examine the specific interaction of two features of the home environment, availability of toys and amount of maternal involvement. The researchers found that higher locomotor, eye-hand coordination, and general developmental quotients were associated with the additive combination of more 'optimal play materials' and 'high level of maternal involvement'. When examining the independent contribution of the factors, appropriate play materials were associated with more favorable eye-hand coordination. Goyen and Lui (2002) examined the relationship between the HOME and motor development for children ages 18 months and 3- to 5-years, in groups of "apparently normal" high-risk infants. They concluded that the development of gross- and fine-motor skills appeared to be differently influenced by the home environment. Infants with a lower HOME score consistently scored poorer on *Peabody* motor scores, however, the difference was only significant for the gross-motor skills.

Abbott, Bartlett, Fanning and Kramer (2000) used three subscales of the HOME inventory (Maternal Responsivity, Provision of Appropriate Learning Materials and Maternal Involvement) and the *Alberta Infant Motor Scale* (AIMS) to assess homes and their 8-month-old children's motor development. Results did not show any significant correlations between HOME and AIMS scores. One of the problems was that most children scored high on the AIMS and on the HOME [that is, there were few low HOME scores]. According to researchers, lack of sensitivity in the HOME inventory (ceiling effect), questionable validity of the HOME inventory to support infant motor development, homogeneity of family aspects (median and high SES) and significantly high motor scores with the AIMS, could have combined to reflect the results. The general problem with a ceiling effect is not uncommon in this line of research based on the difficulty with identifying homes that score in the extreme low range.

During the day (but only referring to the time spent in your house):	YES	NO
24. My child plays with other children as a usual and ordinary every day event.	☐	☐

On a typical day, how would you describe the amount of awake time your child spends in each of the situations below? *(Read carefully each question and mark the box respective to your answer)*

33. Carried in adult arms, attached to caregiver's body or in some carrying device.

No time ☐ *Very little time* ☐ *Some time* ☐ *A long time* ☐

Fig. 12.1 Examples of dichotomic and Likert-type scale questions provided by the Affordances in the Home Environment for Motor Development – Self Report (AHEMD-SR)

The researchers concluded that although the home environment is surely within the host of subsystems that contribute to infant motor development, little research exists examining this relationship. Furthermore, at the time of the report they strongly emphasized that, "a valid measure reflecting aspects of the home environment that support infant motor development needs to be created" (p. 66).

Since that recommendation, three contemporary assessment instruments have been created and reported in the literature – tools that were designed to examine the multidimensional effects of the home on infant and early childhood motor development.

Affordances in the Home Environment for Motor Development – Self Report (AHEMD-SR)

Based in large part on the propositions of ecological (affordance) theory noted earlier, the AHEMD-SR is a reliable and valid parental self-report assessment instrument that addresses the home opportunities for infants' motor development from 18- to 42 months (Rodrigues, Saraiva, & Gabbard, 2005; applications of the instrument were described by Gabbard, Caçola, & Rodrigues, 2008 and summarized in a subsequent section here).

The instrument consists of five factors (subscales: Inside Space, Outside Space, Variety of Stimulation, Fine Motor Toys and Gross Motor Toys) plus a section on Child and Family Characteristics. Three types of questions are used: simple dichotomic choice, 4-point Likert-type scale, and description-based queries; representing 20 variables and 67 items. Fig. 12.1 provides examples of two types of questions. In addition, pictorial examples with description based queries are provided to help the user identify available categories and specific items (see Fig. 12.2).

Readability was established at an approximate fourth grade reading level. Although the AHEMD-SR is reliable as a self-report by parents/caregivers, in some cases, direct administration by an examiner (in the home) is appropriate. In essence, the AHEMD-SR is a valid and reliable instrument for assessing how well home environments afford movement and potentially promote motor development. To date,

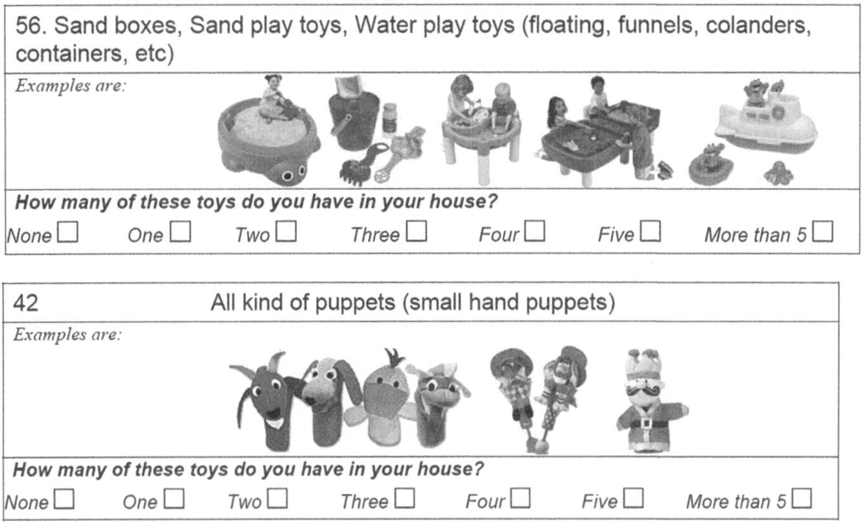
56. Sand boxes, Sand play toys, Water play toys (floating, funnels, colanders, containers, etc)
Examples are:
How many of these toys do you have in your house?
None One Two Three Four Five More than 5
42 All kind of puppets (small hand puppets)
Examples are:
How many of these toys do you have in your house?
None One Two Three Four Five More than 5

Fig. 12.2 Examples of description-based queries provided by the Affordances in the Home Environment for Motor Development – Self Report (AHEMD-SR)

the AHEMD-SR has been translated into eight languages other than English, used in a variety of research and clinical settings, and reported in several scientific journals. As a general note, parents' reports have been described to be a sensitive, accurate and reliable source of information in a naturalistic environment (Bartlett et al., 2008; Sirard, Nelson, Pereira, & Lytle, 2008; Wilson, Kaplan, Crawford, Campbell, & Dewey, 2000).

Research Findings

In 2009, Haydari, Askari, and Nezhad (2009) examined validity of the AHEMD with an Iranian sample of children aged 18–42 months. They found that the instrument was valid and reliable. Furthermore, there were strong and significant multi-relationships between motor development and AHEMD scores. The best predictor of the AHEMD for overall motor ability was fine-motor toy availability.

Temple, Naylor, Rhodes, and Wharf-Higgins (2009) were interested in examining physical activity levels in family childcare. The AHEMD was used to assess whether the family childcare environment afforded movement. The researchers assessed 65 3- to 5-year-olds representing 23 childcare homes. Results indicated that the majority of homes (80–90%) provided good or very good affordances in respect to inside space, variety of stimulation, gross motor toys, fine motor toys and outside space.

In 2011, Hsieh, Hwang, Liao, Chen, Hsieh and Chu examined the reliability and validity of the Chinese version of AHEMD and compared results to the widely used HOME inventory. They assessed homes of 106 typically developing infants and of 45 infants with motor delays; mean ages 28 and 24 months respectively. Results demonstrated adequate reliability and convergent validity with the HOME inventory. However, the Outside Space subscale did not correlate significantly with the HOME. We wish to note once more that the HOME inventory, although widely used, was not designed to assess specific movement affordances in the home.

More recently, using a Japanese version of the AHEMD-SR, Mori, Nakamoto, Mizuochi, Ikudome, and Gabbard (2013) with children ages 18–42 months, found that home environment score was associated with level of motor function. That finding was most evident for availability of fine- and gross-motor toys (subscales). The researchers also found, using a separate parental physical activity questionnaire, that higher activity level was correlated with higher AHEMD-SR scores.

Affordances in the Home Environment for Motor Development – Infant Scale (AHEMD-IS)

Since the reporting and use of that instrument, several comments have been noted on the need for a tool that addresses earlier development. Due to the dramatic changes in motor behavior from the first months of life to the achievement of independent walking (up to 18 months), a younger version of the instrument needed to be created to address factors in the home environment that potentially affect infant motor development (Caçola, Gabbard, Montebelo, & Santos, 2015). In addition, it is generally understood by the medical and therapy community that interventions may be most effective if begun early in life, and delays may have long lasting effects (Nordhov, Rønning, Ulvund, Dahl, & Kaaresen, 2012). With that in mind and considering the growing interest of this topic in research and clinical communities, the AHEMD for infants, named the AHEMD – Infant Scale (*AHEMD-IS*) was created.

Since its creation, the AHEMD-IS (Caçola, Gabbard, Santos, & Batistela 2011; Caçola et al., 2015) has gained in popularity as a research and clinical tool. Furthermore, the AHEMD-IS has been noted in recent studies of infant development, with general findings supporting the idea that environmental factors are associated with infant's motor development and motor affordances can have a positive impact on future motor ability and later cognitive behavior (a brief summary of selected reports follows).

The AHEMD-IS is a self-administered parental tool designed to accurately measure the availability of opportunities for infants between 3- and 18 months of age, with a separation for infants between 3- and 11 months of age and between 12- and 18 months (additional toys for the older age range). There are a total of 35 items divided into 4 dimensions (Physical Space, Variety of Stimulation, Fine-Motor Toys, Gross-Motor Toys) and a total AHEMD score that can be categorized into 4 descriptions of home motor affordances (scoring system): Less than adequate,

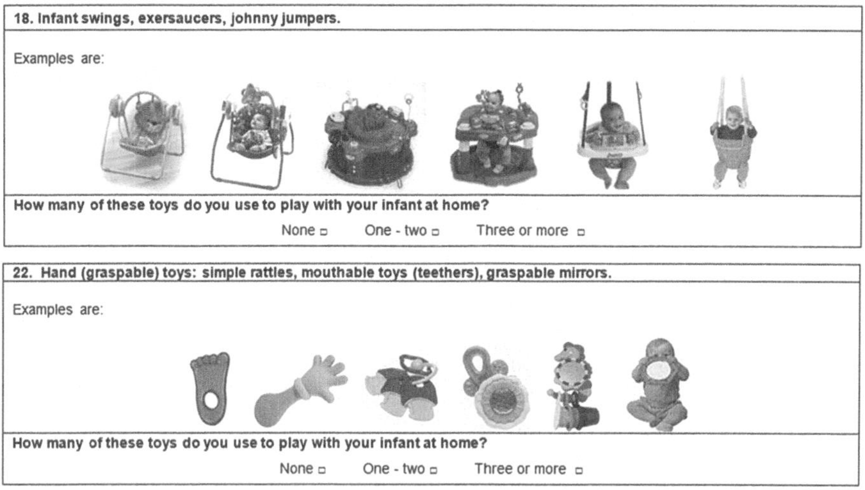

Fig. 12.3 Examples of description-based queries provided by the Affordances in the Home Environment for Motor Development – Infant Scale (AHEMD-IS)

Moderately adequate, Adequate, and Excellent. With that, it is important to note that the items of the Fine-Motor Toys and Gross-Motor Toys dimensions aim to measure the quantity and quality of toys in each category; a sample is shown in Fig. 12.3.

The AHEMD-IS dimensions that are specific to play materials comprise the biggest part of the questionnaire, with nine items for the Gross-Motor Toys and 11 for the Fine-Motor Toys. The instrument, especially in regards to play materials, functions as an inventory to assess the quantity, variety, and quality of toys present in the home, and it follows the assumption that availability of affordances represents the real use of these opportunities by infants (Correr, Ouro, Caçola, Almeida, & Santos, 2014).

Research Findings

In 2008, Schobert and Valentini explored the context of affordances and events in infant motor development using the original AHEMD. The author examined the relationship between the home, nursery school environment, and motor development of 6- to 18-month-olds using the Alberta Infant Motor Scale. Results demonstrated that infants whose homes had higher AHEMD scores displayed significantly better motor scores; 19% had lower home scores and lower motor scores. Using an infant sample assessed over time, Miquelote, Santos, Caçola, Montebelo, and Gabbard (2012) examined the association between motor affordances in the home and infant motor and cognitive behavior. They assessed the sample using the Bayley Scales and AHEMD-IS at age 9 months and 6 months later with the inclusion of cognitive ability. For motor ability, there was an overall improvement in performance from the 1st to the 2nd assessment, with significant positive correlations between the dimensions of the home (daily activities and play materials) and global motor performance (1st assessment) and fine-motor performance on the 2nd assessment. In regard to cognitive behavior (2nd assessment), results indicated a positive association with fine-motor performance. The results suggested that motor affordances can have a positive impact on future motor ability and speculatively, later cognitive behavior in infants.

A study interested in the relationship between infant health characteristics and the home environment was reported by Saccani, Valentini, Pereira, Müller, and Gabbard (2013). The sample was over 500 infants ages newborn to 18 months. Using the AHEMD-IS, Alberta Infant Motor Scale, and selected biological/medical factors (prematurity, APGAR score, birthweight, birth length, cephalic perimeter, and duration of infant stay in intensive care), the researchers found that the home environment predicted infant status as well as some typical biological risk factors. That is, during the first year of life, home factors were significantly associated with infant motor development, as much as or even more than some biologic factors. Currently, the AHEMD-IS is also being used as part of a study that is exploring the impact of perinatal different intrauterine environments on child growth and development in the first six moths of life (Bernardi et al., 2012). Also in 2013, Freitas, Gabbard, Caçola, Montebelo, and Santos reported significant and positive associations between availability of Physical Space, Toys (AHEMD-IS subscales), and SES indicators (income and parents' level of education) using a sample of 300 infants ages 3–18 months. The most interesting outcome was that Daily Activities were not influenced by any of the SES indicators. That is, parents of low SES status attended to their child's daily activities in a similar manner to those of higher SES status. The researchers concluded that for many families, income and education are not major environmental constraints that can have a negative impact on that aspect of the home environment in promoting infant motor development.

Daily Activities of Infants Scale (DAIS)

The DAIS (Bartlett, Fanning, Miller, Conti-Becker, & Doralp, 2008) is a parent-completed measure of opportunities parents provide infants for development of postural control and movement. The theoretical perspective driving the design of this instrument was dynamic systems theory as it has been applied to infant motor development. Its creation underscores the general idea is that development occurs through the interaction between intrinsic dynamics and a task performed in context if the assembly of all components is fluid to allow for exploration and selection of adaptive solutions. Thus, exploration is key for motor change to occur and a primary subsystem critical to movement is postural control.

The instrument is based on evaluation of 1300 photographs of typical activities from families with infants aged 4–11 months. The researchers established nine dimensions of activities (feeding, bathing, dressing, carrying, playing with others, quiet play, active play, outings, and sleeping) graded across three levels of opportunity for development. Following pilot testing that supported content validity, parents of infants born preterm ages 4- to 11 months participated in psychometric testing. The researchers found that completion of the DAIS over 1 day was representative of data collected over 3 sequential days. Older infants obtained significantly higher DAIS scores than younger infants, providing preliminary evidence for discriminant validity. DAIS scores demonstrated a significant part-correlation of 0.20 with scores on the *Alberta Infant Motor Scale* obtained concurrently, providing some evidence for convergent validity. The intraclass correlation coefficients reflecting interrater reliability and test–retest reliability of the total DAIS score were 0.76 and 0.77 respectively. In summary, the DAIS is a valid and reliable instrument for use in clinical practice and research.

The creators of the instrument note that the DAIS is currently being used as a mediating construct in a study to explore explanatory models of early motor development, including personal and environmental factors, first with infants born at term, and subsequently with infants born preterm. The instrument has been translated into Dutch and Norwegian, and cross-cultural variations in parental childrearing practices and perceptions of their infants' vulnerability are being investigated. And, ultimately, like the AHEMD-SR and AHEMD-IS, one of the goals is to determine the effectiveness of using the DAIS as an intervention tool.

Currently, the DAIS is being used as part of several studies related to high risk infants. For example, it is one of the tools evaluating the effectiveness of a newly developed physiotherapeutic intervention that has educational and motor goals, the COPCA (Coping with and Caring for infants with special needs – a family centered program), in a randomized controlled trial for infants at very high risk for cerebral palsy (Hielkema et al., 2010). Furthermore et al. (2011) utilized the DAIS to help determine differences in parents' perceptions of vulnerability of their infants born preterm and their childrearing practices across different cultures.

Applications

In addition to their use in research, the instruments described have clinical and parental use applications. As a follow-up to assessing the home using either the AHEMD versions or DAIS, the environment can be modified to include developmentally appropriate play materials and recommendations to the parents for implementation. In addition to typically developing children, this may be especially applicable with high-risk and special populations.

Parental involvement in the home with intervention is an ideal setting. This notion underscores the belief that providing early intervention services in naturalistic settings facilitates the child's access to opportunities for learning that occur throughout the day as well as providing opportunities for children to learn by interacting with typically developing peers (Kellar-Guenther, Rosenberg, Block, & Robinson, 2014).

Bartlett et al. (2008) note that early intervention service providers, such as physical therapists working with at-risk infants (born preterm or very low birth weight), often suggest activities for families to do with their children throughout the day. For example the DAIS can provide specific information on how daily routine activities can be more stimulating for motor development, such as moving arms and legs while taking a bath and playing with toys while maintaining the seated position in the bath tub. In addition, specific practical recommendations are made about ways to handle young children through daily activities and to our favor, much of the interaction involves 'play' activities. This approach is consistent with contemporary thoughts with respect to theories of child and human development, determinants of good health and the perspective that family-centered care is vital to long-time positive outcomes. This approach complements the medical model supporting comprehensive program that includes a variety of medical staff and family interaction.

Abbott et al. (2000) recommended the use of measures that evaluate specific aspects of the home environment that afford motor development primarily to identify what kinds of situations can and should be modified in order to enhance motor development. For example, for a typically developing child, therapists can determine what types of toys parents should acquire for their children, as well as making specific recommendations on how to use the toys to improve fine- and gross motor skills.

Iltus (2006) suggested that one of the important steps in the process of establishing intervention protocols is encouraging the engagement of parents in activities that involve toys and use of equipment that is provided by the physical space, in their own home environment. Also, the frequency in which parents are involved in games and playing with toys should be considered and emphasized in intervention protocols. In high-risk populations, toys and situations that reinforce movements used in daily-living skills can be identified and recommended by clinicians to be administered by a professional or parent.

Obviously, as with any developmental assessment, there are limitation with their use. For example, these questionnaires did not include certain areas of an infant's experience such as activities outside of the home. In addition, these reports should be considered only a snapshot of an environment that may be constantly changing. Another limitation is that while these questionnaires identify affordances in the home, they do not provide insight as to the amount or quality of time spent on items. Moreover, the quantity and quality of affordances could be related to socioeconomic status. Whereas that observation may apply, as noted in the Freitas et al. (2013) study using the AHEMD-IS, Daily Activities were not influenced by SES factors. It was speculated that for many families, income and education are not major environmental constraints in terms of promoting infant motor development.

Summary

Contemporary theory and practice views suggest quite convincingly that the home environment is a primary agent for learning and development – including motor development. The research findings described here support the contention that there is a close interrelation between affordances in the home environment, motor, and cognitive development. Complementing this acknowledgement, the literature indicates that there is a resurgence of interest in the role of early motor development in cognitive ability and academic performance. Level of fine- and visual-motor ability has been associated with daily-living skills, movement proficiency, and cognitive ability (Piek et al., 2008; Murray et al., 2006). Findings from these two studies suggest that motor development acts as a 'control parameter' for further development, in that motor abilities are essential for the acquisition or practice of other developmental functions such as perceptual or cognitive ability (Bushnell & Boudreau, 1993).

One reason and practical first step in acting on this idea is the need for assessing the home for motor affordances, family characteristics, and parent behaviors that are conducive to facilitating infant and early childhood development. And, as noted in a few of the studies described, the development of motor skills via home stimulation has a positive impact on future cognitive and social behavior. In addition to their research applications, the instruments described show promise in helping the practitioner improve the developmental status of the child via parental education and intervention.

References

Abbott, A., Bartlett, D., Fanning, J., & Kramer, J. (2000). Infant motor development and aspects of the home environment. *Pediatric Physical Therapy, 12*, 62–67.

Adolph, K. E., & Berger, S. E. (2006). Motor development. In W. Damon & R. Lerner (Eds.), *Handbook of child psychology* (pp. 161–213). New York, NY: Wiley.

Bartlett, D., Fanning, J., Miller, L., Conti-Becker, A., & Doralp, S. (2008). Development of daily activities of infants scale: A measure supporting early motor development. *Developmental Medicine and Child Neurology, 50*, 613–617. https://doi.org/10.1111/j.1469-8749.2008.03007.x

Bartlett, D. J., Der Sanden, N. G. M. W., Fallang, B., Fanning, J. K., & Doralp, S. (2011). Perceptions of vulnerability and variations in childrearing practice of parents of infants born preterm. *Pediatric Physical Therapy, 23*(3), 280–288. https://doi.org/10.1097/PEP.0b013e318227cc6b

Bernardi, J. R., Ferreira, C. F., Nunes, M., Silva, C. H., Bosa, V. L., Silveira, P. P., & Goldani, Z. (2012). Impact of perinatal different intrauterine environments on child growth and development in the first six months of life – IVAPSA birth cohort: Rationale, design, and methods. *BMC Pregnancy and Childbirth, 12*(25), 1–11. https://doi.org/10.1186/1471-2393-12-25

Bornstein, M. H., & Bradley, R. H. (2012). *Socioeconomic status, parenting, and child development, Monographs in Parenting Series*. New York, NY: Taylor & Francis Group.

Bradley, R., Caldwell, B., Rock, S., Ramey, C., Barnard, K., & Gray, C. (1989). Home environment and cognitive development in the first 3 years of life: A collaborative study involving six sites and three ethnic groups in North America. *Developmental Psychology, 25*, 217–235.

Bronfenbrenner, U. (2005). *Making humans being humans: Bioecological perspectives of human development*. Thousand Oaks, CA: Sage.

Bryck, R. L., & Fisher, P. A. (2012). Training the brain: Practical applications of neural plasticity from the intersection of cognitive neuroscience, developmental psychology, and prevention science. *The American Psychologist, 67*(2), 87–100. https://doi.org/10.1037/a0024657

Bushnell, E., & Boudreau, J. (1993). Motor development in the mind: the potential role of motor abilities as a determinant of perceptual development. *Child Development, 64*, 1005–1021.

Caçola, P., Gabbard, C., Montebelo, M., & Santos, D. (2015). Further development and validation of the affordances in the home environment for motor development – infant scale (AHEMD-IS). *Physical Therapy, 95*(5), 1–23.

Caçola, P., Gabbard, C., Santos, D. C. C., & Batistela, A. C. (2011). The development and application of the Affordances in the Home Environment for Motor Development – Infant Scale (AHEMD-IS). *Pediatrics International, 53*(6), 820–825. https://doi.org/10.1111/j.1442-200X.2011.03386.x

Caldwell, B., & Bradley, R. (1984). *Home observation for measurement of the environment*. Little Rock, AR: University of Arkansas at Little Rock.

Correr, M. T., Ouro, M. P. C., Caçola, P. M., Almeida, T. G. A., & Santos, D. C. C. (2014). A disponibilidade de brinquedos no ambiente domiciliar representa oportunidades para o desenvolvimento motor de lactentes? *Temas sobre Desenvolvimento, 20*(108), 25–29.

Davidson, R. J., & McEwen, B. S. (2012). Social influences on neuroplaticity: Stress and interventions to promote well-being. *Nature Neuroscience, 15*(5), 689–695. https://doi.org/10.1038/nn.3093

Freitas, T. C. B., Gabbard, C., Caçola, P., Montebelo, M. I. L., & Santos, D. C. C. (2013). Family socioeconomic status and the provision of motor affordances in the home. *Brazilian Journal of Physical Therapy, 17*(4), 319–332. https://doi.org/10.1590/S1413-35552013005000096

Gabbard, C., Caçola, P., & Rodrigues, L. P. (2008). A new inventory for assessing affordances in the home environment for motor development (AHEMD-SR). *Early Childhood Education Journal, 36*(1), 5–9. https://doi.org/10.1007/s10643-008-0235-6

Gibson, E. J. (2002). *Perceiving the affordances: a portrait of two psychologists*. Mahwah, NJ: Erlbaum.

Gibson, J. J. (1979). *An ecological approach to perception*. Boston, MA: Houghton Mifflin.

Goyen, T., & Lui, K. (2002). Longitudinal motor development of "apparently normal" high-risk infants at 18 months, 4 and 5 years. *Early Human Development, 70*, 103–115.

Haydari, A., Askari, P., & Nezhad, M. Z. (2009). Relationship between affordances in the home environment and motor development inchildren ages 18–42 months. *Journal of Social Sciences, 5*(4), 319–328. https://doi.org/10.3844/jssp.2009.319.328

Hielkema, T., Hamer, E., Reinders-Messelink, H. A., Maathuis, C. G. B., Bos, A. F., Dirks, T., & Hadders-Algra, M. (2010). LEARN 2 MOVE 0-2 years: Effects of a new intervention program in infants at very high risk for cerebral palsy; a randomized controlled trial. *BMC Pediatrics, 10*(76), 8. https://doi.org/10.1186/1471-2431-10-76

Hirose, N. (2002). An ecological approach to embodiment and cognition. *Cognitive Systems Research, 3*, 289–299.

Hsieh, Y. H., Hwang, A. W., Liao, H. F., Chen, P. C., Hsieh, W. S., & Chu, P. Y. (2011). Psychometric properties of a Chinese version of the home environment measure for motor development. *Disability and Rehabilitation, 33*(25–26), 2454–2463. https://doi.org/10.3109/09638288.2011.574775

Iltus, S. (2006). *Significance of home environments as proxy indicators for early childhood care and education* (Background paper for EFA Global Monitoring Report 2007).

Kellar-Guenther, Y., Rosenberg, S. A., Block, S. R., & Robinson, C. C. (2014). Parent involvement in early intervention: What role does setting play? *Early Years: An International Research Journal, 34*(1), 81–93. https://doi.org/10.1080/09575146.2013.823382

La Veck, B., & Hammond, M. (1982). Performance on the motor scale of the McCarthy scales of children's abilities as related to home environment and neonatal reflexes. *Perceptual and Motor Skills, 54*, 1265–1266.

Miquelote, A. F., Santos, D. C. C., Caçola, P. M., Montebelo, M. I. L., & Gabbard, C. (2012). Effect of the home environment on motor and cognitive behavior of infants. *Infant Behavior & Development, 35*, 329–334.

Mori, S., Nakamoto, H., Mizuochi, H., Ikudome, S., & Gabbard, C. (2013). Influence of affordances in the home environment on motor development of young children in Japan. *Child Development Research, 89*(8406), 1–5. https://doi.org/10.1155/2013/898406

Mundfrom, D., Bradley, R., & Whiteside, L. (1993). A factor analytic study of the infant-toddler and early childhood versions of the HOME inventory. *Educational and Psychological Measurement, 53*, 479–489.

Murray, G. K., Veijola, J., Moilanen, K., Miettunen, J., Giahn, D. C., Cannon, T. D., et al. (2006). Infant motor development is associated with adult cognitive categorization in a longitudinal birth cohort study. *Journal of Child Psychology and Psychiatry, 47*, 25–29. https://doi.org/10.1111/j.1469-7610.2005.01450.x

Nordhov, S. M., Rønning, J. A., Ulvund, S. E., Dahl, L. D., & Kaaresen, P. I. (2012). Early intervention improves behavioral outcomes for preterm infants: Randomized controlled trial. *Pediatrics, 129*, E9–E16. https://doi.org/10.1542/peds.2011-0248

Parks, P., & Bradley, R. (1991). The interaction of home environment features and their relation to infant competence. *Infant Mental Health, 12*, 3–16.

Piek, J. P. (2006). *Infant Motor Development*. Champaign, IL: Human Kinetics.

Piek, J. P., Dawson, L., Leigh, M., & Smith, N. G. (2008). The role of early fine and gross motor development on later motor and cognitive ability. *Human Movement Science, 27*, 668–681. https://doi.org/10.1016/j.humov.2007.11.002

Poresky, R., & Henderson, M. (1982). Infants' mental and motor development: Effects of home environment,maternal attitudes, marital adjustment, and socioeconomic status. *Perceptual and Motor Skills, 54*, 695–702.

Rodrigues, L., Saraiva, L., & Gabbard, C. P. (2005). Development and construct validation of an inventory for assessing the home environment for motor development. *Research Quarterly for Exercise and Sport, 76*(2), 140–148. https://doi.org/10.1080/02701367.2005.10599276

Saccani, R., Valentini, N. C., Pereira, K. R. G., Müller, A. B., & Gabbard, G. (2013). Associations of biological factors and affordances in the home with infant motor development. *Pediatrics International, 55*, 197–203. https://doi.org/10.1111/ped.12042

Schobert, L., & Valentini, N. C. (2008). Infants' motor development and the environment: Daycare nurture. In *Human Movement: Research issues* (1st ed., pp. 155–177). Erechin, RS: Edifapes.

Sirard, J. R., Nelson, M. C., Pereira, M. A., & Lytle, L. A. (2008). Validity and reliability of a home environment inventory for physical activity and media equipment. *International Journal of Behavioral Nutrition and Physical Activity, 5*, 24. https://doi.org/10.1186/1479-5868-5-24

Son, S. H., & Morrison, F. J. (2010). The nature and impact of changes in home learning environment on development of language and academic skills in preeschool children. *Developmental Psychology, 46*, 1103–1118. https://doi.org/10.1037/a0020065

Spencer, J. P., Blumberg, M. S., McMurray, B., Robinson, S. R., Samuelson, L., & Tomblin, B. (2009). Short arms and talking eggs: Why we should no longer abide the nativist-empiricist debate. *Child Development Perspectives, 3*(2), 79–87.

Stoffregen, T. A. (2000). Affordances and events. *Ecological Psychology, 12*, 1–28.

Temple, V. A., Naylor, P., Rhodes, R. E., & Higgins, J. W. (2009). Physical activity of children in family child care. *Applied Physiology, Nutrition, and Metabolism, 34*(4), 794–798. https://doi.org/10.1139/H09-061

Treyvaud, K., Inder, T. E., Lee, K. J., Northam, E. A., Doyle, L. W., & Anderson, P. J. (2012). Can the home environment promote resilience for children born very preterm in the context of social and medical risk? *Journal of Experimental Child Psychology, 112*, 326–337. https://doi.org/10.1016/j.jecp.2012.02.009

Walker, S. P. (2010). Commentary: Early stimulation and child development. *International Journal of Epidemiology, 39*(1), 294–296.

Wilson, B., Kaplan, B., Crawford, S., Campbell, A., & Dewey, D. (2000). Reliability and validity of a parent questionnaire on childhood motor skills. *American Journal of Occupational Therapy, 54*, 484–493. https://doi.org/10.5014/ajot.54.5.484

Carl Gabbard is Director of the Child Motor Development Laboratory and a Fellow in the National Academy of Kinesiology. In addition to numerous research publications, he is the author of the popular textbook, *Lifelong Motor Development, 7th edition, Wolters Kluwer Health (2017).*

Priscila Caçola is Director of the Developmental Motor Cognition Laboratory. In addition to being a well-published researcher, she was honored with the Lolas E. Halverson Motor Development Young Investigator Award, a distinction given in recognition of outstanding contributions to her research in motor development and learning.

Part III
Physical Education Programs and Preservice/Inservice Teacher Education

Chapter 13
Break for Physical Activity: Incorporating Classroom-Based Physical Activity Breaks into Preschools

Danielle D. Wadsworth and E. Kipling Webster

Physical Activity and Preschoolers

Participation in regular physical activity is important for the health and wellness of young children. Participating regularly in physical activity exudes positive health benefits including improved bone and joint health, increased muscular strength and endurance, reduced risk of developing chronic diseases and positive psychological health outcomes such as improved self-esteem confidence and reduced stress and anxiety (Daniels, 2006; Physical Activity Guidelines Advisory Committee, 2008). Preschool years represent a critical time for promoting physical activity (Timmons et al., 2012), prompting a number of initiatives such as Active Start and Healthy People 2020 advocating for physical activity opportunities within preschool curriculums.

The Institute of Medicine (2011) recommends that preschoolers should engage in at least 60 min and up to several hours per day of daily, unstructured physical activity and should not be sedentary for more than 60 min at a time except when sleeping. While this measure does not delimit the intensity of physical activity, the Australia, Canada, and the UK recommends that preschool children participate in physical activity of any intensity (light, moderate, or vigorous) in order to achieve a minimum of 3 h of physical activity every day (Department of Heath, Physical Activity, Health Improvement and Protection, 2011; Department of Health and Ageing, 2010; Tremblay et al., 2012). Nonetheless, studies of objectively measured physical activity and sedentary behavior in preschool children show low levels of

D. D. Wadsworth (✉)
School of Kinesiology, Auburn University, Auburn, AL, USA
e-mail: wadswdd@auburn.edu

E. Kipling Webster
School of Kinesiology, Louisiana State University, Baton Rouge, LA, USA
e-mail: kipwebster@lsu.edu

H. Brewer, M. R. Jalongo (eds.), *Physical Activity and Health Promotion in the Early Years*, Educating the Young Child 14,
https://doi.org/10.1007/978-3-319-76006-3_13

physical activity and high amounts of sedentary behavior (Pate et al., 2015; Tucker, 2008). A systematic review of the physical activity levels of preschool-aged children representing a total of 10,316 participants from seven countries has reported that nearly half of preschool-aged children do not engage in sufficient physical activity (Tucker, 2008). Another study shows that only 50% of preschoolers are meeting the guidelines for physical activity (Pate et al., 2015). In fact, studies such as those by Brown et al. (2006) have reported that preschool aged children spend approximately 80% of their day participating in sedentary activity. Another study by Cardon & de Bourdeaudhuij (2008) found that preschoolers spent 85% of their time during the school day in sedentary activities. Others have found similar results reporting high levels of sedentary behavior in preschool settings and low levels of moderate-to-vigorous physical activity (Logan et al., 2016; MVPA; Wadsworth, Robinson, Beckman, & Webster, 2012; Wadsworth et al., 2014). This is concerning because young children's sedentary patterns have been shown to affect their physical activity patterns later in life. Pate, Baranowski, Dowda, and Trost, (1996) report that 3- to 4-year-old children who participate in less physical activity than their peers remain less active after the age of three. Furthermore, this trend of physical activity decline continues into adolescence and adulthood (Kwan, Cairney, Faulkner, & Pullenayegum, 2012).

Although many factors contribute to a preschoolers' physical activity participation, such as gender, age and seasonality, the largest source in variability in a preschoolers' physical activity level is the preschool center itself (Finn, Johanssen, & Specker, 2002; Pate, Pfeiffer, Trost, Ziegler, & Dowda, 2004). Preschools that have adequate outdoor and indoor play places (Boldemann et al., 2006), planned curriculum (Wadsworth et al., 2014; Wadsworth et al., 2013) opportunities for physical activity (Bower et al., 2008) and teacher reinforcement for being active (Wadsworth et al., 2014) show higher levels of physical activity. Currently, preschool teachers have no required formal training in physical activity programming, but are often responsible for promoting and implementing physical activity programs for their classroom. Early childhood educators typically provide unplanned free play at preschool or daycares (Stork & Sanders, 2008) as physical activity programming. While free play may allow children many benefits such as imaginative play and participation in gross and fine motor skill practice, free play does not result in MVPA (Brown et al., 2006; Wadsworth et al., 2014). A study by Wadsworth et al. (2014) showed during a 45-min free play condition children spent only 3 min or 7% of their time in moderate physical activity and 3 min or 7% of their time in light activity, with the remaining 86% of their time in sedentary pursuits and no time was spent in vigorous physical activity. Due to the fact that currently preschoolers participate in low levels of physical activity and high levels of sedentary behavior, as well as, the link between physical activity and growth and development of young children it is imperative to implement effective intervention strategies that are low cost and can be easily implemented.

Physical Activity and Fundamental Motor Skills

Fundamental motor skills (FMS) are basic movement skills, like running, hopping, throwing, and catching, that are believed to be the foundation for more advanced movements and physical activity pursuits (Clark & Metcalfe, 2002; NASPE, 2009). The combination of these basic skills allows children to interact with their environment and peers (Haywood & Getchell, 2014). These FMS develop early in childhood and create a wide-ranging base of movements that are influential in future physical activities (Clark, 2007; Clark & Metcalfe, 2002). Unlike typical perceptions, these skills are not naturally developing, rather they need to be taught at an early age and children should be allowed time to practice and reinforce these skills (Goodway, Crowe, & Ward, 2003). Inadequate development of FMS competency in early childhood has been shown to negatively influence physical activity longitudinally (Barnett, van Beurden, Morgan, Brooks, & Beard, 2009); therefore, it is important to develop FMS in young children and to identify interventions that are effective for all levels of motor skill competency.

Physical Activity and Time On-Task

In order for physical activity to become a priority in preschool curriculum it is critical to highlight the connection between physical activity and academic behaviors (e.g., learning, classroom behavior, cognition). Although the importance of physical activity for overall health is well known, the positive impacts of physical activity on increasing concentration, mental cognition, and academic performance, as well as, reducing self-stimulatory behaviors (e.g. fidgeting) or school-related stress are not as well understood. A positive association between physical activity and several facets of cognitive functioning in children has been established (CDC, 2010; Diamond, 2015; Hillman, Kamijo, & Scudder, 2011; Hillman et al., 2009).

One behavioral outcome that has received empirical consideration is the effect of physical activity on attention (i.e. on-task behavior) in the classroom, specifically after shorts bouts of activity from classroom-based physical activity breaks. Time on-task measures a child's ability to be engaged and participate in the lesson planned in a classroom. In elementary-age children, short bouts of activity in the classroom have been shown to be an effective method of bolstering time on-task in the classroom (Grieco, Jowers, & Bartholomew, 2009; Mahar, 2011; Mahar et al., 2006; Mullender-Wijnsma et al., 2015a, 2015b). However, these studies were conducted with elementary and secondary age school children. For preschoolers, time on-task represents the child's ability to pay attention, follow directions and engage in lesson play activities. One concern of the implementation of physical activity programs is the child's ability to return and settle after the opportunity to be physically active in the classroom. Thus, physical activity programming must show that a child's time on-task is not decreased.

Break for Physical Activity

An emerging strategy to increase daily physical activity is the implementation of structured, classroom-based physical activity breaks. A typical break consists of 10–15 min of activities designed to promote MVPA. These breaks are easy to implement and require no equipment. Activity breaks can be used to reinforce academic concepts, such as reading or spelling, and children generally find them more enjoyable than traditional sedentary lessons (Vazou & Smiley-Oyen, 2014). This strategy was first utilized for school-age children and shown to significantly increase physical activity participation during school. Research found that approximately 10 min of classroom-based activity increased physical activity measured through pedometer or accelerometer step counts (Donnelly et al., 2009; Mahar et al., 2006; Murtagh, Mulvihill, & Markey, 2013; Stewart, Dennison, Kohl, & Doyle, 2004), MET levels (Stewart et al., 2004), direct observation (Grieco et al., 2009; Whitt-Glover, Ham, & Yancey, 2011), and heart rate monitoring (Mullender-Wijnsma et al., 2015a, 2015b). Additionally, long-term adoption of activity breaks has been shown to help maintain a healthy body mass index over a 3-year period (Donnelly et al., 2009). These breaks are conducive for the preschool population as physical activity patterns are characterized as short in duration and omnidirectional (Bailey et al., 1995). Young children don't have the capacity to sustain long bouts of cardiovascular activity so periods of activity accumulated throughout the school day may be an ideal way of increasing physical activity behaviors (Haywood & Getchell, 2014). The evidence strongly suggests that the implementation of a short bout of activity in elementary classrooms positively influences school-day physical activity participation.

Over the past several years the Exercise Adherence and Obesity Prevention Laboratory within the School of Kinesiology at Auburn University has implemented researcher-led and teacher-led physical activity breaks for preschoolers (Logan et al., 2016; Wadsworth et al., 2012; Webster, Wadsworth, & Robinson, 2015). It was initially important to ensure that a preschool-age population would reap similar benefits as their older peers. Therefore, the first two studies implemented researcher-led classroom-based activity breaks. Wadsworth et al. (2012) showed that physical activity breaks can effectively increase physical activity as well as time on-task. Logan et al. (2016) found that physical activity breaks effectively increased time spent in moderate and vigorous physical activity regardless of intervention site or level of motor skill. Webster et al. (2015) found that physical activity and time on-task is increased following teacher implemented physical activity breaks. In fact, following a teacher led 10-min activity break, the most off-task children improved by 30 percentage points; these results were similar to what has been previously shown in elementary age children (Mahar et al., 2006). Benefits of classroom based physical activity breaks for preschoolers are summarized in Table 13.1. Our findings suggest that classroom based physical activity breaks are an effective strategy to increase physical activity across levels of motor competence, while improving time on task.

Table 13.1 Benefits of physical activity breaks

Physical activity – Activity breaks are an effective method to increase physical activity during the school day and break up long bouts of sedentary time. Depending on the content of the breaks you can increase *MVPA*, *flexibility* (through yoga exercises and stretching), and *muscular endurance* (through FMS exercises like hopping and jumping).
Fundamental motor skills (FMS) – As FMS development is so critical in early childhood, activity breaks are an opportunity to teach students new skills (like hopping on one foot or skipping) and allow them time to reinforce and practice these abilities. Since FMS do not develop naturally, this is an ideal way to incorporate motor skill development.
Academic behaviors – Activity breaks are an established way to increase time on-task for preschool-age children, which can be critical after prolonged sedentary activities or when students begin to lose attention and increase fidgeting behaviors. Research has also shown a strong relationship between acute bouts of exercise and cognitive benefits such as improved executive functioning which can help children be ready to learn. Breaks may also be used to reinforce academic concepts through kinesthetic approaches, like tracing the alphabet with your feet or a relay race for spelling; physical activity may also be used to reinforce lessons for counting, reading, and science.

Considerations for Implementing Classroom Physical Activity Breaks

Based on our findings, classroom based physical activity breaks are for everyone, regardless of body shape (Webster et al., 2015), preschool center (Logan et al., 2016) and fitness level. The following section details how to implement classroom based physical activity breaks into preschools.

Getting Started

Preschool policies, type of activities, adequate space, when and how often are several factors that need to be considered prior to implementing the breaks. Table 13.2 provides a checklist to follow prior to break implementation.

Preschool Policies and Physical Activity Breaks

Prior to implementing the breaks it is important to identify how the classroom physical activity breaks can supplement policies, procedures and children's learning. For example, one preschool center utilized the breaks to help transition children from one area of the preschool to the next (i.e, homeroom to art center). This implementation was not feasible at other preschools where students needed to be quiet in the hallways. Additionally, breaks have supported reiteration of school procedures. For example, one center had a "plan, do, recall" program aimed at encourage children to exhibit forethought and planning prior to action. At this center, teachers allowed

Table 13.2 Pre-break checklist

Prior to implementing the physical activity breaks ask yourself:
What is the best strategy to implement the breaks?
Are there policies that will be affected by the implementation of the breaks?
Can the breaks support the preschool curriculum?
Where is the best place to implement the breaks?
What is the best time to implement the breaks?
How often should the breaks be implemented?
What activities would be best for your preschool?
How can your preschool get parents involved?

the children to plan the activities, followed by participating in the activities and discussing how the activities felt to them. Another aspect to consider is parental involvement. Parents provide key reinforcement to continue or discontinue physical activity outside of preschool. Informing parents of your new strategies to increase physical activity and improve the academic learning environment may be beneficial to your efforts.

Choosing Activities for Your Physical Activity Breaks

To choose your exercises think of the break in three different sections: warm-up, physical activity and cool down. Activities for the warm-up are designed to increase breathing and heart rate; remind children about the rules and prepare them for the physical activity portion. The physical activity portion should promote age appropriate movement activities that encourage children to move as much as possible. Learning concepts such as listening, memory, math and language skills can be incorporated into the break. The cool-down portion should be used to slowly return the children to a resting state. We like to incorporate emotional control exercises, such as breathing, into the cool-down so that children can begin to practice these skills. Table 13.3 details exercises to utilize for the warm-up, physical activity portion and cool-down activities. In terms of time components, the warm-up should represent 25% of the break, the physical activity portion 50% and the cool-down 25% of the break. Activity breaks can be easily pieced together by creating a rotation of activities (approximately 30 s to 1 min each; See Table 13.4) of a specific exercise or tasks. We have found that teachers are able to implement physical

Table 13.3 Physical activity break activities

Warm-up: Are designed to increase breathing and heart rate; remind children about the rules and prepare them for the physical activity portion.
1. March in place – Alternate lifting the arms and legs in a swinging motion.
2. Elbow to knee- alternate lifting the knees, touching each knee with the opposite elbow
3. Slow jumping jacks – Stand with your feet and arms together at your side. Bend your knees and jump moving your feet apart and arms overhead. Pause, then jump again bring your hands and feet back to the start
4. Arm-circles – Extend the arms out to the side. Circle the arms slowly in small circles. Extend the circles to become bigger. Repeat and go the opposite direction.
5. Tree-twists – Stand with your hands on your hips or in the air as a tree. Twist from side to side.
6. Inch worms: From a standing position, slowly roll forward until your hands touch the ground. Walk your hands out away from your feet until you extend as fall as possible. Inch your feet towards your hands until you come to a forward folded position. Roll slowly up to a standing position.
Activity portion: Designed to promote age appropriate movement activities that encourage children to move as much as possible
1. Bunny hops – Jump up and down like a bunny with your feet together.
2. Scissor kicks – Stand with your legs spread apart one foot in front of the other in a staggered stance. Jump and switch the position of your feet.
3. Fancy football feet – With your hands up, feet shoulder width apart move on the balls of your feet as fast as you can go.
4. Frog jumps – Bend down like a frog, explode from the floor extending your arms straight up. Land with your knees bent.
5. Skipping – Alternate brining one knee up at a time while hopping on the other foot.
6. Crab walk – Sit on your bottom and lift your bottom off of the floor balancing on your hands and feet. Walk backwards using your hands and feet.
Cool-down: Designed to slowly return children to resting state.
1. Tip-toeing – Walk around the room while balancing on your tip-toes
2. Balancing act – Balance on one foot, than close your eyes. Switch to the other side
3. Balloon breathing – Inhale blowing up your stomach like a balloon. Hold the breath. Slowly release as if the balloon is deflating.
4. Love sway – Wrap your arms around your chest as if you are giving yourself a hug, sway from side to side. Repeat, switching the position of your arms.
5. Tree pose – Balance on one foot with the heel of your other foot on your calf or inner thigh. Bring your hands palm to palm in front of your chest. Repeat on the other side.
6. Forward fold – Cross your arms over your chest and slowly roll forward as far as you can, bringing your chest towards your knees. Exhale and slowly roll back up.

activity breaks when provided with a binder full of activities divided by color into warm-up, physical activity and cool-down activities. For example, red is for the warm-up, green is for the exercises and blue is for cool down. Teachers are than able to choose 3 to 4 exercises for each portion that fits their time frame, schedule and space. Once students have learned a few exercises provide some autonomy and have them choose and lead the exercises as well.

Table 13.4 10-min sample activity break divided into 30-s increments

Time	Activity
Warm-up (min 0–2:30)	
:00	March in place
:30	Elbow to knee
1:00	Slow jumping jacks
1:30	March in place
2:00	Elbow to knee
Activity portion (min 2:30–7:30)	
2:30	Jumping jacks
3:00	Bunny hops
3:30	Skipping
4:00	Frog jumps
4:30	Jumping jacks
5:00	Bunny hops
5:30	Skipping
6:00	Frog jumps
6:30	Crab walk
7:00	Crab walk
Cool-down (min 7:30–10:00)	
7:30	Tip toe
8:00	Love sway
8:30	Love sway
9:00	Breathing
9:30	Breathing
10:00	Tip-toe to next activity

Space Considerations for Activity Breaks

In terms of space, children need enough room to move freely without hitting objects or each other. Typically, we ask children to open their arms wide as if they are plane wings and turn a circle, if they do not touch anything than they have adequate space.

When and How Often to Implement Breaks

Typically the best time to implement a classroom based physical activity break is prior to an indoor activity that requires children to pay attention for long periods of time, such as read aloud time. Breaks can also be incorporated in transition from one indoor activity to the next, such as moving from morning activities to centers. How often breaks can be incorporated is greatly dependent on teachers schedules, however, we recommend at least twice a day. Breaks can be offered more on days when children are indoors longer or less when able to go outdoors more. Structured activities result in more moderate-to-vigorous physical activity for preschoolers than free play (Wadsworth et al., 2014), so consider an outdoor break as well.

It's Time to: Break for Physical Activity!

Implementing the breaks should be a fun experience for the children and the teacher. At the beginning of the break remind the children of the rules that have been established. If you are able display the activities so that children know what to do next. To reinforce participation, teachers should actively participate in the break with the children. This is the time for fun, silliness and exploring how our bodies move. If possible, avoid excessively correcting children and prompting sedentary pursuits. If children begin to break the rules, stop the break, reiterate the rules and then return to the break. The breaks are very flexible in how they are structured in the classroom, so use your imagination and adjust the breaks to suit your needs. Although work has primarily examined academic behaviors improving after 10 min of activity, breaks can be catered to meet the classrooms needs and time constraints. Breaks can be implemented once or multiple times during the day or broken into smaller segments. They may also be used for extended transition times between activities or as an early morning energizer or an afternoon round-up.

Sustainability

After you have implemented your breaks, reflect on the experience and determine how the breaks can become a sustainable activity within your curriculum. Consider changes to maximize time spent being physically activity, as well as, changes to improve break efficiency. For example, do you need to reconsider your space or the time of day you complete the break? Would you prefer for the children to select the exercises or would it be more beneficial for the teacher to select the exercises? Do your preschool policies need to adapt to accommodate the breaks? Reflecting on your experience will provide insight for the teachers and preschools to successfully implement the physical activity breaks over time.

Conclusions

Research centered on classroom-based activity breaks has found this to be a useful avenue to increase physical activity in young children and improve time on-task in the classroom. The breaks are easily implemented, require little or no resources, applicable to all preschools and children of all abilities are able to participate. Teachers should think of activity breaks as an experience that children will enjoy, as well as, improve student's health through physical activity behaviors and help reinforce classroom goals through reinforcement of academic concepts.

References

Bailey, R. C., Olson, J., Pepper, S. L., Porszasz, J., Barstow, T. J., & Cooper, D. M. (1995). The level and tempo of children's physical activities: An observational study. *Medicine & Science in Sports & Exercise, 27*(7), 1033–1041.

Barnett, L. M., van Beurden, E., Morgan, P. J., Brooks, L. O., & Beard, J. R. (2009). Childhood motor skill proficiency as a predictor of adolescent physical activity. *Journal of Adolescent Health, 44*, 252–259.

Boldemann, C., Blennow, M., Dal, H., Mårtensson, F., Raustorp, A., Yuen, K., & Wester, U. (2006). Impact of preschool environment upon children's physical activity and sun exposure. *Preventive Medicine, 42*, 301–308.

Bower, J. K., Hales, D. P., Tate, D. F., Rubin, D. A., Benjamin, S. E., & Ward, D. S. (2008). The childcare environment and children's physical activity. *American Journal of Preventive Medicine, 34*(1), 23–29.

Brown, W. H., Pfeiffer, K. A., McIver, K. L., Dowda, M., Almeida, J. M., & Pate, R. R. (2006). Assessing preschool children's physical activity: The observational system for recording physical activity in children-preschool version. *Research Quarterly for Exercise and Sport, 77*, 167–176.

Cardon, G. M., & de Bourdeaudhuij, I. M. M. (2008). Are preschool children active enough? Objectively measured physical activity levels. *Research Quarterly for Exercise & Sport, 79*(3), 326–332.

Centers for Disease Control and Prevention [CDC]. (2010). *The association between school-based physical activity, including physical education, and academic performance*. Atlanta, GA: U.S. Department of Health and Human Services.

Clark, J. E. (2007). On the problem of motor skill development. *Journal of Physical Education, Recreation, and Dance, 78*(5), 39–44.

Clark, J. E., & Metcalfe, J. S. (2002). The mountain of motor development: A metaphor. In J. E. Clark & J. H. Humphrey (Eds.), *Motor development: Research and review: Vol. 2* (pp. 62–95). Reston, VA: National Association for Sport and Physical Education.

Daniels, S. R. (2006). The consequences of childhood overweight and obesity. *Future of Children, 16*, 47–67.

Department of Health and Ageing. (2010). *National physical activity guidelines for Australians. Physical activity recommendations for 0–5 year olds*. Canberra, Australia: Commonwealth of Australia.

Department of Heath, Physical Activity, Health Improvement and Protection. (2011). *Stay active, stay active: A report on physical activity for health from the four home countries; chief medical officers*. London, UK: Department of Health, Physical Activity, Health Improvement and Protection.

Diamond, A. B. (2015). The cognitive benefits of exercise in youth. *Current Sports Medicine Reports, 14*(4), 320–326.

Donnelly, J. E., Greene, J. L., Gibson, C. A., Smith, B. K., Washburn, R. A., Sullivan, D. K., … Williams, S. L. (2009). Physical activity across the curriculum (PAAC): A randomized controlled trial to promote physical activity and diminish overweight and obesity in elementary school children. *Preventive Medicine, 49*, 336–341.

Finn, K., Johanssen, N., & Specker, B. (2002). Factors associated with physical activity in preschool children. *The Journal of Pediatrics, 140*, 81–85.

Goodway, J. D., Crowe, H., & Ward, P. (2003). Effect of motor skill intervention on fundamental motor skill development. *Adapted Physical Activity Quarterly, 20*, 298–314.

Grieco, L. A., Jowers, E. M., & Bartholomew, J. B. (2009). Physically active academic lessons and time on task: The moderating effect of body mass index. *Medicine & Science in Sport & Exercise, 41*, 1921–1926.

Haywood, K., & Getchell, N. (2014). *Life span motor development* (6th ed.). Champaign: Human Kinetics.

Hillman, C. H., Kamijo, K., & Scudder, M. (2011). A review of chronic and acute physical activity participation on neuroelectric measures of brain health and cognition during childhood. *Preventine Medicine, 52*, S21–S28.

Hillman, C. H., Pontifex, M. B., Raine, L. B., Castelli, D. M., Hall, E. E., & Kramer, A. F. (2009). The effect of acute treadmill walking on cognitive control and academic achievement in preadolescent children. *Neuroscience, 159*, 1044–1054.

Institute of Medicine [IOM]. (2011). *Early childhood obesity prevention policies*. Washington, DC: The National Academies Press.

Kwan, M. Y., Cairney, J., Faulkner, G. E., & Pullenayegum, E. E. (2012). Physical activity and other health-risk behaviors during the transition into early adulthood: A longitudinal cohort study. *American Journal of Preventive Medicine, 42*(1), 14–20.

Logan, S. W., Wadsworth, D. D., Robinson, L. E., & Webster, E. K. (2016). Influence of classroom-based physical activity breaks on physical activity and on-task behavior in preschool children. *Journal of Education and Human Development, 4*(4), 39–46.

Mahar, M. T. (2011). Impact of short bouts of physical activity on attention-to-task in elementary school children. *Preventive Medicine, 52*, S60–S64.

Mahar, M. T., Murphy, S. K., Rowe, D. A., Golden, J. A., Shields, T., & Raedeke, T. D. (2006). Effects of a classroom-based program on physical activity and on-task behavior. *Medicine & Science in Sports & Exercise, 38*(12), 2086–2094.

Mullender-Wijnsma, M. J., Hartman, E., de Greeff, J. W., Bosker, R. J., Doolaard, S., & Visscher, C. (2015a). Improving academic performance of school-age children by physical activity in the classroom: 1-year program evaluation. *Journal of School Health, 85*(6), 365–371.

Mullender-Wijnsma, M. J., Hartman, E., de Greeff, J. W., Bosker, R. J., Doolaard, S., & Visscher, C. (2015b). Moderate-to-vigorous physically active academic lessons and academic engagement in children with and without a social disadvantage: A within subject experimental design. *BMC Public Health, 15*, 404–412.

Murtagh, E., Mulvihill, M., & Markey, O. (2013). Bizzy break! The effect of a classroom-based activity break on in-school physical activity levels of primary school children. *Pediatric Exercise Science, 25*, 300–307.

National Association for Sport and Physical Education. (2009). *Active start: A statement of physical activity guidelines for children from birth to age 5* (2nd ed.). Oxon Hill, MD: AAHPERD Publications.

Pate, R. R., Baranowski, T. O. M., Dowda, M., & Trost, S. G. (1996). Tracking of physical activity in young children. *Medicine and Science in Sports and Exercise, 28*, 92–96.

Pate, R. R., O'Neill, J. R., Brown, W. H., Pfeiffer, K. A., Dowda, M., & Addy, C. L. (2015). Prevalence of compliance with a new physical activity guideline for preschool-age children. *Childhood Obesity, 11*, 415–420.

Pate, R. R., Pfeiffer, K. A., Trost, S. G., Ziegler, P., & Dowda, M. (2004). Physical activity among children attending preschools. *Pediatrics, 114*(5), 1258–1263.

Physical Activity Guidelines Advisory and Committee. (2008). *Physical activity guidelines advisory committee report* (p. 683). Washington, DC: US Department of Health and Human Services.

Stewart, J. A., Dennison, D. A., Kohl, H. W., & Doyle, J. A. (2004). Exercise level and energy expenditure in the TAKE 10! In-class physical activity program. *Journal of School Health, 74*(10), 397–400.

Stork, S., & Sanders, S. W. (2008). Physical education in early childhood. *The Elementary School Journal, 108*(3), 197–206.

Timmons, B. W., LeBlanc, A. G., Carson, V., Connor Gorber, S., Dillman, C., Janssen, I., … Tremblay, M. S. (2012). Systematic review of physical activity and health in the early years (aged 0–4 years). *Applied Physiology, Nutrition, and Metabolism, 37*, 773–792.

Tremblay, M. S., LeBlanc, A. G., Carson, V., Choquette, L., Connor-Gorber, S., Dillman, C., … Timmons, B. W. (2012). Canadian physical activity guidelines for the early years (aged 0–4 years). *Applied Physiology, Nutrition, and Metabolism, 37*, 345–356.

Tucker, P. (2008). The physical activity levels of preschool-aged children: A systematic review. *Early Childhood Research Quarterly, 23*, 547–558.

Vazou, S., & Smiley-Oyen, A. (2014). Moving and academic learning are not antagonists: Acute effects on executive function and enjoyment. *Journal of Sport & Exercise Psychology, 36*, 474–485.

Wadsworth, D. D., Robinson, L. E., Beckman, K., & Webster, K. (2012). Break for physical activity: Incorporating classroom-based physical activity breaks into preschools. *Early Childhood Education Journal, 39*(6), 391–395.

Wadsworth, D. D., Robinson, L. E., Rudisill, M. E., & Gell, N. (2013). The effect of physical education climates on elementary students' physical activity behaviors. *Journal of School Health, 83*, 306–313.

Wadsworth, D. D., Rudisill, M. E., Hastie, P. A., Boyd, K. L., & Rodriguez-Hernandez, M. (2014). Preschoolers' physical activity and time on task during a mastery motivational climate and free play. MHSalud. *Revista Ciencias del Moviment Humando y Salud, 11*(1), 26–34.

Webster, E. K., Wadsworth, D. D., & Robinson, L. E. (2015). Preschoolers' time on-task and physical activity during a classroom activity break. *Pediatric Exercise Science, 27*(1), 160.

Whitt-Glover, M. C., Ham, S. A., & Yancey, A. K. (2011). Instant recess: A practical tool for increasing physical activity during the school day. *Progress in Community Health Partnerships: Research, Education, and Action, 5*(3), 289–297.

Danielle D. Wadsworth is an associate professor at Auburn University in the School of Kinesiology and Director of the Exercise Adherence and Obesity prevention laboratory. Her research focuses on identifying environmental, psychological and social underpinnings of exercise adherence and translating these findings to effective evidence based interventions, primarily for women and children. Dr. Wadsworth has served as a co-investigator on National Institutes of Health and Robert Wood Johnson Foundation grants aimed at examining the impact of physical activity policies on children's physical activity levels at school and during physical education. Her research has been published in peer-reviewed journals and presented at international and national conferences.

E. Kipling Webster is an Assistant Professor at Louisiana State University. Her research interests are focused on physical activity behaviors and motor skill competency in pediatric populations. Her research primarily examines school-based programs that target positive health-related outcomes, such as reducing childhood obesity and increasing physical activity, fitness, motor skill competency, and psychological variables related to health. Her research has been published in peer-review journals and presented at international and national conferences.

Chapter 14
Active Designs for Movement in Early Childhood Environments

Serap Sevimli-Celik

Introduction

Children are naturally born to be active and ready to discover different ways of moving. Movement helps children to develop physical skills that are necessary for the discovery of their immediate environment. While running, jumping, hopping, skipping, or galloping, children actively involved in exploring and experimenting movement capabilities and limitations of their bodies. Children also start to be aware of (a) what their bodies can do, (b) where their bodies can move, and (c) with whom their bodies can move. Thus they start to control their bodies effectively and purposefully (Gallahue & Ozmun, 1998). Piaget (1964) considers movement as one of the primary sensory experiences helping children to gain physical knowledge about their surroundings. For him, it is also through the active engagement and interaction with the environment children start to identify their bodies in time and space. In this way, children secure information about themselves, the environment, and the topological properties of objects around them (Athey, 2007). It is a way for children to relate the world through their physical senses by moving, doing, interacting, and exploring (Olds, 2000).

As children actively discover, they also refine and develop the fundamental movement skills necessary for being proficient in complex motor abilities in childhood and later in life (Haywood & Getchell, 2009). Thus opportunities to run, jump, hop, swing, pull, push, throw, catch, and kick are considered the ABCs of movement (Vidoni & Ignico, 2011). When children feel competent in those skills early in life, they are likely to remain active throughout childhood and into adulthood (Gallahue & Ozmun, 1998). Environments that accommodate and encourage movement and offer diverse and stimulating design elements for movement in particular would

S. Sevimli-Celik (✉)
Department of Elementary & Early Childhood Education, Middle East Technical University, Ankara, Turkey

H. Brewer, M. R. Jalongo (eds.), *Physical Activity and Health Promotion in the Early Years*, Educating the Young Child 14,
https://doi.org/10.1007/978-3-319-76006-3_14

thus be primary settings for children to acquire necessary physical skills for life. It is therefore essential to provide various opportunities for children to use their bodies actively during the day by creating high quality environments that have a sense of movement, exploration, experimentation, and discovery.

Form and Function in Actively Engaging Environments

Schools are one central avenue to offer environments where children are encouraged to be physically active and challenged to discover different ways of moving. To that end, school environment should be arranged in such a way that it could afford a variety of physical skills from walking to running, hopping to jumping, or skipping to sliding. It is therefore essential to "consider the individual and the environment as an interactive system" (Cosco, 2006, p. 17). Similarly, Heft (1988) offers a descriptive framework for conceptualizing the environment in terms of its functional possibilities. Children engage in physical activities more in school grounds that include natural and built elements, such as shelters, rock amphitheaters, trees, shrubs, wildflower meadows, ponds, grassy berms and food gardens (Dyment & Bell, 2008). Relatively smooth surfaces in school grounds, for instance, can afford walking, running, cycling, or skating; and relatively smooth slopes can afford rolling, sliding, or running down. Such adapted forms of grounds encourage physical activity by offering complex and rich stimuli for being active. Based upon that perspective, understanding the relational and functional properties of the environment would help to inform environmental design for schools.

The variations in the functional properties of children's environment also associate with having different physical activity behaviors among children. Having dynamic elements (e.g., curves, loops, ramps, or pathways) in the environment increases the sense of active exploration and discovery. For instance, environments with pathways and open areas with different ground surfaces offer perceptual complexity while increasing the likelihood of being physically active. (Cosco, Moore, & Islam, 2010). In addition to the aforementioned dynamic qualities, environments that offer natural and multi-sensory experiences improve children's outdoor play opportunities and as well as their gross motor abilities. A good example of such an improvement is that, Fjortoft (2001) highlighted an increase in children's physical activity levels after playing around natural elements in the forest (e.g., trees for climbing; shrubs for hide and seek; shelters for role-playing; cliffs for sliding and crawling; dense snow for thumbing, rolling and other acrobatics). The study results exemplified a significant relationship between the landscape diversity and the affordance of active play opportunities. Thus, inclusion of natural elements would be an effective strategy to motivate and encourage children to be more active while engaging them in different forms and amount of play.

The environments that have dynamic qualities also provide the means of movement for children to boost confidence in physical capabilities while giving them some control over their actions. For instance, when certain activities (e.g., gross motor movements) are performed repetitively, the body's natural motivators, noradrenalin and dopamine, are released (Filer, 2008; Jensen, 2000) that could in return improve physical and emotional well-being of children. In a study investigating the effects of ecologically diverse environments on children's well-being, Moore and Wong (1997) reported a decrease in the stress levels of children and an increase in 'intense peace'. Similarly, environments with trees, shrubbery, and broken grounds afford preschoolers dynamic play opportunities and create new physical opportunities of varying interests and abilities (Boldemann et al., 2006). Yet, despite the numerous benefits such dynamic environments offer, there is an apparent change in children's play shifting from outdoors to indoors and active to more sedentary (Clements, 2004; Frost, 2010; Gray, 2011; Singer, Singer, D'Agostino, & DeLong, 2009).

Design Considerations for School Environments

The decline in the time spent outside reveals the need of reconsidering and redesigning school environments to support children being physically active. In the design process, environment should be considered as a place for exploring, discovering, and developing environmental awareness for children (Dudek, 2007). It is also necessary to consider (a) how children would use the space, (b) what they would see from their perspective, and (c) what kinds of experiences they would have in that space (Head Start Design Guide, 2005). That is simply *designing through the eyes of a child* and allocating ample space to children to position their bodies in the environment comfortably. In a book entitled Personal Space, Sommer (1969) talks about the importance of being sensitive from children's perspective:

> Movement in and out of the classrooms and the school building is rigidly controlled. Everywhere one looks there are "lines"–generally straight lines that bend around corners before entering the auditorium, the cafeteria, or the workshop (or, I might add, the bathroom). The straight rows (of the classroom) tell the student to look ahead and ignore everything except the teacher; the students are so tightly jammed together that psychological escape, much less physical separation, is impossible. The teacher has 50 times more free space than do the students with the mobility to move around… teacher and children may share the same classroom but they see it differently. From a student's eye level, the world is cluttered, disorganized, and full of people's shoulders, heads and body movements. His world at ground level is colder than the teacher's world. (Sommer, 1969, p. 99)

For school environments, flexibility is one of the most prevalent characteristics of being physically active, and requires complex spaces for active play and movement. When children have open and quick indoor-outdoor flow, they move freely between in and out of the classroom (Cosco & Moore, 2009). Such flexibility aspects of an environment encourage play opportunities that are active, challenging, self-directed, and exploratory. In addition, flexibility allows children to perceive their environment from various dimensions and become familiar with the environmental contrasts in everything they experience (Olds, 2000). For instance, elevated spaces that have both high and low levels enable children to experience "up" and "down". Similarly, concave and convex-shaped spaces help children to feel secure and move freely and expansively (Olds, 2000). Through these spatial contrasts, children can see things from different perspectives and explore their bodies in different dimensions (Curtis & Carter, 2003).

The sense of freedom and invitation to movement are other considerations in designing environments for children. Early years are the critical time periods to develop fundamental movement skills (e.g., running, jumping, balancing, throwing, catching), however, there is a tradition for not recognizing movement as part of the curriculum. Additionally, although the educational trend is shifting from teacher-directed to child-centered and from passive learning to active engagement; many school environments fail to keep up with the new educational trends. In Dudek's (2007) terms, this is a "dysfunctional relationship" between space and pedagogy. It is necessary to make that relationship more functional because how we design school environments determines children's perceptions toward movement and being physically active. Torelli and Durrett (1996) argue that, for example, when there is no affordance for children to climb on, they would find ways climb onto tables and chairs. In response to that behavior, teacher might redirect children off the piece of equipment which could restrict children's sense of freedom for movement.

When the amount of time children spend in schools nowadays is considered, designing environments for children to expend their surplus energy during the day has become of utmost importance. For that reason, environment designs should be responsive to the daily physical needs of children by supporting everyday movement activities that are fundamental for active and healthy life styles. A good example of such design considerations is creating different pathways in and out of the classroom that would encourage physical stimulation, perceptual complexity, circular motion, and sense of exploration (Cosco et al., 2010). Likewise, National Learning Initiative suggests a system of "hierarchical pathways" to make mobility more efficient and effective for children. For example, while primary paths that are hard surfaced and wide would allow children to use wheeled toys or carts, secondary paths with hard or soft surfaces would allow social interaction with peers, and tertiary paths with soft surfaces or stepping-stones would encourage mobility and physical exploration.

The landscape variations contribute children's mobility and also provide continuous exploration and expansion of territorial limits through which different sensorial experiences would be enriched. Such variations could be exemplified by lower and higher hills, stairs, platforms, or pathways which encourage active play opportunities while increasing the ability of children to position their body in space (e.g., height and complexity variations stimulate vestibular sense). In this way, children can both test their physical capabilities and maintain strong spatial skills necessary for being aware of oneself in space. Climbing, for instance, stimulate vestibular sense by allowing children to decide where to put their feet and hands and how to position their bodies. Such physically challenging experiences make children competent in moving and help them to "improve their ability to recognize and cope with potentially hazardous conditions later in life" (Frost, 2010, p.17).

Creating and maintaining environments that are stimulating, natural, complex, and challenging is an essential component for providing broader context and various levels of movement skills and active play. Particularly, open spaces with portable and multi-purpose play materials were associated with higher physical activity levels among children (Hannon & Brown, 2008; Trost, Ward, & Senso, 2010). When play materials can be moved, carried, combined, or redesigned in multiple ways, children stay active physically and intellectually. This type of active involvement in creating and modifying the play space would give children freedom to determine the nature of their own play and control their environments (Patte & Brown, 2011; Play England, 2009). Moreover, providing spaces and materials that vary in degree of complexity and structure could hold the attention longer and add value to children's play. A loft, for instance, has high mobility elements in it and invites children for climbing, sliding, hanging, or swinging. While supporting motor exploration, it can also be a great "get-away" space for children (Torelli, 2002).

Thoughtful Environments and Sensory Experiences

Designing environments where children have a sense of physical well-being requires embracing space as an essential component of the curriculum. In the pedagogical philosophy of considering the environment as "the third teacher", Reggio Emilia approach inspires environmental design principles of exploration and discovery by designing aesthetically complex and enriching environments for children. According to Gandini (1993), children's natural sense of exploration needs to be supported through the sense of touching, smelling, hearing, seeing, and tasting. A variety of sensory inputs and first-hand experiences make the environment more dynamic and interactive for children. The more dynamic the environment, the more freedom children get to actively use their bodies in space. For example, bushes offer sensory stimulation of vision and tactile interaction and also encourage games that are physically active (e.g., chasing, hide and seek) (NLI, 2009). Similarly, tree stumps or logs stimulate vestibular sense while offering balancing, climbing, jumping, or simply sitting and standing.

Stimulating variety of senses provides a meaningful learning interaction between the environment and the child. Such an interaction is a key for planning and creating an environment where curiosity, wonder, and intellectual engagement are awaken and the movement needs of children are maintained at the same time (Curtis & Carter, 2003). Environments including visual elements help children to internalize movement more as part of their daily routines. For instance, presence of books, posters, and pictures in the classrooms related to movement were associated with higher levels of physical activity (Henderson, Grode, O'Connell, & Schwartz, 2015). That way, movement becomes one central avenue for children to engage in active play in an integrated manner (Henniger, 2009). When movement is integrated into math, literacy, or science; physical activity levels, concentration skills, and self-regulation abilities of children improve significantly (Trost, Fees, & Dzewaltowski,

2008). For instance, asking children to count how many balloons they kicked in 1 min or march around a circle of letters offer both physically and intellectually stimulating experiences that are purposeful, relevant, holistic, and engaging for children. Such integrated approach may improve children's perceptual skills, verbal achievements, and academic readiness as well (Sibley & Etnier, 2003).

Architecturally thoughtful environments also create meaningful connections between the child and the architectural structure of the building itself. For instance, high ceilings give a sense of spaciousness and invite children for active play opportunities. On the other hand, in the building level, for example, circular shaped buildings generate more energy and dynamism that boost movement in terms of walking or running (Dudek, 2007). Contrary to rigid lines that produces less-stimulating atmosphere for movement, fluid lines offer continuous movement flow in and outside of the building (Apps & MacDonald, 2012). The horizontality of the buildings also creates a sense of freedom of movement while encouraging children to go out and explore their surroundings. Additionally, for example, placing an external canopy across the play area both extent the space terrains and help ease the use of play area in extreme weather conditions (Dudek, 2007). Consequently, thoughtful environments that include aforementioned qualities and elements potentially motivate children to be more active and stay connected with the world outside.

Outdoor Environments for Movement and Active Play

Similar indoor architectural attributes are applicable to outdoor environments as well. In the examination of the physical factors that contribute gross motor play and spontaneous exploration, Herrington and Lesmeister (2006) identified seven architectural criteria for encouraging active play of children aged three to five years: character, context, connectivity, change, chance, clarity, and challenge. The researchers point all of them out as essential criteria for evaluating outdoor play area. The clarity criteria, for instance, is closely related to landscape design and defined as the physical legibility and perceptual image-ability of play space. The researchers also stated that when an environment contains modular or pre-fabricated equipment placed in the center of the play area, the flow of movement and the nature of play are interrupted by the play structure. As a result, children have a difficulty to engage in active play opportunities because of the disconnected peripheral spaces. On the other hand, organic-shaped play areas containing natural materials (e.g., trees, shrubs, or rocks) and circular layouts are more related to the scale and the movement of children (Herrington & Lesmeister, 2006).

Considering design as an integral part of child development is essential to create playful environments where the daily physical needs of young children and their active play agendas are supported simultaneously. Outdoor play environments, in particular, offer a variety of sensory integration, contact with nature, and physical diversity. For example, outdoor landscapes varied in size, color, texture, line, form, or pattern not only promote early sensory experiences, but also make children more responsive players toward their environments and playmates as well. Such variety also helps children to identify the patterns and processes of the natural world around them (Wulsin, 2013). Children can observe, understand, and experience seasonal changes of plants in terms of height, color, and texture. As children grow physically, the growth of small trees or bushes around the play area might serve as a reference point for them to understand the concept of time. It is therefore essential to have trees, shrubs, or lawns that are close to each other in the play area; thus children can visually observe the differences in shape or color in time (Cosco & Moore, 2009). Ultimately, stimulating the senses by natural diversity would help children to effectively navigate and orient their whole bodies in the play area, enable them to fully engage in the natural world, and that is the first essential step toward caring for it.

Along with the physical benefits, natural elements and materials also help to create meaningful and challenging play destinations, and to make play more personal and memorable for children. As children actively engage in nature, they can manipulate and modify their surroundings, leave their play imprints on the play area, and free themselves from adults' agendas. The idea of giving children control over their environments was first introduced with the adventure playgrounds where children *"are empowered to shape and develop"* and have a sense of ownership (Play England, 2009). When children have such control, they may challenge themselves physically and discover risk-taking during play. For instance, placing stepping stones, stumps, wooden beams, or rope ladders in the playgrounds would encourage children to test the limits of their physical abilities, and to take reasonable risks (Herrington & Lesmeister, 2006). However, since the physical growth and development occur at different rates among young children, a variety of natural elements and materials should be available to try in the play area. The child, for example, may not feel competent to climb on a rope ladder; yet a grassy hill could be an alternative to practice climbing skills. Accordingly, developmentally appropriate design elements and materials would serve to improve the physical skills of children with varying levels of abilities.

Design for Active and Healthy Relationships

Generally, early years of life are associated with frequent exploration, discovery, and mobility of young children; hence, maintaining spaces that are physically nurturing leverages the possibility of creating a positive atmosphere in and outside of the classroom. When an environment restricts the mobility and self-directed play opportunities of children, aggressive behaviors or bullying problems may become a concern in the classrooms (Siraj-Blatchford & Sylva, 2004; Torelli, 2002). According to the surplus energy theory developed by Spencer in 1873, active play is considered as one of the most effective ways for children to get rid of surplus energy for preventing possible classroom management problems over time (Bogden & Vega-Matos, 2000; Evans & Pellegrini, 1997; Hartle et al., 1994). Therefore, designs with a strong emphasis on mobility and exploratory play contribute physical and social-emotional needs of children. That then may allow children and teachers to direct their attention to the joy of moving, exploring, and discovering rather than focusing on maintaining classroom safety, functionality, and order.

The way we design environments also influences the intensity and the types of active play opportunities. It is generally accepted that indoors are associated with limited mobility when compared to outdoors. When children are in classrooms, they are required to engage in activities that are less bodily expressive and dynamic, children thus may not get rid of their surplus energy due to the inadequate space allocated to them. Compared to outdoors, there is a strict adult control on children's mobility indoors as well. Stephenson (2002) observed differences in child-adult interactions over a period of five months in a childcare setting. One of the observations was that while playing outside, children drew adults' attention to what they were physically doing. That is what Stephenson referred to as *"look at me"* However, when children were inside, they drew adults' attention on what they made (*"look what I have made"*), rather than the actual physical action they engage in. Hence, identifying the mobility and active play opportunities of the indoors and outdoors would be a starting point of the design process to accommodate a variety of active play for any school setting. Afterwards, imposing appropriate active design strategies would help to create spaces where children are motivated to move, explore, investigate, and play actively in and outside of the classroom.

Active Design Strategies and Ideas

A thoughtfully designed environment would enable to meet the daily physical needs of children and encourage them to perform big and small movements regardless of the school setting. Incorporating active living strategies into the classroom routine would be one of the promising efforts to reduce sedentary time and increase the mobility levels. Usually, having a separate room for play and movement may not be achievable due to the limitations imposed by the school's land size, facilities and building capacity thus having a movement center in the classroom would help to achieve the daily-recommended physical needs of children. Also, specifying the location of the movement center in the classroom would enable teachers to allow children to test their skills and boundaries in a safe and controlled environment. It is therefore essential to make the movement center accessible, engaging, and effective to keep the flow of movement in the classroom. The movement center, which may include, for example, movement cards, books, posters, or pictures related to active living styles, would assist children to engage in active play for achieving to their fullest potential. In addition to those aforementioned ones, larger elements such as portable climbers or slides with shock absorbent surfaces would enable to perform big movements indoors (Carlson, 2011). It is also critical to clearly define the boundaries of the movement center to create an effective and efficient traffic flow that would permit children to play without interrupting his/her peers.

As children need environments with sufficient spaces for moving and playing, the overall classroom layout should be responsive to children's movement needs. Yet traditional educational view usually separates the mind from the body and sees the mind superior to the body (Lisahunter, 2011). For that reason, the room layouts mostly ignore active learning opportunities and physically restrain children to orient their bodies in an environment which is less dynamic, much predictable, less flexible, and unchallenging. Changing the classroom set up and arranging the furniture layout in terms of children's movement needs may facilitate active learning with more engaging, meaningful, and experiential ways. For instance, movable chairs and tables give more sense of movement freedom, help better meet individual needs, and create functional learning areas for small and large group activities, fine and gross motor activities, and quiet and noisy activities. Movable furniture gives children sense of change and dynamism beneficial for maintaining and stimulating interest as well.

Considering its easy access and high mobility value, hallways could also be used as an alternative movement space inside the buildings. Hallways serve as a critical transition zones between indoors and outdoors and give children a reference point about exiting from the present setting and entering to another one. Therefore, decorating the hallways with visual, tactile, or auditory signs (e.g., green wall paintings, pictures of trees, real flowers and plants, grassy floors) not only offers sensory stimulation but also helps to indicate the entry to outdoor play area. Moreover, children could engage in such physical activities as obstacle courses, relay races, hula-hoop games, or soccer games even in indoors by using the hallways. Further, placing stepping-stones or big wooden blocks in hallways may stimulate jumping, balancing, climbing, stepping, or directional skills.

Spaces designated for active play should be spacious enough for children to practice their spatial awareness. To establish such an enabling environment, it is necessary to create open spaces and make room to prevent circulation and movement related issues in the classroom. Installing furniture that has flexible qualities could provide ease of space while nurturing the ever-changing needs of young children. Hammocks or balcony/bay windows, for instance, maximize floor space and offer a sense of spatial variety (Dudek, 2007; Torelli & Durrett, 1996). Thus children benefit from places of "prospect and refugee" where they feel secure, relaxed, supported, and connected to their environment (Dosen & Ostwald, 2013; NLI, 2009). Removing excess furniture contributes to make room for children to explore and understand how they move their bodies in general and personal space. Children's participation in such activities as moving their bodies from one location to another, balancing and maintaining postural control, handling and controlling objects would help children to realize what their bodies can do and where their bodies can move. As children begin to improve their spatial awareness, they learn to move efficiently and become aware of other's space. Learning to maintain personal boundaries may thus prevent behavioral problems that emerge due to moving and working together in a limited space.

Furthermore, understanding the spatial relationships helps children to perceive their environment physically, visually, and intellectually. According to the Space

Syntax Theory, environment influences people's perception and the activities they engage in, thus maintaining a connection between space and people is one of the essential considerations for design purposes (Hillier & Hanson, 1984). Maximizing the connectivity through the building increases the mobility levels and creates a sense of belonging. For example, transparent doors and floor-to-ceiling glass windows in the classrooms and along the corridors provide higher visual connection and easy access to outdoor play areas. Likewise, ramps are often practical in multi-storey buildings and frequently stimulate children to use their locomotion skills (e.g., walking, running, hopping, skipping, galloping) in the sense of discovery and curiosity. Especially, circular-shaped ramps both connect floors for travelling up and down and encourage children to actively circulate around the building. Besides connectivity, ramps also maintain visual continuity of movement through elevations in the building.

Summary

A high quality environment increases active and effective usage of space. Such qualities as physical layout, architectural connectivity and flow between indoors and outdoors, and spatial variety are vital in influencing movement and active play opportunities of children. To the extent that children benefit from enabling environments depends on the availability and variety of stimulating experiences. Namely, creating movement centers, arranging the furniture, transforming unused or underused spaces into active areas, providing natural and sensory-rich elements, and creating multi-level and complex spaces are some helpful strategies for indoors and outdoors to accommodate the daily physical needs of children, encourage children to move and play actively, and give freedom to children to discover their capabilities. Additionally, for outdoor play environments, pathways, elevated areas, planting, floor surfaces, and natural equipment would extend the play value for children and promote physical activity and independent mobility (see Appendix A for a list of online resources and Appendix B for a detailed list of effective designs that encourage physical activity).

Space is one of the fundamental considerations for physical, sensory, and vestibular stimulations, designing environments with the knowledge of how children move and play actively would thus help promote active behaviors and to reduce sedentary lifestyles in young children. Designing environments that engage the senses, create meaningful connections, stimulate curiosity and wonder, provide flexibility and mobility, afford physical challenge and complexity, and maintain open-ended and natural elements should spark children's desire to move and play actively. Besides, designing environments with well-defined boundaries, easy access to active play areas, and movable equipment and furniture would contribute to the physical, intellectual, and emotional well-being of children and the quality of interactions they have in that space. With particular emphasis on the aforementioned design strategies, movement and active play could be an intrinsic part of children's daily life.

Appendices

Appendix A: Additional Online Resources

- Early Childhood Environment Rating Scale. Retrieved from http://ers.fpg.unc.edu/early-childhood-environment-rating-scale-ecers-r

The website gives information about the Early Childhood Environments Rating Scale, a set of criteria for assessing the early childhood environments.

- Evaluating the effects of the Lunchtime Enjoyment Activity and Play (LEAP). (2014, March). Retrieved from http://www.londonplay.org.uk/resources/0000/1229/BMC_Public_Health.pdf

The document informs about the positive long-term effects of introducing movable/recycled materials into the school playground on the physical activity levels in children.

- Danks, S. G. (2014). The Green schoolyard movement. Retrieved from http://nebula.wsimg.com/2df79d6da2c6f1f929ba284abe3a3dfc?AccessKeyId=065718B828D697FE7ED3&disposition=0&alloworigin=1

In this document, the author provides information about transforming school grounds into active and vibrant spaces for children where they can engage in nature while learning and playing at the same time.

- Moore, R. (2014). Nature Play & Learning Places. Creating and managing places where children engage with nature. Retrieved from https://naturalearning.org/nature-play-and-learning-places-creating-and-managing-places-where-children-engage-nature.

In this document, Moore talks about creating, managing, and promoting natural environments for children in urban/suburban communities.

- Moore, R. & Cosco, N. (2014). Growing up Green: Naturalization as a health promotion strategy in early childhood outdoor learning environments. Retrieved from https://naturalearning.org/growing-green-naturalization.

In this document, the authors talk about research in which a cost effective naturalization approach that improve the quality of outdoor learning environments and physical activity levels of children.

- School Health Guidelines. (2015, August 19). Retrieved from http://www.cdc.gov/healthyschools/npao/strategies.htm

The website includes guidelines and additional resources for more active and healthy lifestyles.

- The Built Environment and Physical Activity. (2006). Retrieved from http://futureofchildren.org/publications/journals/article/index.xml?journalid=36&articleid=97&sectionid=599

The document focuses on the effects of built environments on the physical activity levels in children and adolescents.

Appendix B Effective Designs that Encourage Physical Activity

Characteristics of environment	Encourage
Form & function	
Smooth surfaces	Walking/running/cycling
Smooth slopes/cliffs	Rolling/sliding/running down/crawling
Trees	Climbing/swinging/hanging/sitting
Bushes/shrubs	Chasing/hiding/sitting
Shelters	Playing hide and seek/role playing
Pathways:	Perceptual complexity
Hard-surfaced paths	Riding wheeled toys/bicycles
Soft-surfaced paths	Sitting/interacting socially
Tree stumps/logs/rope ladders	Balancing/climbing/jumping/sitting/swinging/risk taking/managing risk/testing physical limits
Building considerations	
Easy indoor/outdoor flow	Moving freely between in and outside the classroom
Elevated surfaces	Experiencing "up" and "down"
Concave and convex layouts	Feeling secure and free to move
High ceilings	Sense of spaciousness
Ramps	Sense of discovery and curiosity/visual connectivity of movement
Clarity	Physical legibility/perceptual image-ability
Circular layouts	Sense of energy and dynamism/flow of movement
Transparent doors/floor to ceiling glass windows	Sense of belonging/visual connection to outside/easy access to outside
Hallways	Reference points/sensory stimulation/directional skills
Organic-shaped layouts	Diverse play opportunities/creativity/related to the scale and movement of children/uninterrupted play
Strategies & ideas	
Moveable furniture	Sense of change and dynamism/sense of ownership, belonging and control/functional learning areas
Hammocks/lofts/balcony/bay windows	Sense of spatial variety/maximizing floor space/prospect and refuge areas
Portable climbers/slides	Big movements/spatial awareness/experience "up" and "down"
Movement center	Daily physical needs in a safe and controlled environment/freedom from adult control

References

Apps, L., & MacDonald, M. (2012). Classroom aesthetics in early childhood education. *Journal of Education and Learning, 1*, 49–59.

Athey, C. (2007). *Extending thought in young children. A parent-teacher partnership*. London, UK: Sage Publication.

Bogden, J. F., & Vega-Matos, C. A. (2000). *Fit, healthy, and ready to learn: A school health policy guide. Part I: Physical activity, healthy eating, and tobacco-use prevention*. Alexandria, VA: National Association of State Boards of Education.

Boldemann, C., Blennow, M., Dal, H., Martensson, F., Raustorp, A., Yuen, K., & Wester, U. (2006). Impact of preschool environment upon children's physical activity and sun exposure. *Preventive Medicine, 42*, 301–308.

Carlson, F. (2011). *Big body play: Why boisterous, vigorous, and very physical play is essential to children's development and learning*. Washington, DC: National Association for the Education of Young Children.

Clements, R. (2004). An investigation of the status of outdoor play. *Contemporary Issues in Early Childhood, 5*, 68–80.

Cosco, N. (2006). *Motivation to move: Physical activity affordances in preschool play areas*. Unpublished doctoral thesis, Edinburgh College of Art, School of Landscape Architecture, ECA/Heriot-Watt University.

Cosco, N., & Moore, R. (2009). Sensory integration and contact with nature: Designing outdoor inclusive environments. *North American Montessori Teachers Association Journal, 34*, 159–177.

Cosco, N. G., Moore, R. C., & Islam, M. Z. (2010). Behavior mapping: A method for linking preschool physical activity and outdoor design. *Medicine & Science in Sports & Exercise, 42*, 513–519.

Curtis, D., & Carter, M. (2003). *Designs for living and learning: Transforming early childhood environments*. St. Paul, MN: Redleaf Press.

Dosen, A. S., & Ostwald, M. J. (2013). Prospect and refuge theory: Constructing a critical definition for architecture and design. *The International Journal of Design in Society, 6*, 9–23.

Dudek, M. (2007). *A design manual schools and kindergartens*. Basel, Switzerland: Birkhauser.

Dyment, J. E., & Bell, A. C. (2008). Grounds for movement: Green school grounds as sites for promoting physical activity. *Health Education Research, 23*, 952–962.

Evans, J., & Pellegrini, A. (1997). Surplus energy theory: An enduring but inadequate justification for school break-time. *Educational Review, 49*, 229–336.

Filer, J. (2008). *Healthy, active and outside. Running an outdoors program in the early years*. New York, NY: Taylor & Francis.

Fjortoft, I. (2001). The natural environment as a playground for children: The impact of outdoor play activities in pre-primary school children. *Early Childhood Education Journal, 29*, 111–117.

Frost, J. L. (2010). *A history of children's play and play environments: Toward a contemporary child-saving movement*. New York, NY: Taylor & Francis.

Gallahue, D., & Ozmun, J. (1998). *Understanding motor development infants, children, adolescents, adults*. New York, NY: McGraw-Hill.

Gandini, L. (1993). Fundamentals of the Reggio Emilia approach to early childhood education. *Young Children, 49*, 4–8.

Gray, P. (2011). The decline of play and the rise of psychopathology in children and adolescents. *American Journal of Play, 3*, 443–463.

Hannon, J. C., & Brown, B. B. (2008). Increasing preschoolers' physical activity intensities; an activity-friendly preschool playground intervention. *Preventive Medicine, 46*, 532–536.
Hartle, L., Campbell, J., Becker, A., Harman, S., Kagel, S., & Tiballi, B. (1994). Outdoor play: A window on social-cognitive development. *Dimensions of Early Childhood, 23*, 27–31.
Haywood, K. M., & Getchell, N. (2009). *Life span motor development*. Champaign, IL: Human Kinetics.
Head Start Design Guide. (2005). *A guide for building a head start facility*. Washington, DC: U.S. Department of Health and Human Services.
Heft, H. (1988). Affordances of children's environments: A functional approach to environmental description. *Children's Environments Quarterly, 5*, 29–27.
Henderson, K. E., Grode, G. M., O'Connell, M. L., & Schwartz, M. B. (2015). Environmental factors associated with physical activity in childcare centers. *International Journal of Behavioral Nutrition and Physical Activity, 12*, 1–10.
Henniger, M. L. (2009). *Teaching young children: An introduction*. Upper Saddle River, NJ: Prentice Hall.
Herrington, S., & Lesmeister, C. (2006). The design of landscapes at child-care centres: Seven Cs. *Landscape Research, 31*, 63–82.
Hillier, B., & Hanson, J. (1984). *The social logic of space*. New York, NY: Cambridge University Press.
Jensen, E. (2000). *Learning with the body in mind*. Thousand Oaks, CA: Corwin Press.
lisahunter. (2011). Re-embodying (pre-service middle years) teachers? An attempt to reposition the body and its presence in teaching and learning. *Teaching and Teacher Education, 27*, 187–200.
Moore, R. C., & Wong, H. (1997). *Natural learning: The life history of an environmental schoolyard*. Berkeley, CA: MIG Communications.
National Learning Initiative. (2009). *Creating and retrofitting play environments: Best practice guidelines*. Chattanooga, TN: Collage of Design, NC State University.
Olds, A. (2000). *Child care design guide*. New York, NY: McGraw-Hill.
Patte, M. M., & Brown, F. (2011). Playwork: A profession challenging societal factors devaluing children's play. *Journal of Student Wellbeing, 5*, 58–70.
Piaget, J. (1964). Cognitive development in children: Development and learning. *Journal of Research in Science Teaching, 2*, 176–186.
Play England. (2009). *Developing an adventure playground: The essential elements*. London, UK: The National Lottery.
Sibley, B. A., & Etnier, J. L. (2003). The relationship between physical activity and cognition in children: A meta analysis. *Pediatric Exercise Science, 15*, 243–256.
Singer, D. G., Singer, J. L., D'Agostino, H., & DeLong, R. (2009). Children's pastimes and play in sixteen nations: Is free play declining? *American Journal of Play, 1*, 283–312.
Siraj-Blatchford, I., & Sylva, K. (2004). Researching pedagogy in English preschools. *British Educational Research Journal, 30*, 713–730.
Sommer, R. (1969). *Personal space: The behavioral basis of design*. Bristol, UK: Bosko Books.
Stephenson, A. (2002). Opening up the outdoors: Exploring the relationship between the indoor and outdoor environments of a center. *European Early Childhood Research Journal, 10*, 29–38.
Torelli, L. (2002). Enhancing development through classroom design in early Head Start: Meeting the program performance standards and best practices. *Children and Families, 8*, 44–50.
Torelli, L., & Durrett, C. (1996). Landscape for learning: The impact of classroom design on infants and toddlers. *Early Childhood News, 8*, 12–17.
Trost, S. G., Fees, B., & Dzewaltowski, D. (2008). Feasibility and efficacy of a "move and learn" physical activity curriculum in preschool children. *Journal of Physical Activity Health, 5*, 88–103.

Trost, S. G., Ward, D. S., & Senso, M. (2010). Effects of child care policy and environment on physical activity. *Medicine & Science in Sports & Exercise, 42*, 520–525.
Vidoni, C., & Ignico, A. (2011). Promoting physical activity during early childhood. *Early Child Development and Care, 181*, 1261–1269.
Wulsin, L. R. (2013). *Classroom design-Literature review*. Retrieved from https://www.princeton.edu/provost/space-programming-plannin/SCCD_Final_Report_Appendix_B.pdf

Serap Sevimli-Celik is an Assistant Professor of Elementary & Early Childhood Education in the College of Education at the Middle East Technical University (METU). She teaches courses on movement education, play, creativity and visual arts at the undergraduate level and embodied learning at the graduate level. Her research interests center on movement education, embodied learning, movement-friendly designs for indoors & outdoors, play pedagogy & crosscultural play, and creative thinking.

Chapter 15
Teaching Pre-service Early Childhood Educators About Health and Wellness Through Educational Movement

Traci D. Zillifro and Marybeth Miller

Children Need to Move

A teacher opens the doors to an empty gymnasium and allows a class full of children to enter without giving any specific directions. What do the children do? They run! They have nowhere to go, they have no goal in mind, they are doing what their bodies need and want to do....run...move!

Human bodies were designed to move. This fact is never as obvious as it is in childhood. Movement not only helps maintain health, it helps to prepare the body to learn, and when movement is combined with learning, it helps the brain retain and recall information (Ratey, 2008). This chapter will explore a dynamic of how Early Childhood educators may nest health and wellness in an educational movement framework using experiential or active learning.

Globally speaking, a fundamental tenet of well-functioning societies rests upon the health and education of its people. Health and education affects individuals in shaping their ability to optimally contribute, in a collaborative manner, to the workforce and help build a vibrant economy.

Nevertheless, different opinions exist concerning the best setting to promote both health and education. The Association for Supervision and Curriculum Development (ASCD), a global leader in educational leadership, considers schools to be the perfect setting for the interaction and collaboration of health and education (ASCD.org). No longer limited to health services and education working in their own silo,

T. D. Zillifro (✉)
Slippery Rock University, Slippery Rock, PA, USA
e-mail: traci.zillifro@sru.edu

M. Miller
Slippery Rock University of Pennsylvania, Slippery Rock, PA, USA
e-mail: marybethmiller@comcast.net

H. Brewer, M. R. Jalongo (eds.), *Physical Activity and Health Promotion in the Early Years*, Educating the Young Child 14,
https://doi.org/10.1007/978-3-319-76006-3_15

schools today are embracing a newer, comprehensive model called Whole School, Whole Community, Whole Child (WSCC). WSCC represents a coordination of policy, process and practices toward improving learning as well as physical and social-emotional health. This model operates on a Whole School collaboration of health and education that draws upon its Whole Community resources to meet the needs of the Whole Child. In the United States of America, ASCD,–along with the Centers for Disease Control,–promote schools to adopt the WSCC as a framework to improve students' learning and health. Attention to this detail reaches beyond K-12, and extends itself to the youngest citizens, preschool-age children to be offered the opportunity for early childhood education.

Nationwide, the movement for early childhood education is reaching, and continues to expand a groundswell of programs in schools and community settings, led by highly trained administrators and teachers. Who, more than family, has the most significant influence upon a young child, than his or her teacher? Teachers of young children are called upon to provide best-practice approaches to deliver information and provide experiences that build skills and understanding to the context of daily routines using intentional play-based opportunities that stimulate exploration, discovery, and the curiosity to want to know more. Research confirms that play is the primary medium for young children's learning. Early childhood educators learn to design intentional play opportunities to stimulate the psychomotor, cognitive, and affective learning domains. The WSCCC standards framework can be used as a guide. Its key learning areas include, among others, Approaches to Learning through Play, and Health, Wellness and Physical Development. The standard Health, Wellness, and Physical Development has a primary focus, learning about my body (pp. 71–77). This standard has five learning concepts: (1) concepts of health, (2) healthful living, (3) Safety and Injury Prevention, (4) Physical Activity – Gross Motor Coordination, and (5) Concepts, Principles, and Strategies of Movement – Fine Motor Coordination organized to guide early childhood educators to intentionally plan play experiences that cultivate the learning of healthy and safe practices. Preparing individuals studying to become an educator of pre-school age children (3–5 year olds) includes coursework addressing how children learn about their bodies through educational movement experiences. Educational movement has a framework of four elements:

1. body awareness (what the body can do)
2. space awareness (where the body moves),
3. quality (how the body moves),
4. relationship (to whom and to what the body relates).

In the authors' professional experience, the elements and concepts involving body awareness, space awareness and relationship are initially addressed with preservice teachers. Educational movement that involves a service-learning program of pre-school age children is studied and practiced.

The National Association for Education of Young Children (NAEYC) in 2010 published the Standards for Initial Early Childhood Professional Preparation.

Standard 5: Using Content Knowledge to Build Meaningful Curriculum has three key elements that (1) identify candidates understand content knowledge and resources inclusive of creative movement, physical activity, physical education, health and safety (5a), (2) know and use the central concepts, inquiry tools and resources (5b), (3) then use their knowledge, academic standards and resources to plan, teach and evaluate developmentally appropriate and challenging curriculum. Together, standards provide the branding of health and wellness as important academic content in early childhood education curriculum. The catalyst for implementation may be through meaningful creative and educational movement experiences.

Learning about health and wellness learning outcomes for young children through a concept-based educational movement framework can be an eye-opening experience for pre-service early childhood educators. The movement paradigm explored is not commonly in a pre-service educator's comfort zone. The question regarding a pre-service teacher's willingness to go forward and take the time to plan quality standards-based learning experiences to support health, wellness and physical development, reflects if their physical activity/education learning experience was positive, and therefore value health and wellness enough to act as a role model to children and believe that learning to be healthy and well is important to young children's education. A plethora of research has been published stating the benefits of physical activity to a child's physical, emotional, and cognitive well-being. The Department of Health and Human Services published in 2008 Physical Activity Guidelines for Americans. Activity Guidelines for Children and Youth state that children should be physically active for at least 60 min each day to promote heart health, muscle and bone strength (Department of Health and Human Services, 2008). Make no mistake – organized sports do not play a role in this framework for pre-kindergarten children. The WSCC model promotes the health and education, school-wide, throughout the school day involving activities that are age-appropriate, enjoyable, and offer variety.

The theory of experiential learning (Kolb, 1984) supports the premise of learning by doing. The experiential approach to learning skills and concepts is believed to reach a deeper level of processing information that is converted to knowledge. Key understandings to be addressed and developed with pre-service early childhood education teachers include: foundation of movement, ways to incorporate movement throughout the school day, how to maintain an educational environment in large spaces when children are moving and using props, how to maintain safety, both physical and emotional, when children are engaging in physical activity, and incorporating games, interdisciplinary learning and rhythmic activities to achieve a more comprehensive approach to educating the whole child.

Foundational Content

Academic content in physical activity and physical education starts with a study of learning what to teach. This begins with an overview of fundamental motor skill development, and educational movement concepts of Laban's Movement Education Framework. Adults often forget that just as students must learn addition and subtraction before learning calculus, children must learn and practice fundamental motor skills before they become skilled at more complex motor skills. Teachers learn to become comfortable and confident in modeling these skills when providing physical activity instruction. These skills can easily blend with exploratory and creative movement experiences centered upon educational movement concepts, all-the-while, integrating language arts, mathematics, health and safety, social development (Character Counts), and rhythmics.

Fundamental Motor Skills

Teachers of young children need to have an understanding of what fundamental motor skills are (Fig. 15.1) and their patterns of development. All fundamental motor skills progress from immature to mature patterns through active play and quality instruction. These skills are used in combination with each other to form higher level movements used in dance and sporting activities. Their application at the early childhood level is with creative movement, rhythmics, and exploratory play involving various types of materials (e.g. balloons, paddle, balls, beanbags, low level balance benches and more). With frequent opportunities for active play and quality instruction by teachers, these skills gradually mature in movement form as young children grow through the elementary school years (Haywood & Getchell, 2005). Table 15.1 illustrates an aggregated percent of children 3–5 years of age progressing toward a level of maturity for the fundamental locomotor and manipulative skills. The trend of increased percentages across age for each skill may reflect, in combination, children receiving quality instruction in a wide variety of movement experiences where these skills are used along with growth in height and weight therefore becoming stronger. Research involving stages of development for locomotor and manipulative skills peak around age 11 years (Ulrich,

Locomotor	Manipulative	Axial
walk	toss	twist
run	throw	turn
slide	kick	swing
gallop	catch	sway
hop	strike	stretch

Fig. 15.1 Three categories of fundamental movement

Table 15.1 Percent of children demonstrating mastery on locomotor and manipulative subtest skills

Fundamental motor skills	Age in years for pre-kindergarten		
	3 years	4 years	5 years
Locomotor skills:			
Run	75	82	86
Gallop	23	44	62
Hop	20	43	64
Horizontal jump	35	47	49
Slide	40	54	63
Leap	29	47	51
Manipulative skills:			
Strike a stationary ball	42	54	58
Stationary dribble (hand)	14	27	41
Catching (tossed ball)	31	45	68
Kick (run to stationary ball)	51	57	69
Overhead throw (one hand)	22	35	40
Underhand roll	21	41	45

2000). Studying the progressions and patterns of fundamental motor skills and knowing their developmental trends of mastery may assist early childhood educators on how to intentionally plan activities for their use. Children moving leads to children becoming more fit and healthy for their developmental level. The next section will explore types of fitness, describe which one is of best fit for early childhood, and why.

Fitness and Health

There are two types of physical fitness, (1) Skill-Related Fitness (also known as Motor Fitness) and (2) Health-Related Physical Fitness. Through a lens of fitness involving early childhood, a developmental direction starts with skill-related fitness because its components of balance, coordination, agility, reaction time, speed and power begin as underpinnings of the motor milestones within the first 12 months of life. Skill-related fitness continues its journey of developmental progression into the middle childhood years where fundamental motor skills (locomotor, non-locomotor, and manipulative skills) develop to a mature pattern with greater engagement in physical activity. The skill-related fitness component of power is not to be thought of as "power lifting" rather, in the early childhood timeframe, power is developed through the functional activities of being able to push, pull, lift and lower objects. An example of this may include using the legs to push a tricycle, or the arms to move forward on a scooter.

Scaled to developmental appropriateness, the components of Health-Related Physical Fitness, cardiorespiratory endurance, muscular strength, muscular endurance, body composition, and flexibility (1) may be introduced in the early childhood years through an educational movement concept called Body Awareness (what the body can do). For example, as children between 3–5 years of age begin to learn about their large and small body parts the health-related fitness awareness can be addressed with the start of learning about their heart (location, size and general function) and the major muscles underlying the skin. Developmentally appropriate physical activities aid in strengthening the muscular system but it is in no way thought of as strength training. To avoid the misconception of engaging young children in physical fitness activities to produce an athletic child with hopes of an athletic scholarship as the child grows, individuals teaching young children must have the knowledge and understanding of human growth and development in childhood, and this does not advocate or encourage early fitness training. Before puberty, children do not have the hormone development (testosterone) to influence muscle strength and cardiovascular endurance such as in distance running. Physical fitness training of this nature only becomes developmentally appropriate at and after puberty. Teachers of young children (preschool and elementary) can provide the education to them of the value of physical activity, its importance to enjoying life with family and friends, and its importance to being healthy. A good starting point for young children to learn about their body is to organize physical activities around a theme of Body Awareness which focuses upon what the body can do (balance, transfer of weight, creating shapes). The use of interactive animated educational PowerPoint technology (Parette, Hourcade & Blum, 2011) is a medium central to this direction of education which is grounded in early childhood learning standards (Pennsylvania Learning Standards for Early Childhood, 2014). This technology, paired with developmentally appropriate physical activity, can bring the concepts of heart health, strong muscles and bones and their enhancement through active play to life.

Concept-Based Learning: Movement Concepts and Skills

In 1974 Rudolph Laban created a classification system that allows movement to be identified and analyzed. This classification is based on movement concepts and skills grouped under four elements of body awareness, space awareness, qualities (effort), and relationships. Body awareness refers to what the body can do – the way it balances, the shapes it can make and the transfer of weight from one body part to another body part. Space awareness refers to where the body moves – moving in general and personal space, different directions, at different levels and across different pathways. "Qualities" refers to how the body moves – with different speeds, force and flow of movement. Relationship refers to whom and what the body relates to e.g. leading and following someone, or sitting on a carpet square at circle time. These four elements form the basis of Movement Education (Kirchner & Fishburne,

1998) which is being coined in this chapter as Educational Movement. Teaching movement through a concept-based approach builds physical literacy (gross motor skill development) and vocabulary of these movement concepts (language and literacy). Scaffolding health concepts into educational movement experiences helps children to understand why movement is important to being healthy.

Young children are very curious about their own body awareness. As they begin to identify large and small body parts, they explore their use in various movement formats such as balancing on different body parts, number of body parts, right side up and upside down (body awareness). As they travel from one location to another using locomotor skills of running, galloping, sliding, jumping, hopping or skipping they travel with the ability to move skillfully enough to not fall (an example of dynamic balance). They learn to travel in different ways, changing directions (forward, backward, sideways), changing their levels in space from low, to medium to high (space awareness) and moving among others and obstacles by going around, over, under, and between exploring their relationship to others and objects.. These are examples of concept-based movement illustrating how movement is transformed to an educational format. Table 15.1 provides an illustration of movement concepts and their supporting themes and examples of physical activities associated with each concept. Educational movement applies a guided discovery and exploratory approach to its pedagogy, thus upholding the best-practice learning environment of being child-centered.

Physical Activity Learning Environments: Indoors and Outdoors

Indoors

Due to space limitations in a classroom filled with tables and chairs, there may be designated places to promote play involving fine motor skills (small muscle movement such as pushing a toy car) as opposed to gross motor movements. One exception may be during circle time located at a designated space in the classroom/limited spaces. Using circle time, teachers may guide gross motor activities while children stand on their carpet square or pre-determined spot acting out movement to a story involving Readers Theatre. This format may be applied for rhythmic movement to music. Teachers may search resources that are specific to guiding movement in the classroom. In a language and literacy lesson as children learn to print letters, and in a mathematics lesson as children learn to write numbers, they may create them with their body on the floor at the circle or with their arms at their table. This active learning approach, otherwise known as kinesthetic learning encourages the body to move, the heart rate to increase, the blood to circulate and to bear weight on muscles and bones (Table 15.2).

Teachers who have the opportunity to move to a larger space such as the school gymnasium or multipurpose room may create a routine as shown in Fig. 15.1.

Table 15.2 Crosswalk of physical activities by motor skills, educational movement concepts, health and safety concepts

Physical activity examples (Source: SPARK 3-5)	Gross motor skills	Educational movement concepts	Concepts of health & safety (Source: Pennsylvania Department of Education Health Wellness and Physical Development 10.1-10.4)
Rhythmics:			
Hokey Pokey	Walk	Balance	Identify and locate body parts
Chicken Dance	Gallop	Transfer of weight	Coordination of body movements
Head Shoulders Knees and Toes	Bending and stretching	General and personal space	
		Change of direction	
		Pathways shapes	
Explore with manipulatives:			
Hula hoops		Balance	Exhibit balance while moving on the ground or using equipment
Large balls		General and personal space	Recognize safe and unsafe practices
Yarn balls		Directions	Identify specific practices that support development and function (physical activity)
Lollypop paddles		Levels	
Fat plastic bats		Force	
		Relationship to equipment	
Explore with large equipment:			
Scooters	Pushing/pulling	Balance	Exhibit balance while moving on the ground or using equipment
Benches	Traveling on feet/hands and feet	Transfer of weight	Recognize safe and unsafe practices
Low balance beam	Climbing	Shapes	Identify specific practices that support development and function (physical activity)
Flat ladders	Rolling	Direction	Exhibit balance while moving on the ground or using equipment
Trestles/trees to climb	Making shapes/balances	Levels	
	Pushing/pulling	Relationship to equipment	

Figure 15.1 is an example of an intentionally planned physical activity session where fundamental motor skills are integrated with Laban's educational movement concepts of Body Awareness and Relationship to materials. What's more, it is standards-based and evidence based, coming from a credible resource. Developmentally appropriate activities like, and with greater variety, can be found in numerous resources listed at the end of this chapter.

Outdoors

To work on building health-related fitness in children during school recess and in community playgrounds, one must consider the types of supervised physical activities that they enjoy. Short bursts of rapid running, climbing stairs to a slide, or pedaling a tricycle are all great activities to strengthen a child's heart, muscles, and bones. You may ask, "If the children do this already, why is instruction necessary?" There are many reasons, such as: (1) not every child will engage in physical activity without prompting, (2) inappropriate movement patterns may be developed without proper instruction, (3) to insure the physical and emotional safety of the students; (4) activities should be developmentally appropriate and age -related, planned, varied, and inclusive, and (5) children may not feel comfortable enough to participate among their peers.

In order to be "healthy" one must move their body. Children need to learn to be "skilled movers". Of course the vast majority of children learn to walk, run, and play without any specific instruction, however, in order to move beyond the basic movement patterns, to improve muscular strength, endurance, and coordination, to engage in activities that require a specific skill set, beyond the basics, children must learn to control their bodies.

Teacher Expectations for Management and Safety

New teachers starting their field experiences or student teaching lack the experience and confidence to be firm, fair and consistent with class management. Modeling, cueing and positively reinforcing desired behaviors as they occur in the physical activity sessions is vital to maintaining a physically and emotionally safe learning environment.

1. Establish simple rules for following directions and model them.
2. Create visual and verbal cues for gaining and sustaining attention and use them
3. Develop consistent formats of a lesson/session and be consistent with them
4. Direct supervision: keep your back-to-the-wall and eyes on the entire group at all times
5. Implement a Character Counts Program – to teach personal and social responsibility

Children's safety is paramount. Teachers must know how to maintain a controlled atmosphere in a large, open space, with equipment and many children moving at one time. This is a skill that is learned. The way to begin this process is by teaching and solidifying a few class structures that can form the basis of all class activities. Two common class organizations include general space and personal space. In addition to class structures posting and reviewing class rules, actively supervising activity at all times, and giving clear and consistent commands will create an organized and safe atmosphere.

Emotional Safety During Physical Activity

The importance of maintaining emotional safety throughout instructional time in physical activity cannot be understated. Just as the child in math class does not want the teacher to display his or her grade on a test in which they did poorly, the child that does not excel physically does not want their ability, or lack thereof, to be on display. The goal of teacher-planned learning experiences should be to teach children how to live a healthful life that includes physical activity and to help inspire a love of physical activity within each child so that they will continue to be active throughout their lifetime. The goal of including physical activity throughout the school day assists children in achieving their goal of moderate to vigorous physical activity for 60 min each day.

Teachers should not put students who are struggling with a physical task in the awkward situation of performing in front of peers. Pitting two students against each other in front of the class is another situation to avoid, as this tends to result in one feeling competent and the other, quite embarrassed. Humiliating experiences in early childhood can cause a person to avoid physical activity for a lifetime, which works against the goal of physical activity in the schools.

Students must learn to be accepting of each other. This should be stated and reinforced in class. Techniques to help this work can include the implementation of blending elements of a nationally known character development program developmentally appropriate for Pre-K through 12, such as Character Counts 5.0. This framework is commonly used in early childhood education and K-12 schools to foster character development (http://charactercounts.org).

Fostering the development of character in a physical activity environment intentionally planned by teachers translates into choosing developmentally appropriate activities that include maximum participation for every child. Elimination games, such as traditional tag games, Duck-Duck-Goose, and Steal the Bacon, where as few as one student moves while the others are still simply do not align with the goal of maximum physical activity. Traditional elimination games can easily be made appropriate through a few simple rule changes to get and keep all students active for the entire extent any game is played.

Conclusion

Why Discuss Health and Wellness in Early Childhood Education?

Most pre-service early childhood educators, by the end of their college career, are well-versed in what content should be delivered and how to deliver that content…. on reading, writing, mathematics, science, and social studies, to children sitting at desks in a classroom. But with the plethora of studies highlighting the childhood obesity epidemic, showing how movement can enhance learning and how sitting for extended periods of time is detrimental to health, there needs to be more. We have all heard the phrase that "without our health, we have nothing". Children need to learn how to be and stay healthy.

References

Association for Supervision and Curriculum Development. (2016). *Whole school, whole community, whole child: A collaborative approach to learning and health.* Retrieved January 31, 2016, from http://www.ascd.org/programs/learning-and-health/wscc-model.aspx

Haywood, K. M., & Getchell, N. (2005). *Life span motor development* (4th ed.). Champaign, IL: Human Kinetics.

Josephson Institute. (2015). *Character counts!* Retrieved January 31, 2016, from charactercounts.org

Kirchner, G., & Fishburne, G. (1998). *Movement concepts and skill in physical education for elementary school children* (10th ed., pp. 91–101). Boston, MA: McGraw Hill.

Kolb, D. A. (1984). *Experiential learning: Experience as the source of learning and development.* Englewood Cliffs, NJ: Prentice- Hall.

National Association for the Education of Young Children. (2010). *2010 standards for initial and advanced early childhood professional preparation programs.* Washington, DC: NAEYC.

Office of Child Development and Early Learning. (2014). *Pennsylvania learning standards for early childhood: Pre-kindergarten* (3rd ed.). Harrisburg, PA: Pennsylvania Department of Human Services, Pennsylvania Department of Education.

Parette, H. P., Hourcade, J., & Blum, C. (2011). Using animation in Microsoft Powerpoint to enhance engagement and learning in young learners with developmental delay. *Teaching Exceptional Children, 43*(4), 58–67.

Ratey, J. (2008). *Spark: The revolutionary new science of exercise and the brain.* Boston, MA: Little, Brown and Company.

Ulrich, D. (2000). *Test of gross motor development – 2* (2nd ed.). Dallas, TX: Pro-Ed.

US Department of Health and Human Services. (2008). *2008 physical activity guidelines for Americans.* Retrieved January 31, 2016, from http://health.gov/paguidelines/guidelines/chapter3.aspx

Traci D. Zillifro has been teaching for over 15 years and has taught physical activity courses at all levels. She teaches pre-service early childhood educators in teaching and leading health and fitness activities for young children. Traci has conducted research and workshops on promoting physical activity in early childhood at the state and national level. She has also published in peer-reviewed journals on topics related to fitness among young children and lifelong physical activity.

Marybeth Miller taught adapted physical education for 11 years prior to entering higher education teacher education. Marybeth specializes in teacher education training having an emphasis in motor development and early childhood physical activity. Her book *Service-Learning in Physical Education and Related Professions: A Global Perspective* (Jones & Bartlett) connects scholars world-wide with expertise in service-learning.

Chapter 16
Increasing Children's Participation in Physical Activity Through a Before School Physical Activity Program

Keri S. Kulik and Justin R. Kulik

The goal of this chapter is to review current recommendations for physical activity and discuss specific strategies to increase children's physical activity in the school based setting beyond that of traditional physical education. Worldwide, there are several leading organizations including the World Health Organization (WHO) and the Centers for Disease Control and Prevention (CDC) that have developed recommendations and programs to promote physical activity in children. The initiatives include a multifaceted approach whereby children are provided increased opportunities for physical activity to achieve the recommended amount of daily physical activity. The successful implementation of these initiatives depends on several factors including a basic understanding of physical activity, fitness and health outcomes, knowledge of the recommendations for physical activity in children and specific program design.

Physical Activity, Physical Fitness and Health

The terms physical activity and physical fitness are sometimes used interchangeably to describe how a specific population remains active. However, while related, these terms are not interchangeable. According to the World Health Organization, "Physical activity is any bodily movement produced by skeletal muscles that requires energy expenditure"(World Health Organization, 2015). This definition

K. S. Kulik (✉)
Department of Kinesiology, Health, and Sport Science, Indiana University of Pennsylvania, Indiana, PA, USA
e-mail: kskulik@iup.edu

J. R. Kulik
Blairsville-Saltsburg School District, Blairsville, PA, USA

H. Brewer, M. R. Jalongo (eds.), *Physical Activity and Health Promotion in the Early Years*, Educating the Young Child 14,
https://doi.org/10.1007/978-3-319-76006-3_16

provides some insight into what it means to be physically active, but it could also be misinterpreted. For example, in a classroom setting physical activity could be easily mistaken by something as simple as a student raising their hand to answer a question. While not excessive in energy expenditure, skeletal muscles were involved in this movement and therefore physical activity occurred. This is not the intention of increasing physical activity in the school system. The intention is to increase physical activity in a planned and structured manner so that it produces a specific positive physical fitness outcome. Engaging in physical activity in a manner that improves personal physical fitness and health outcomes is referred to as exercise (WHO, 2015).

Physical fitness is the development of attributes that are improved through both planned and unplanned physical activity. These attributes include cardiorespiratory endurance (aerobic power), skeletal muscle endurance, skeletal muscle strength, skeletal muscle power, flexibility, balance, speed, reaction time, and body composition (Centers for Disease Control, 2010).

Participation in regular physical activity and improved physical fitness has been shown to help maintain healthy bones and muscles, control weight and improve body composition, and decrease the incidence of chronic diseases such as cardiovascular disease, hypertension and diabetes mellitus in children (CDC, 2010). When compared to physically inactive children, physically active children may be less likely to experience chronic disease risk factors, to become overweight and may be more likely to remain active throughout adulthood (Fulton, Garg, Galuska, Rattay, & Caspersen, 2004). In addition to the improved health outcomes, participation in physical activity also creates many positive benefits for young children and provides an opportunity for play activity and environmental exploration. Regular physical activity facilitates the development of motor skills and increases energy expenditure (Batch, 2005; American Heart Association, 2013). Improved fitness as a result of increased physical activity can also increase self-esteem and may reduce anxiety and stress (Calfas & Taylor, 1994). Improved academic performance, classroom behavior, and mental focus have also been associated with participation in physical activity (Pontifex, Saliba, & Hillman, 2013).

Physical Activity Participation Recommendations for Children

The global recommendation is for children to participate in 60 min of moderate to vigorously intense physical activity every day. The physical activity should include both aerobic exercise and activities to strengthen bone and muscle. It is also recommended that daily participation exceeding 60 min will provide additional health benefits (WHO, 2011). Although some countries have developed their own specific recommendations for physical activity among children, most recommendations are consistent with regards to time, type and intensity. Table 16.1 provides examples of recommendations that have been developed by individual countries.

Table 16.1 Example recommendations by individual countries

Organization	Recommendations
Canadian Physical	Children should accumulate at least 60 min of moderate-to vigorous-intensity physical activity daily
	Vigorous-intensity activities should be included at least 3 days per week
	Activities should include those that strengthen bones and muscle at least 3 days per week
	More daily physical activity provides greater health benefits
World Health Organization	Children and youth should accumulate at least 60 min of moderate to vigorous physical activity every day
	Amounts of physical activity greater than 60 min provide additional health benefits
	Most of the daily physical activity should be aerobic. Vigorous activity should be incorporated, including activities to strengthen bone and muscle
SHAPE America	Age and developmentally appropriate activity
	Accumulate at least 60 min, and up to several hours, on all or most days, including moderate and vigorous physical activity with majority of time spent in intermittent activity
	Several bouts lasting 15 min or more each day
	Variety of age-appropriate physical activity to achieve optimal health, wellness, fitness and performance benefits
	Discourage extended periods of inactivity ≥2 h
Centers for Disease Control	Children should do 60 min (1 h) or more of physical activity each day
	Aerobic activity should make up most of the 60 or more minutes of physical activity each day. This can include either moderate-intensity aerobic activity, such as brisk walking, or vigorous-intensity activity, such as running. Be sure to include vigorous-intensity aerobic activity on at least 3 days per week.
	Include muscle strengthening activities, such as gymnastics or push-ups, at least 3 days per week as part of the 60 or more minutes.
	Include bone strengthening activities, such as jumping rope or running, at least 3 days per week as part of the 60 or more minutes.

Although the benefits of physical activity are well established and the guidelines for participation are clear, many young children do not participate in regular physical activity (CDC, 2010; Kalman et al., 2015). Recently it was reported that 80% of the world's youth population is physically inactive (WHO, 2015). Moreover, the percentage of children who meet the recommendations decreases as age increases (Nader, Bradley, Houts, McRitchie, & O'Brien, 2008).

To reverse this alarming health trend, global initiatives have been developed to provide national and regional policy makers with guidance and strategies for increasing physical activity among children. In addition to the global initiatives, several countries have developed their own initiatives. For example, the United States developed the Healthy 2020 national physical activity objectives to help improve levels of physical activity among children (United States Department of Health and Human Services, 2010). Included in these objectives are specific goals targeting schools and policies related to recess and physical education.

The Role of Early Learning Facilities and Schools

Schools and early childhood education centers have played a central role in providing opportunities for children and adolescents to participate in physical activity (Pate et al., 2006). Traditionally, students have engaged in physical activity during physical education, recess breaks, by walking or biking to and from school, and participation in school sports. However, as we move through the twenty-first century, alarming health trends are emerging suggesting that schools may need to reevaluate and expand their role in providing physical activity to children (Pate et al., 2006).

Currently, schools have an opportunity to influence and encourage participation in physical activity, promote healthy weight and provide education for a healthy lifestyle (Story, Kaphingst, & French, 2006). The WHO identifies the school environment as a key setting to implement programs and strategies designed to address the prevalence of overweight and obesity because most children spend a large portion of time in school. Schools provide many opportunities to engage children in healthy eating, through school breakfast and lunch programs, and physical activity during physical education and recess. Schools also provide many opportunities to reinforce healthy messages related to nutrition and physical activity.

Within the school setting, physical education has been identified as the primary place to deliver healthful messages and provide students with opportunities to participate in physical activity. Physical education has been a part of the school curriculum since the late 1800s and school sports have been a component of educational institutions since the early 1900s (Pate et al., 2006). Unfortunately many children do not participate in regular physical activity. Most schools are not able to provide children with opportunities to achieve the 60 min of daily physical activity. This trend may be caused in part by recent legislation and policies that provide school incentives and funding based on the results of standardized academic testing (Rentner et al., 2006). In an attempt to improve test scores, schools are reducing the physical education instruction time in favor of providing more classroom instruction in core areas such as reading and math. The reduction in allotted instruction time for physical education and physical activity is alarming as obesity rates continue to rise in children and adolescents. If children are not provided opportunities to participate in physical activity during the school day, they may not be able to reach the recommended activity time per day and may not be receiving the improved health benefits.

Strategies for Increasing Physical Activity Within Schools

To combat this trend and shift the focus back on the importance of physical activity, schools are looking for ways to increase opportunities for physical activity outside of the traditional physical education classes. The CDC developed the Comprehensive School Physical Activity Program (CSPAP) to provide schools with a model to increase opportunities for physical activity before, during and after school. This model includes a multi-component approach to physical activity that includes quality physical education, physical activity before, during and after school, staff involvement and family and community engagement (CDC, 2015). Implementation of this model provides schools with a framework to offer students increased opportunities to achieve the recommended 60 min of physical activity each day. In the next section, specific strategies for creating a before school physical activity program for young children will be explained.

Starting a Before School Physical Activity Program

A before school physical activity program can be a powerful tool in developing students both physically and academically. As indicated by current recommendations, the combination of improved health, decreased risk of developing non-communicable diseases, and the potential improvement in academic success warrants the inclusion of additional physical activity for children. A successful program is dependent upon proper planning and implementation to achieve desired results. Consideration should be given to factors such as the intended participants, available resources and personnel needed to implement the program.

Participants

The first consideration when designing a before school program is the participants. This includes the specific number of participants as well as their age and ability. The number of students in any given school limits the number of participants involved in the program. In addition, the number of participants impacts both the scheduling as well as available resources and needs consideration for a successful program. This becomes a scheduling issue as well as an issue for available resources. Both of these areas will be addressed in the upcoming sections.

Regardless of the number of students participating in any before school program, they will most likely vary in age due to multiple age groups or grades participating. Because of this, it is important to understand that young children of varying ages will also have varying degrees of ability. Program design should reflect this fact through the use of strategies that allow maximum participation for any specific skill or activity regardless of ability. This also permits students to work within their individual comfort level, which will lead to a greater enjoyment of the activity. An example of this strategy can be illustrated with one of the most natural movements in which nearly all children participate, running.

A common practice among teachers is to set a specific distance and then have all students complete that same distance regardless of the amount of time it takes to complete. This is an extrinsic motivator and can sometimes make students feel inadequate about their individual abilities or it can promote competition between students. While competition is not inherently bad, when physical activity and fitness improvement is the intended outcome, it should be avoided between children. Instead, competition against ones self is a better strategy. Using intrinsic motivation as a strategy, the aforementioned running activity could be executed by determining a specific time frame for which everyone will run. In the following scenario, the teacher provides brief instruction and alters the activity yet keeps the focus on running:

> After students complete an appropriate warm-up activity, the teacher informs the students that today they will be working on improving their cardiovascular fitness levels through a running activity. After organizing students in a safe manner to complete the activity, the teacher informs the students that they will be trying to run as fast as they are able in a straight pathway back and forth across the gymnasium for 45 seconds and then they will be taking a 30 second rest. This pattern will repeat itself five times. The student's main goal during this activity will be to minimize the number of times they need to walk.

This example is only one of the many different ways to plan physical activity to elicit physical fitness gain. Physiological response to physical activity is beyond the scope of this chapter and as a result will not be covered. More important to this chapter are the organizational strategies to increase student engagement while participating in a before school physical activity program. In this example, all students will still be performing the same physical activity; only now the focus is off of the specific distance covered and is placed upon the individual student to attempt to run for the desired amount of time. Organized in this manner, students are less likely to be singled out due to either inferior or superior performance and as a result, they are required to focus on their own performance during the activity. In addition, planning an activity in this manner involves all students simultaneously and provides maximum participation for the entire group of students. This alteration in strategy individualizes the activity and allows students of varying abilities and ages to enjoy success without a focus on any one student. This particular strategy can be utilized in a number of ways with a variety of skills, games and activities. Additional examples of program design are provided in the following section.

Scheduling

Each educational setting is unique and as a result, each scheduling situation is just as unique. When planning a program, consider the total amount of daily time needed for program implementation. This will include the participant arrival, physical activity program and dismissal procedures to the regular classroom or homeroom setting. Consideration of these factors will help to determine the total daily program length and establish a program start time. Table 16.2 provides an example of a potential daily schedule that provides 25 min of structured activity and 10 min of unstructured activity. This design yields over half of the recommended physical activity time for the day. In addition to the daily schedule, consideration needs to be

Table 16.2 Typical daily schedule

Time	Activity
7:50–8:00	Drop off and free play
8:00–8:05	Daily agenda, attendance, and warm-up or running related activity
8:05–8:15	Fitness based skill of the week
8:15–8:25	Game or team activity
8:25	Dismissal for regular school day

given to the duration of the program during the school year. As an example, there could be a 12–15 week program in the fall semester and a 12–15 week program in the spring semester.

As illustrated in the table above, consideration and time will need to be devoted to student arrival and dismissal from the program. Student arrival is a critical time and includes student check-in by the parent or guardian and unstructured physical activity time. The check-in procedures may be determined by the school safety policy to ensure that each student is accounted for and safely admitted to the school. Once checked-in, students will be immediately engaged in unstructured physical activity. This will ensure that students are on-task in a meaningful and appropriate activity and will serve as a pre-warm-up for the structured physical activity component of the program. One strategy is to have pre-determined activities set-up and ready for students as they arrive or to allow the students to engage in free play for a specific amount of time. As an example, when students enter the gymnasium, they will have their choice of 4 different station activities: jumping skills activity, a bean-bag target toss game, a low balance beam station, and an animal movement station. It is important to have the physical space set-up prior to student arrival. This will reduce time off task and minimize any potential behavior issues. After all students have arrived and been checked-in, the structured physical activity program portion may begin.

The structured physical activity component of the program will account for the largest amount of time in the schedule. This component includes a warm-up activity, physical fitness skill, game play and cool-down. The warm-up activity takes place immediately following the unstructured physical activity time. A properly developed age appropriate warm-up may include running based activities and total body gross motor movement activities such as skipping, hopping, jumping, and jumping jacks. This design will prepare the body for the moderate- to vigorous activities included in the fitness skill and game play sections. The physical fitness skill component includes higher intensity activities to improve the health-related and skill related fitness components and includes both cardiovascular and strength based skills. The game play component of the physical activity program provides students an opportunity to apply the skills developed during the previous activities in a fun and engaging game. Examples of the game play are tag games, relay races, obstacle courses and invasion games. Following the game play, students participate in a cool down, which includes flexibility and range of motion activities. Table 16.3 provides a more detailed example of a daily plan.

Table 16.3 Structured physical activity components daily plan

Program section and time	Focus area and activity
Warm-up – 5 min	**Focus**: General total body activation and upper body specific exercises to prepare for the fitness based skill
	Activity: Perimeter walks/jog/run
	While moving around the perimeter of the gym, students perform upper body movements to prepare for the upcoming fitness based skill
Fitness based skill – 10 min	**Focus**: Upper body strength
	Activity: Pushups: Technique will be modified to accommodate multiple ability levels to allow for maximum participation
Game play – 10 min	**Focus**: To improve general fitness levels and reinforce fitness based skills
	Activity – Pushup tag: All students are considered taggers. Each student is trying to tag all other students. If any student gets tagged twice, they must move to the fitness area, perform 3 pushups of their choice and then may re-enter the tag game
Cool down, flexibility and range of motion – 5 min	**Focus**: Allow for closure on the activities of the day and perform range of motion activities to improve future movements
	Activity: Upper body arm/shoulder flexion and extension activities

Equally as important as the arrival procedures are the dismissal procedures. There should be ample time for students to transition to their regular schedule just as they would when they arrive at the school at a regular time. The transition should not be disruptive to the regular organization of the school day. A simple strategy is to dismiss students by age groups, grade levels, or individual classrooms. Utilizing this method minimizes large groups of students moving to classrooms at the same time and instead creates a manageable flow of students through hallways or around school campuses. Recruiting additional faculty and staff within the school to help with the dismissal procedures will help to ensure a smooth and efficient transition.

Facilities and Equipment

In addition to the individual needs and abilities of the children participating in the program, it is important to consider the space(s) available for the program as well as the available resources and physical fitness equipment. The space available for the program may be indoors, outdoors or a combination of both. If using an outdoor space, weather may impact program planning/design and implementation may be limited to specific months or seasons. Other considerations for space include size and general condition of the space. The space available may limit the number of children who can participate in the program. One strategy to address a small space may be to divide the students in half and offer the program to small groups on opposite days. For example, grades K-1 participate in the program on Monday, Wednesday and Friday, while grades 2–3 participate on Tuesday and Thursday. The group then

Table 16.4 Example Program Implementation Schedule

Month	Week	Day
September	**Week1**	**Monday/Wednesday/Friday**
		Group A – 50 children
		Tuesday/Thursday
		Group B – 50 children
	Week 2	**Monday/Wednesday/Friday**
		Group B – 50 children
		Tuesday/Thursday
		Group A – 50 children
	Week 3	**Monday/Wednesday/Friday**
		Group A – 50 children
		Tuesday/Thursday
		Group B – 50 children
	Week 4	**Monday/Wednesday/Friday**
		Group B – 50 children
		Tuesday/Thursday
		Group A – 50 children

alternates the following week so that grades 2–3 have the program on Monday, Wednesday and Friday and grades K-1 have the program on Tuesday and Thursday. This same strategy may be used by schools with limited access to equipment. Table 16.4 provides an example schedule for program implementation and is based on 100 participants, divided into two groups represented as group A and group B. There are many different ways to organize a program and this serves as one example. Organizational strategies may be adjusted to meet the needs of individual schools.

This program design allows a maximum number of students to participate and have access to adequate physical space for a safe program and sufficient use of the equipment available.

Staff Involvement

A key component of any program is the individuals needed to implement the program (McKenzie, Neiger, & Thackeray, 2013). Faculty and staff involvement is essential for sustaining before or after school physical activity programs (Beets, Beighle, Erwin, & Huberty, 2009). Recruiting the help of additional classroom teachers, administration, paraprofessionals and custodial staff for the program will help to create excitement about the program and contribute to developing a healthy school environment. Although these individuals may not have specific training in physical education or physical activity, they may be able to assist with student arrival, program management and dismissal procedures. Additionally, faculty and staff who assist with the program will serve as positive role models for students and demonstrate the importance of adopting healthful habits and behaviors.

Parental Support

Parents play and important role in influencing the physical activity levels of children (Gustafson & Rhodes, 2006). Therefore, a critical element to the success of the before-school physical activity program is parental support. Because the program occurs before the regular school day, parents may be responsible for transporting students to the school for the program. Parental support is also needed to encourage students to rise earlier than normal and arrive to school before their regular school day. Strategies for increasing parental support may include letters mailed home to each of the families targeted for participation, a school newsletter and/or social media.

Summary

Implementation of a before-school physical activity program can provide increased opportunities for children to participate in physical activity and assist in achieving the recommended 60 min of daily physical activity. Implementation of a program requires carful planning and preparation to ensure program success. To increase success in before or after-school physical activity programs, early childhood educators and physical education teachers must consider (1) participants, (2) scheduling, (3) facilities and equiptment, (4) staff involvement, and (5) parental support. This chapter described the importance of physical fitness in children, reviewed the health benefits of physical activity, and provided strategies for increasing physical activity within early childhood and K-12 settings through structured before school programs.

References

American Heart Association (AHA). (2013). *The AHA's recommendations for physical activity in children*. Retrieved from: http://www.americanheart.org/presenter.jhtml?identifier=4596

Batch, J. A. (2005). Benefits of physical activity in obese adolescents and children. *Internal Medicine Journal, 35*, 446.

Beets, M. W., Beighle, A., Erwin, H. E., & Huberty, J. L. (2009). After-school program impact on physical activity and fitness: A meta-analysis. *American Journal of Preventive Medicine, 36*(6), 527–537.

Calfas, K. J., & Taylor, W. C. (1994). Effects of physical activity on psychological variables in adolescents. *Pediatric Exercise Science, 6*, 406–423.

Centers for Disease Control and Prevention. (2010). *Division of nutrition, physical activity, and obesity: Facts about physical activity*. Retrieved from: http://www.cdc.gov/physicalactivity/data/facts.htm

Centers for Disease Control and Prevention. (2015). *Comprehensive school physical activity program (CSPAP)*. Retrieved from: http://www.cdc.gov/healthyschools/physicalactivity/cspap.htm

Fulton, J., Garg, M., Galuska, D., Rattay, K., & Caspersen, C. (2004). Public health and clinical recommendations for physical activity and physical fitness: Special focus on overweight youth. *Sports Medicine, 34*(9), 581–599.

Gustafson, S. L., & Rhodes, R. E. (2006). Parental correlates of physical activity in children and early adolescents. *Sports Medicine, 36*(1), 79–97.

Kalman, M., Inchley, J., Sigmundova, D., Iannotti, R. J., Tynjala, J. A., Hamrik, Z., ... Bucksch, J. (2015). Secular trends in moderate-to-vigorous physical activity in 32 countries from 2002 to 2010: A cross-national perspective. *European Journal of Public Health, 25*(2), 37–40.

McKenzie, J., Neiger, B., & Thackeray, R. (2013). *Planning, implementing, & evaluating health promotion programs* (6th ed.). Boston, MA: Pearson.

Nader, P. R., Bradley, R. H., Houts, R. M., McRitchie, S. L., & O'Brien, M. (2008). Moderate-to-vigorous physical activity from ages 9–15 years. *Journal of American Medical Association, 300*(3), 295–305.

Pate, R. R., Davis, M. G., Robinson, T. N., Stone, E. J., McKenzie, T. L., & Young, J. C. (2006). Promoting physical activity in children and youth: A leadership role for schools. *Circulation, 114*, 1214–1224.

Pontifex, M. B., Saliba, B. J., & Hillman, C. H. (2013). Exercise improves behavioral, neurocognition, and scholastic performance in children with ADHD. *Journal of Pediatrics, 162*(3), 543–551.

Rentner, D.S., Scott, C., Kober, N., Chudowsky, N., Chudowsky, V., Joftus, S., & Zabala, D. (2006). *From the capital to the classroom: Year 4 of no child left behind.* Washington, DC: Center for Education Policy. Retrieved from http://www.cep-dc.org/displayDocument.cfm?DocumentID=301

Story, M., Kaphingst, K. M., & French, S. (2006). The role of schools in obesity prevention. *Childhood Obesity, 16*(1), 109–142.

United States Department of Health and Human Services. (2010). *Office of disease prevention and health promotion. Healthy people 2020 topics and objectives: Physical activity.* https://www.healthypeople.gov/2020/topics-objectives/topic/physical-activity/objectives

World Health Organization. (2011). *Global recommendations on physical activity for health.* Retrieved from: http://www.who.int/dietphysicalactivity/publications/physical-activity-recommendations-5-17years.pdf?ua=1

World Health Organization. (2015). *Fact sheet: physical activity.* Retrieved from: http://www.who.int/mediacentre/factsheets/fs385/en/

Keri S. Kulik has been teaching for over 16 years in both public school and higher education. She has conducted research and workshops on promoting physical activity and physical education in the K-12 setting. She has also published in peer-reviewed journals and presented at national conferences on topics related to physical activity and physical education.

Justin R. Kulik is an elementary Physical Education Specialist with more than 18 years experience working with pediatric populations in educational, fitness and sport settings. He has published in peer-reviewed journals and has presented at local, state and national conferences.

Chapter 17
The Role of Service-Learning in Preparing Teachers and Related Professionals to Promote Health and Physical Activity in Early Childhood

Marybeth Miller

Defining Service-Learning

Every Thursday morning, in a university campus gymnasium, there is music, laughter and an energetic atmosphere of over 55 pre-school age children, with and without disabilities who come from pre-school programs and the surrounding communities to participate in Moving Concepts, a free physical activity program offered through an undergraduate teacher preparation course taught in the Department of Physical and Health Education. Every session begins at the Friendship Circle where pre-service teachers in physical education, special education and early childhood education meet their assigned mentor child. The opening gets the large group moving to music, such as the Hokey Pokey, followed by teachers rotating through four learning centers where children climb tressle trees, walk on low-level balance beams, roll balls, and participate along with an animated PowerPoint. The Powerpoint is interactive, and children identify major body parts used to run, bat, throw and catch. After 40 minutes of active play, pre-service teachers and young children return to the Friendship Circle to close the program by singing the Good-Bye song. In this inclusive learning environment, children make new friends, develop social skills, develop gross motor skills, learn about having a healthy body, and learn to interact appropriately with others.

Grounded in Experiential Learning Theory (Kolb, 1984), service-learning is an evidence-based educational experience that connects academic curriculum content to a service-in-need and reflection done by service providers. Service-learning is a teaching and learning strategy that integrates meaningful community service with instruction and reflection to enrich the learning experience, teach civic responsibility, and strengthen communities (Learn and Serve America's National Clearning House, n.d.). In the example above, university pre-service teacher candidates

M. Miller (✉)
Slippery Rock University of Pennsylvania, Slippery Rock, PA, USA
e-mail: marybethmiller@comcast.net

H. Brewer, M. R. Jalongo (eds.), *Physical Activity and Health Promotion in the Early Years*, Educating the Young Child 14,
https://doi.org/10.1007/978-3-319-76006-3_17

enrolled in a professional activity course study educational movement content and early learning standards, apply the content to design developmentally appropriate activity plans and teach the activities to pre-school age children. Following their teaching, they reflect upon their experience to draw the connection between the academic coursework and the service provided.

Service Learning at a Glance: A High Impact Practice

Erickson and Anderson (1997) define service-learning "as a pedagogical technique for combining authentic community service with integrated academic outcomes (p.1). Service-learning is dually thought of as a teaching method to reach course goals and a philosophy of learning, cultivated through well thought out and purposefully planned intentional program designs. Being directly connected to academic course outcomes, both the provider and those being served benefit in learning which is a key component to differentiating service-learning from volunteerism (Duncan & Kopperund, 2008, p. 5). A practice of teaching future teachers to learn-by-serving and serving-to-learn may foster high levels of student engagement through experiential learning opportunities, proven through research, to be meaningful and promote successful learning outcomes (leap.aacu.org/toolkit/high-impact (Association of American Colleges & Universities (n.d.)). A contemporary term in higher education for applied learning experiences, such as service-learning, is known as High Impact Practices (HIP). Unto itself, the HIP of service-learning is anchored in theory, and connected by subject area course(s), reflective practice, and serving a need.

Experiential Learning Theory Overview

Service-learning is grounded in Kolb's (1984) Experiential Learning Theory which is based upon the central role experience plays in the process of learning. As shown in Table 17.1, this theory can be explained by Kolb's four-stage learning cycle lead by stage 1 concrete experience (get actively involved) followed by stage 2 reflective observation (process, question, review), then stage 3 abstract conceptualization (study and understand present and past knowledge and experiences for planning), and finally stage 4 active experimentation (plan and provide service practices). This continuous learning cycle is common to service-learning that would be grounded in Kolb's theory. One resource among many I used to steer the cycle's momentum and useful to design and/or evaluate programs are the Seven Elements of High Quality Service Learning.

Table 17.1 Seven elements of high quality service learning

Element	Criteria
Integrated learning	The service project has clearly articulated knowledge, skill or value goals;
	The knowledge, skill or value goals arise from broader classroom and school goals;
	The service informs the academic learning content;
	Life skills learned outside the classroom are integrated back into classroom learning.
High quality service	The service responds to an actual community need;
	The need is recognized by the community impacted by the service;
	The service is age-appropriate
	The service is well-organized;
	The service is designed to achieve significant benefits for students and community.
Collaboration	The service-learning project is a collaboration among as many of these partners as is feasible; students, parents, community-based organizations, businesses, school administrators, teachers, and the people on whose behalf the service is done;
	All partners are involved in the planning of the service-learning project;
	All partners contribute to the service-learning project;
	All partners benefit from the service-learning project;
	Roles and expectations of each partner are clearly defined.
Student voice	Students engage in a process that leads them to define "community" and "need."
	Students are involved in choosing and planning the service project;
	Students participate actively in the collaboration among the project's partners;
	Students are involved in planning the reflection sessions, evaluation, and celebration;
	Student voice is age appropriate.
Civic responsibility	The service-learning project promotes young people's responsibility to care for others and to contribute to the community;
	The service-learning project helps students understand the historical and community context of their actions;
	By participating in the service-learning project, students understand how they can impact their community;
	Students use critical thinking to analyze their project and the related issues;
	The service-learning project provides opportunities for students to connect with adult role models.
Reflection	Reflection occurs before, during, and after the service-learning project;
	Reflection activities utilize multiple techniques so all students can successfully reflect;
	Reflection examines the results, processes and relationships in the service-learning project;
	Reflective activities help participants consider the social and ethical dimensions of their experience;
	Reflection establishes connections between students' service experiences and the academic curriculum.

(continued)

Table 17.1 (continued)

Element	Criteria
Evaluation	The evaluation has a clear purpose and target audience;
	All the partners, especially students, are involved in evaluating the service-learning project;
	The evaluation seeks to measure progress towards the learning and service goals of the service-learning project;
	The evaluation uses tools that respect the diversity of learning styles;
	The evaluation is planned before the project happens, rather than afterwards.

Source: Adapted from Youth Service California 2004, 663 13th St. Oakland, CA 94612 info@yscal.org. Retrieved June 18, 2015, from http://yscal.org/resources/sltools.html

Seven Elements of High Quality Service Learning

A highly useful resource tool used to help develop course-embedded service-learning projects is the document titled Seven Elements of High Quality Service Learning developed in 1995 by the Service Learning 2000 Center at Stanford University in collaboration with experienced service-learning practitioners (Youth Service California, 2000). These seven elements and their descriptors shown in Table 17.1 can be helpful to faculty in providing the structure to design and evaluate a service-learning program as well as guide students on understanding the elements based on their criteria.

The Seven Elements of High Quality Service Learning may be a highly useful tool to guide one's thinking about how to design a service-learning program and all of the critical elements important to its implementation. This may also include becoming familiar with any and all documents related to service-learning such as the Wingspread Special Report (Honner & Poulsen, 1989), Standards of Quality for School-Based and Community-Based Service Learning (Alliance for Service Learning in Education Reform, 1995), the Essential Elements of Effective Service-Learning Practice (National Youth Leadership Council, 2003) and *Service-Learning in Physical Education and Related Professions: A Global Perspective* (Miller & Nendel, 2011). In the initial phase of becoming familiar with service-learning as a pedagogy, it is important to understand that it is theory based, has a learning cycle framework, different from volunteerism because learning is anchored to academic rigor such as when service-learning is embedded within a course and/or when a component of a society/club belonging to a program of professional preparation. In either case, central to the success of a service-learning program is its developmentally appropriate design and practice.

Appropriate Practices for Early Childhood Movement Programs

Learning how to learn through physical activity is a means of how children build knowledge and social development. Early childhood is the critical period for optimal learning that builds the foundation for future development. Recent attention to the importance of educating the whole child begins in early childhood when developmentally appropriate programs to cultivate conceptual learning through active engagement includes movement and health education. To cultivate the culture for developmentally appropriate health and physical education/activity programs is to understand how children develop and learn in the early years.

In the year 2000, The Council on Physical Education for Children (COPEC) of the National Association for Sport and Physical Education, published a document titled *Appropriate Practices in Movement Programs for Young Children Ages 3–5 (National Association for Sport and Physical Education*, 2000). Written for teachers, parents, school administrators, policy makers and other individuals responsible for the educational programs for 3-to-5-year-olds, it provides guidelines for developmentally appropriate best practice (and examples of inappropriate practice) for early childhood movement programs in the following contexts (1) making curricular decisions, (2) designing learning experiences, (3) developing movement skills and concepts, (4) facilitating maximum participation, (5) promoting success for all children, (6) incorporating fine and gross motor activities, (7) teaching rhythmical experiences and dance, (8) teaching educational gymnastics (educational movement framework), (9) teaching games, (10) integrating movement programs and play, (11) scheduling activity, (12) providing an adequate and safe environment, (13) limiting class size, (14) facilitating gender equity, and (15) fostering parent-teacher communication. This is an excelling starting point for faculty and students who desire to provide service-learning movement programs for early learners. It is one thing to offer programs off the cuff, and another to offer programs that have a clear standards-based scope and sequence designed from a variety of developmentally appropriate evidence-based resources. A sample listing of these are located at the end of this chapter. In short, if this is about fundamental movement then what about health fundamentals?

Integrating Health with Physical Education/Activity

Learning and health are interrelated and fundamental to developing the whole child. The Whole School, Whole Community, Whole Child (WSCC) approach is a new model for health and learning developed in collaboration by the Association for Child Development and the Centers for Disease Control and Prevention (CDC). Prior to the new model, ASCD's direction was perceived by the health community as an educational initiative on academic achievement minus the accountability of health moving minds. The CDC's Coordinated School Health (CSH) model was perceived by educators to focus only on health outcomes with little regard to academic achievement. More recently, each organization recognized and conversed upon the relationship and integration of learning and health. As previously addressed in this chapter, active engagement in the learning process is central to how young children learn. Moreover, this underlying feature of engaging students in active learning is the intention of how students approach their learning and health (CDC, 2015). It is exciting to know that the interrelationship and integration of learning and health through science backing is finally recognized. What is important is to bring this into action and what better way than to infuse health education into early childhood education programs for young learners. To summarize, many, but not all, early education programs do emphasize health and nutrition. When children learn about health and physical activity at an early age, they can develop healthy lifestyle behaviors that potentially last a lifetime (Friedman, Krauss, & Barnett, 2013).

Evidence-Based Service-Learning in Teacher Education

Across the past decade, scholars in professional preparation fields of physical education and other related professions have embedded service-learning as an integrated course component at both the undergraduate and graduate levels, as an application to meet the needs of university students learning in an applied atmosphere. Further, service learning ensures that college students engage in community service. Various models spanning the globe, including Australia, New Zealand, Canada, Great Britain and the United States systematically examined the impact service-learning had upon those serving and those being served. Globally, service-learning is embraced as a viable pedagogy (method of teaching-learning) as evidenced by the research examining the effectiveness of integrating service-learning in university professional preparation courses in physical education and related fields identifies service-learning to be a highly effective pedagogy in preparing teachers (Miller & Nendel, 2011). Research examining a service-learning approach (a physical activity program for pre-school age children with and without disabilities embedded in a motor development course) for first-year pre-service teachers in physical education would have an impact upon their calling to become a teacher. Results supported the hypothesis that service-learning can provide a positive impact upon one's calling to the vocation of teaching. Participants of the study (the first-year pre-service teachers) noted that the program helped them identify that they wanted to teach young children. Another series of studies conducted by Miller (2009) investigated service-learning pedagogy to facilitate early childhood physical activity as a high quality service and a viable teacher-training method. Pre-service teachers in physical education, early childhood education and special education, all participants of the studies served as mentor teachers to pre-school age children attending a model on-campus educational movement program. Framed within the Seven Elements of High Quality Service-Learning (see Table 17.1), pre-service teachers completed structured weekly journal logs on their service as well as a survey. The results of this series of studies identified the positive impact service-learning had on them as the service providers preparing to become teachers and their perceptions of high quality of service experienced by the young children attending. These findings complement those of others examining service-learning as an effective means to prepare teachers and related-service professionals (Meaney, Bohler, Kopf, Hernandez, & Scott, 2008; Watson, Crandall, Hueglin, & Eisenman 2002).

University Application

Physical educators and pre-service early childhood educators in service-learning programs may use their national and state learning standards specific to children's learning. In the United States for the Commonwealth of Pennsylvania, physical education and early childhood programs utilize the Pre-Kindergarten Pennsylvania Learning Standards for Early Childhood (Office of Child Development and Early Learning, 2009) as one of the primary resources to plan, prepare, and guide children to learn about their body through guided play integrated with information on health concepts. Teacher candidates help children to construct and understand knowledge about healthy lifestyles (e.g. fundamentals of good health, body part identification, ways to stay healthy, safe practices, nutrition) as they develop gross motor (large muscle) and fine motor (small muscle) coordination, strength, body awareness (balance, weight transfer, shapes) and space awareness (location, direction, pathways, levels).

Overall, the literature on health and learning overwhelming supports the early childhood period as highly formative for teaching about healthy lifestyles, forming health habits, eating properly and getting the opportunity for daily physical activity to support being healthy. A service-learning approach can meet this need in schools and communities by teachers and professionals providing opportunities for children to be active and learn how to be healthy. With the rising concern about childhood obesity throughout the United States (CDC, 2015), professional teacher preparation programs in health and physical education, early childhood education, and related professions, may consider cultivating a culture of high impact practice through service-learning initiatives, allowing teacher candidates to make contributions toward a healthier society through civic engagement. What follows is one example of an early childhood education model for integrating service-learning and teacher education in the discipline of physical and health education professional activity course.

Moving Concepts: A Model Course-Embedded Service-Learning Program

*It's Thursday morning and 56 young children are entering the gymnasium to meet their university-student mentors. A variety of learning centers designed to promote health and physical activity are already set up across the gymnasium, and the young children are excited to see the new equipment and familiar faces. The university student mentors are excited for the children's arrival and greet them as they find their spot at the Friendship Circle. They talk to each other and to the children beside them as they wait for the lesson to open by the professor who directs the program. The director gets all children's attention and has them focus on the "word of the day – Responsibility" and provides examples of how they can act responsibly as they play. The music comes on and the children begin to move in general space inside the Friendship Circle to play Cooperative Musical Hoops. Upon completion of the game, each child follows their university-student mentor out onto the gymnasium floor to one of four learning communities, filled with three developmentally appropriate health, wellness and physical development activities that happen to integrate Language and Literacy Development early learning standards concepts and competencies. As Rockin' Reading Readiness (*Schiller, DeVolder, & RONNO, 2005*) plays, these 55 children are developing their body awareness through balances, space awareness by changing levels, moving with effort to change their force in making ripples and waves with a parachute, and relating to others in a lead and follow game of animals movements. When the music pauses, children rotate to the next learning center until all four are completed. Everyone returns to the Friendship Circle for a closing of positive feedback about acting responsibly and singing the Goodbye Song.*

Both a philosophy of learning and pedagogy, I embedded service-learning as a method to reach the learning goals and objectives for an individual undergraduate course I was most familiar with and truly enjoyed teaching, Movement Education. With a framework of study centered upon Laban's educational movement concepts of body awareness (what the body can do), space awareness (where the body can move), effort (quality of movement), and relationship to others and objects, student learning is based upon the learning styles of problem solving, exploration, and guided discovery. These learning styles were a perfect match to what children at the pre-kindergarten level use to learn through free and guided play experiences. Furthermore, a second framework applied to this course was the Seven Elements of High Quality Service Learning, illustrated in Table 17.1, to appropriately capture the element of **integrated learning.**

Steps to Implement the Moving Concepts Program

Professionals interested in implementing a service-learning program implemented with an academic course may find the following steps helpful in the planning process:

- Step one – determine a need for creating and offering a free educational movement program to serve children 3-to-5-years-of-age in the surrounding communities and gather information, consult professionals in the movement and early childhood fields about existing developmentally appropriate physical education/activity programs, including children having special needs. The search shall identify a **community need;**

- Step two – meet with early childhood education program directors in the community as well as the university day care center to present a program proposal that articulates the basis for the need, the integration to their classroom academic content, alignment with the early learning standards (the common language across the preschool and Moving Concepts program), the developmentally appropriate program scope and sequence which would integrate health concepts, the implementation of the Six Pillars of Character, a framework for teaching good character (www.charactercounts.org) and the process of how the Moving Concepts program would operate as a service-learning initiative in preparing physical education, early childhood/special education teachers.
- Step three – create media publications in area newspapers to reach out to families and caregivers to welcome their child or children to the program providing they fit the age range for it. This begins the **collaboration** between the university and community constituents.
- Step four – the design the academic course learning objectives, topical outline of content to be taught and applied to the service (See Appendix A).

Preparing Pre-service Teachers to Lead Educational Movement: Structure and Function

A class of 30 plus teacher candidates may be organized into four learning communities, an organization structure arising from research conducted in the late 1980's and early 1990's on ways to restructure classrooms to promote students being actively involved and more responsible for their own learning and that of their community peers. (Tito, 2003). For the first third of the semester, because all content would be new, lead the service planning with instructor-designed activity plans illustrating education concepts learned in the course, early childhood learning standards and the process of designing developmentally appropriate physical activity plans using developmentally appropriate evidence-based resources. On a weekly basis, each learning community would be assigned to plan physical activities based upon one of the four educational movement concepts as well as a selected appropriate state early learning standard to support and reinforce core content taught in the pre-kindergarten classroom and at home. In Pennsylvania, the standards key learning areas include (1) Creative Thinking and Expression: Communicating Through The Arts, (2) Mathematical Thinking And Expression: Exploring, Processing And Problem Solving, (3) Scientific Thinking And Technology: Exploring, Scientific Inquiry And Discovery, (4) Social Studies Thinking: Connecting To Communities, (5) Language and Literacy Development: English Language Arts (6) Partnerships for Learning: Families, Learning Environments And Communities, (8) Social and Emotional Development: Student Interpersonal Skills, and (9) Health Wellness And Physical Development: Learning About My Body which is applied to each Moving Concepts session.

Planning and Preparation

The sample program outline of learning objectives and topics shown in Appendix A illustrates the flow of course content connected to the embedded service-learning program. Concepts in early childhood health and motor development lay the foundation for developmental appropriateness and an understanding of fundamental motor skill development at a young age. Pre-service teachers are introduced to the early childhood learning standards, the SPARK Curriculum for Early Childhood (SPARK, 2009–2015), and the Character Counts Six Pillars of Character (Trustworthiness, Respect, Responsibility, Fairness, Caring, and Citizenship) developed by the Josephson Institute Center for Youth Ethics that directly relates to the WSCC model, as required resources for planning activity sessions. Many other developmentally appropriate resources are introduced and provided as planning resources for developing activities and "health moments" that are presented though an interactive animated PowerPoint presentation. Students are guided on how to create interactive animated PowerPoint presentations based upon a selected weekly healthy lifestyle/healthy habits topic e.g. handwashing, healthy eating, healthy heart. The integration of technology includes these PowerPoint presentations shown on a large SMART Board wheeled to the gymnasium. Together, the richness of students of different education majors working in learning communities provides a wealth of creative interdisciplinary ideas. The activity plans represent **student voice** with the intention of pre-service teachers having a greater investment into the activity content planned by them and screened for safety and appropriateness. Appendix B illustrates one example of a weekly planning form.

Implementation Process

Tuesdays focus content delivery and planning classes. Thursdays focus on the service-learning Moving Concepts sessions. Children are assigned to university-student mentors. Each session begins at the Friendship Circle with a large group opening activity to music, introduction to the daily Character Counts pillar, then transitioning to learning communities of activities. Each of the four learning communities contained three to four child-centered gross motor activities incorporating language and literacy visuals. The integration of SMART Board technology rotates to a different community each session and, upon arrival to the learning community, children go directly to it for a brief 1 min animated interactive health education moment, then proceed to select an activity to begin within the learning community they arrived to. Four groups rotate to each of the learning communities every 7 min followed by a return to the Friendship Circle to a session closure of the Good-Bye song. An illustration of a floor diagram for this model program is illustrated in Appendix C. The weekly service of **civic engagement** provided by the teacher candidates cultivates a culture of caring for their learning community members and the quality of instruction taking place. This also includes helping each teacher candidate to recognize and understand the important impact they are making in promoting young children's learning and development through developmentally appropriate physical activity.

Technology Integration in Service-Learning

Early childhood educators are encouraged to read Using Animation in Microsoft PowerPoint to Enhance Engagement and Learning in Young Learners With Developmental Delay by H.P. Parette, J. Hourcade & C. Blum (2011) to learn how to create animated PowerPoint slide show technology for teaching and learning. This article provides a clear on concise step-wise procedure on how to create them. Key points to apply these in a physical activity program is to establish a theme relevant to movement concepts (body awareness, space awareness, effort, relationship to others/equipment), health concepts (healthy heart, healthy nutrition, germ-free), safety and injury prevention concepts (safe and unsafe behavior, emergency situations, community helpers). The interactive key is held with children verbally responding to teacher-led questions during the presentation as well as teacher-led gross motor movements following action-based slide animations (e.g. jumping or running in place) along with what is shown on the slides. All interactive PowerPoints should be aligned and documented with learning standards.

Reflective Practice and Assessment

> *"The planning contributions related to my academic discipline." third year early childhood/special education teacher candidate;*
>
> *"The Moving Concepts program is a meaningful way to recognize the civic responsibility of giving" second-year elementary education pre-service teacher candidate*
>
> *"I felt that the academic learning and service were connected" second-year special education pre-service teacher candidate*
>
> *"The Program was highly organized and the learning community culture connected the classroom to the service-learning" third-year early childhood/special education teacher candidate*
>
> *"My learning of education movement concepts was enhanced through the service-learning" second-year physical and health education major*
>
> *"The setting of children with and without disabilities helped me to think about how challenging teaching will be" third-year early childhood major*
>
> *"I felt very satisfied in being able to grow my knowledge by contributing to a worthwhile early childhood learning experience" third year early childhood/special education major*

Critical **reflection** upon the service provided may involve written reflection using a template, to be completed post-program (see Appendix D). Each reflection is read by the course instructor who replies with feedback. Teacher candidate remarks, in the aggregate, include statements of confidence building, enjoyment of working as a learning community, contributing their voice to what they believe matters in the program, taking pride in quality planning and seeing children enjoy the activities, valuing the inclusive direction through the recognition of typically developed peers being role models for age-mates with disabilities, and voicing an appreciation for learning course content in a manner that brings it alive through service. Formatively, critical reflection serves as a mechanism to process information and helps one to organize and understand knowledge gained through service-learning. The final frontier for determining the effectiveness of service-learning involves **evaluation**, and important to this process is student involvement to evaluate the service-learning program. Referring back to the twelve global service-learning models (Miller & Nendel, 2011) the critical reflection component of service-learning, in written (structured journal logs, surveys) and in verbal forms (think-pair-share), transcended the link between academic coursework and the service provided (Eyler, 2002; Hardman & Hardman, 2011).

Summary

Pondering upon service-learning as a professional development practice implies one's adoption of it as a philosophy of learning and a method of teaching. The evidence for service-learning effectiveness is well researched and documented in the service-learning literature inside and outside of education. The central tenants of service-learning are linking it to academic rigor, providing a needed service that links to the academic rigor, and critical reflection, important to differentiating service from service-learning. A tool that can provide structure to frame a program upon can be gleaned from the Seven Elements of High Quality Service Learning that I found to be very useful. Linking a service-learning program to both academic standards and service-learning standards may more fully ensure best-practice engagement for the service providers and those being provided.

This chapter focused on the promotion of health and physical activity to some of our youngest citizens, yearly childhood, through service-learning provided by individuals preparing to be teachers and related professionals. What better foundation than to return to the early-day practice of apprenticeship in the mode of serving the need of more and improved health and physical activity programs for young children. The evidence is out there that the optimal learning window, otherwise known as the critical learning period occurs during the early childhood years. What better opportunity to begin experiential learning opportunities to help young children construct, organize, understand and experience habits of a healthy lifestyle than through either school-based or community-based service-learning.

Appendices

Appendix A

Course Program Outline

Student Learning Objectives

1. Demonstrate the understanding of movement concepts as they are applied to developmentally appropriate learning and performance strategies and tactics upon becoming a physically educated person (SRU Framework 1a, PDE I.A,II.A, NASPE 2);
2. Understand class management structures that are associated with the teaching of basic movement and concepts to support a safe and healthy learning environment (SRU Framework 2c, 2d, 2e, NAEYC 1, NASPE 5, PDE I.H);
3. Apply fundamental locomotor, manipulative and non-locomotor skills to creative movement applications (SRU Framework 1a, NAEYC 5a, NASPE 1, PDE I.D);
4. Construct developmentally appropriate movement experiences for preschool-age children with and without disabilities applied through a service-learning framework (SRU Framework 1a, 1b, 1c, 1f, NASPE Standard 1, NAEYC 5a, PDE II.C);
5. Understand content knowledge and resources of academic disciplines to execute developmentally appropriate interdisciplinary movement experiences involving creative movement, dance, games, brain-breaks, health and safety (SRU Framework 1c,2b,3b,3c,3e, NAEYC 5a and 5 Health, PDE II.D);
6. Articulate developmentally appropriate fitness types, the motor skills of each, and their relationship to the development of children's healthy lifestyle (NAEYC 5 Health, NSAPE 4, PDE10.4.3A);
7. Understand and apply health enhancing principles that promote young children to make healthy choices for themselves including safe play and nutrition (NAEYC 5 Health, PDE 10.2.3D, 10.3.3D);
8. Articulate learning styles that are addressed in developmentally appropriate instructional practices to address differentiated cognitive abilities in the motor learning environment (SRU Framework 1c,2b, 3b,3c,3d, 3e, PDE I.H, PDE II.C);
9. Develop and enhance one's metacognition through the practice of professional reflection related to course embedded service-learning (SRU Framework 4a, NASPE 8, ISTE V b).

Topics Outline

Getting Started:

1. Learning Communities of Practice (CoP)
2. Educational movement framework GRID (on D2L)
3. Seven Elements of High Quality Service Learning
4. Educating the whole child: Movement & brain development
5. Physical fitness: skill-related/health-related
6. Physical activity & the school program

Guiding Concepts: Unit 1

1. **Physical Activity is Critical to Educating the Whole Child**
2. **Motor development and health**
3. **Styles of Learning**
4. **Motor learning environments: Safety and sense of security**
5. **Differentiating Instruction**

BODY AWARENESS (What The Body Can Do: what moves)

1. Class Management Structures: general space, personal space
2. Balance
3. weight transfer: locomotor movements
4. balance & weight transfer sequences
5. SPARK Early Childhood: www.spark.org www.sparkfamily.org

Guiding Concept: 1. Physical Activity Is Critical to Educating the Whole Child

1. Shapes
2. exploring body shapes
3. number/letter shapes: body; ropes

Guiding Concept: 2. Motor Development and Health

SPACE AWARENESS (Where the body moves)

1. Location: personal & general space review
2. Moving in different directions
3. Moving in different levels
4. Moving across different pathways
5. Character Counts Program: 5 Pillars

Guiding Concept 3 Styles of Learning

VARK: visual, auditory, read-write, kinesthetic

Guiding Concept #4 Motor Learning Environments: Safety and Sense of Security

RELATIONSHIP TO OTHERS (to whom and what the body relates)

1. Individuals to each other (partners) – movement prepositions
   (a) Over/under, near/far, meeting/parting, match/mirror, lead/follow
   (b) Individuals to objects: on/off, over/under, beside/between, around

Guiding Concept #5: Differentiating Instruction

FUNDAMENTAL MOVEMENT

Guiding Concepts: Unit 2

1. **Understanding progressions of locomotor development within gross motor development**
2. **Combining locomotor, non-locomotor and manipulative skills for play and physical activity to promote a love of movement leading to healthy and active lifestyles**
3. **Differentiating Instruction**

   Fundamental Motor Skills

1. Locomotor skills (run, jump, gallop, slide, hop, skip, leap)
2. Manipulative skills (roll, toss, catch, throw, kick, strike with hands & implements)
3. The Role of the Classroom Teacher in Physical Activity Programs

Guiding Concepts: Unit 3

1. **Movement as an academic tool: resources in academic disciplines applied to movement school-wide**
2. **Appropriate instructional practices for educating the whole child**
3. **Making healthy choices and prevent hazardous practices**
4. **Healthy nutrition and growing stronger**
5. **High quality movement experiences connecting school, family and community**
1. Mathematical Thinking and Movement
2. Creative Thinking and Expression with Movement
3. Scientific Thinking & Ecology Celebrating Earth Day: Being Green/Nutrition
4. Cultural Determinants of Physical Activity of Young Children: How We Play

Appendix B

Example of the Student Voice: Learning Community Worksheet for Activity Planning

PE 243-04 Movement Education

Today you and your partner are going to create an activity for your learning community that will be applied with children on Thursday March 17. Your movement activity that you create is to also include LANGUAGE AND LITERACY. a) design an activity and give it a name, b) create a developmentally appropriate visual aide that you will use for your activity. When you have completed this, share it with your community members. Afterwards, please give it to your learning community manager who will deliver them to the course instructor who will add it to a master floor plan which will be returned to you on Thursday March 22.

Materials Needed: PDE Learning Standards for Early Childhood: Pre-K
All floor plans I provided to you to date
Textbook: Step by Step & SPARK Early Childhood
Movement Education Grid & Body Awareness handout sheets

Learning Community Center Number 1
Learning Community Theme: **Body Awareness: balance, shape, locomotor skills**
1. Your Created Activity – Give it a Name: ____________________
2. Use this space to draw the activity:
3. The movement education subtheme your activity emphasizes is: ______________
4.**PDE Early Learning Standard Language and Literacy** (pgs.59-66). Illustrate specifically what you would include from this standard for your activity drawn above. I want to be able to see how you have an interdisciplinary approach to learning. **Please list the specific standard and indicator (letter, number and label) you are addressing.**

What materials you will need & amount

Appendix C

Moving Concepts Program General Floor Diagram

Note: On Dr. Miller's verbal cue all groups rotate clockwise to the next learning community (see arrows).

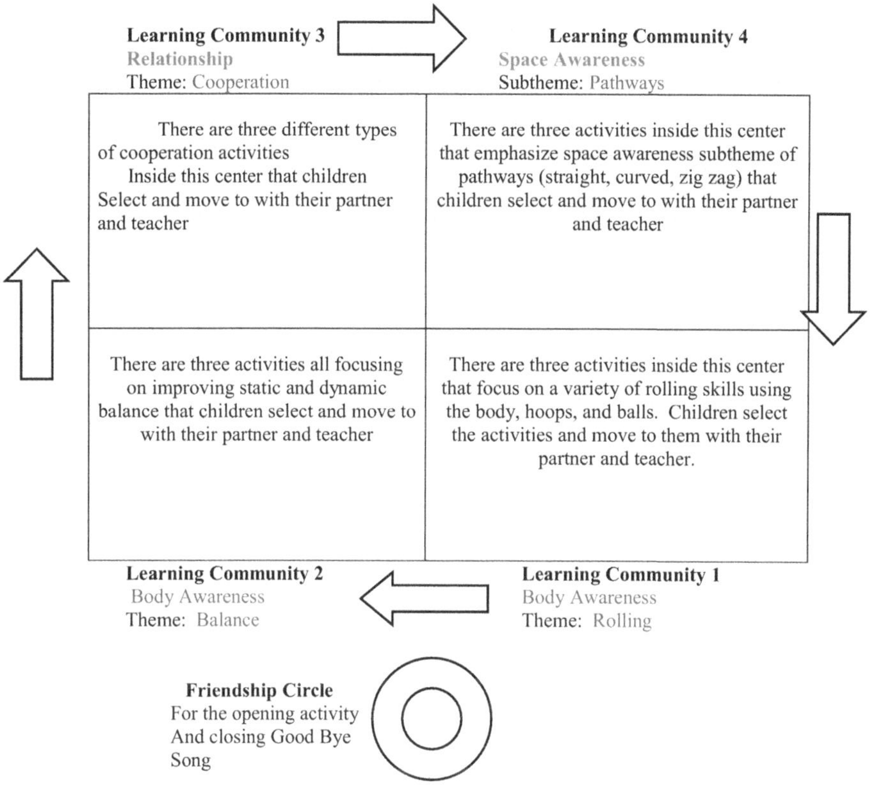

Appendix D

Moving Concepts Service-Learning Program Weekly Reflection

Name ______________________ Date _______ Session Number ______

1. For each learning center, describe the educational movement themes and subthemes that would best match each activity:

Learning Community 1 –
Learning Community 2-
Learning Community 3 –
Learning Community 4-

2. Briefly describe how your child(ren) interacted with each other AND with others in your learning community:
   (a) with each other –
   (b) with other children in your group –
   (c) child's interaction with you
3. Briefly describe any strategies you used to encourage social interaction during any of today's activities:
4. How do you perceive today's service to the children connecting to PE 243 Movement Education classroom learning/content knowledge development?
5. Teacher's Reflections on Emotional States During Moving Concepts
6. What kinds of emotions have you felt while working as a teacher in Moving Concepts today? With each of the emotions listed below, FIRST rate how intensely you felt an emotion (0 = not at all, 1 = low, 2 = moderate, 3 = high) by writing the number on the line. SECOND, please give an example of what caused your emotion.

Emotion	Intensity	Cause of the emotion you felt
Uneasy	______	______________________________
Excited	______	______________________________
Happy	______	______________________________
Discouraged	______	______________________________

References

Alliance for Service-Learning in Education Reform. (1995). *Standards of quality for school-based and community based service learning*. Alexandria, VA: The Close Up Foundation.

Association of American Colleges & Universities. (n.d.). *LEAP campus toolkit: Resources and models for innovation*. Retrieved June 6, 2015, from http://www.leap.aacu.org/toolkit/high-impact-practices

Center for Disease Control and Prevention. (2015). *Whole school, whole community, whole child: A collaborative approach to learning and health*. Retrieved June 19, 2015, from http://www.cdc.healthyyouth/wscc/wsccmodel

Duncan, D., & Kopperund, J. (2008). *Service learning companion*. Boston, MA: Houghton, Mifflin.

Erickson, J. A., & Anderson, J. B. (1997). *Learning with the community: Concepts and models for service learning in teacher education*. Washington, DC: American Association for Higher Education.

Eyler, J. (2002). Reflection: Linking service and learning-linking students to communities. *Journal of Social Issues, 58*(3), 517–534.

Friedman, Krauss, A., & Barnett, W. S. (2013). Early childhood education: Pathways to better health in preschool policy brief, Issue 25. Retrieved June 19, 2015, from www.nieer.org

Hardman, J., & Hardman, A. (2011). Conducing reflection in service-learning. In M. Miller & J. Nendel (Eds.), *Service-learning in physical education and related professions: A global perspective* (pp. 113–149). Sudbury, MA: Jones and Bartlett.

Honner, e. P., & Poulsen, S. J. (1989). *The wingspread special report: Principles of good practice for combining service and learning*. Racine, WI: The Johnson Foundation.

Kolb, D. (1984). *Experiential learning: Experience as the source of learning and development*. Englewood cliffs, NJ: Prentice-Hall.

Learn and Serve America's National Leading Clearinghouse. (n.d.). What is service-learning? Retrieved December 4, 2008, from www.servicelearning.org/what-service-learning

Meaney, K. S., Bohler, H. R., Kopf, K., Hernandez, L., & Scott, L. S. (2008). Service-learning and pre-service educators' cultural competence for teaching: An exploratory study. *The Journal of Experimental Education, 31*(2), 189–208.

Miller, M. P. (2009). *Investigating service learning pedagogy to facilitate early childhood physical activity, poster session accepted for a research consortium presentation at the 2009 American alliance for health*. Tampa, FL: Physical Education, Recreation and Dance National Convention.

Miller, M. P., & Nendel, J. D. (Eds.). (2011). *Service-learning in physical education and related professions: A global perspective*. Sudbury, MA: Jones and Bartlett.

National Association for Sport and Physical Education. (2000). *Appropriate practices in movement programs for young children ages 3–5*. Reston, VA: Author.

National Youth Leadership Council. (2003). *Essential elements of effective service-learning practice*. Retrieved June 22, 2015, from http://www.nylc.org

Office of Child Development and Early Learning. (2009). *Pre-kindergarten Pennsylvania learning standards for early childhood* (3rd ed.). Mechanicsburg, PA: Author.

Parette, H. P., Hourcade, J., & Blum, C. (2011). Using animation in microsoft powerpoint to enhance engagement and learning in young learners with developmental delay. *Teaching Exceptional Children, 43*(4), 58–67.

Shiller, P., DeVolder, B., & RONNO. (2005). *Rockin' reading readiness*. Long Branch, NJ: Kimbo Educational.

SPARK. (2009–2015). *Early childhood curriculum ages 3–5*. San Diego, CA: Author.

Tito, V. (2003). *Learning better together: The impact of learning communities on student success, higher education monograph series, 2003-1, higher education program*. School of Education, Syracuse University. Retrieved June 6, 2015, from, http://www.nhcuc.org/pdfs/Learning_Better_Together.pdf

Watson, D. L., Crandall, J., Hueglin, S., & Eisenman, P. (2002). Incorporating service-learning into physical education teacher education programs. *Journal of Physical Education, Recreation and Dance, 73*, 50–54.

Youth Service California. (2000). *Seven elements of high-quality service-learning*. Oakland, CA: Author.

Marybeth Miller taught adapted physical education for 11 years prior to entering higher education teacher education. Marybeth specializes in teacher education training having an emphasis in motor development and early childhood physical activity. Her book *Service-Learning in Physical Education and Related Professions: A Global Perspective* (Jones & Bartlett) connects scholars world-wide with expertise in service-learning.

Index

H. Brewer, M. R. Jalongo (eds.), *Physical Activity and Health Promotion in the Early Years*, Educating the Young Child 14,
https://doi.org/10.1007/978-3-319-76006-3

The manufacturer's authorised representative in the EU is Springer Nature Customer Service Centre GmbH, Europaplatz 3, 69115 Heidelberg, Germany. If you have any concerns regarding our products, please contact ProductSafety@springernature.com

Printed and bound by CPI Group (UK) Ltd, Croydon, CR0 4YY
05/10/2026
02228135-0011